KU-185-845

C O N C E P T S   O F

Physical Fitness

WITH LABORATORIES

Charles B. Corbin

Arizona State University

Ruth Lindsey

California State University–Long Beach

Brown & Benchmark
PUBLISHERS

Madison, WI Dubuque Guilford, CT Chicago Toronto London
Mexico City Caracas Buenos Aires Madrid Bogotá Sydney

Book Team

Executive Managing Editor *Ed Bartell*
Project Editor *Theresa Grutz*
Production Editor *Patricia A. Schissel*
Proofreading Coordinator *Carrie Barker*
Art Editor *Rita Hingtgen*
Photo Editor *Rose Deluhery*
Production Manager *Beth Kundert*
Production/Imaging and Media Development Manager *Linda Meehan Avenarius*
Production/Costing Manager *Sherry Padden*
Visuals/Design Freelance Specialist *Mary L. Christianson*
Senior Marketing Manager *Pamela S. Cooper*
Copywriter *Sandy Hyde*
Proofreader *Mary Svetlik Anderson*

Basal Text *10/12 Times Roman*
Display Type *Helvetica*
Typesetting System *Macintosh™ QuarkXPress™*
Paper Stock *50# Restorecote*

Brown & Benchmark
PUBLISHERS

Executive Vice President and General Manager *Bob McLaughlin*
Vice President, Business Manager *Russ Domeyer*
Vice President of Production and New Media Development *Victoria Putman*
National Sales Manager *Phil Rudder*
National Telesales Director *John Finn*

A Times Mirror Company

The credits section for this book begins on page C-1 and is considered an extension of the copyright page.

Cover design by Mary Sailer

Cover illustration © Andrew Carson

Proofread by Janet Reuter

Composition by TMHEG Imaging Group; compositor/pager Joann M. Palen

Library of Congress Catalog Card Number: 95–83959

ISBN 0–697–25890–4   2008 1731

Printed in the United States of America by Times Mirror Higher Education Group, Inc., 2460 Kerper Boulevard, Dubuque, IA 52001

10 9 8 7 6 5 4 3 2 1

CONTENTS

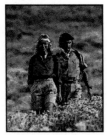
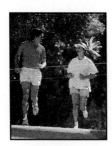
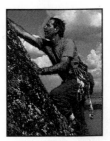
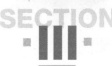
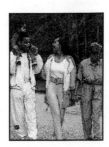
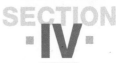

The Labs

Appendices

▪ PREFACE ▪

Looking Forward

Never in history have we had so much scientific information to support the value of healthy lifestyles in the promotion of physical fitness. The recent publication of *The Surgeon General's Report of Physical Activity and Health* provides definitive evidence that physical activity is one of the most important lifestyles that a person can adopt if lifetime fitness is an important goal. This report follows previous documents from the Surgeon General's office including reports on tobacco and nutrition which have had major impacts on our society. *Healthy People 2000* (a statement of national health goals) has focused public attention on healthy lifestyles such as regular physical activity, proper nutrition, controlling use of alcohol and tobacco, and stress reduction to achieve mental health. These reports, and the evidence on which they are based, show that healthy living can increase length of life and improve the quality of life for our extended years. A recent Mid-Decade Update of *Healthy People 2000* goals has shown that national efforts to improve lifestyles are producing results.

As we near the new century we are excited to be a part of the educational effort to promote physical fitness, health, and wellness. The wealth of evidence now available to us far exceeds what was available when we wrote our early editions. This reassures us that what we have presented in the previous eight editions of this text over the past three decades was sound and what we present in this ninth edition of *Concepts of Physical Fitness* will give you the best information available. We are pleased that we can continue our long tradition of providing our readers with information based on the most recent science.

Organization

This text is intended for an introductory college-level course dedicated to promoting healthy lifestyles that result in optimal physical fitness. *Concepts of Physical Fitness* is for teachers and students who want an up-to-date book focusing on physical activity and physical fitness. Section I: Physical Activity, Fitness, and Wellness includes introductory information, concepts on the health benefits of physical activity, preparing for activity, information about how much physical activity and physical fitness are needed to enhance performance and to produce health benefits, plus anatomy and physiology charts to help you identify the major parts of the muscle, skeletal, and circulatory/respiratory systems. **NEW** to this edition is a Physical Activity Pyramid which aids you in identifying the appropriate types of activities for gaining optimal health benefits.

Section II: Health Related Physical Fitness, presents up-to-date information on each of the five health related parts of fitness. The concepts provide the facts about each fitness component, as well as pictures and descriptions of the best exercises and activities for attaining each part of fitness. An attractive light blue color with a dark blue band is used on all pages containing illustrations of exercises. This **NEW** feature will allow you to easily locate exercise illustrations and descriptions. Also **NEW** are a 1 RM strength assessment and charts for determining desirable weight from skinfold measures. (The concept on Questionable Exercises in this section is a classic. Requests for use of this material in books and magazines has been unprecedented. You get the chance to get this information in its most up-to-date form, from its original source.)

Section III: Special Considerations for Physical Activity includes concepts on sports and skill-related fitness, information on care of the back and posture, and planning for lifetime activity.

Section IV: Healthy Lifestyles, includes a wellness overview, and concepts on nutrition, stress management and relaxation, and recognizing quackery. **NEW** to this edition is a discussion of self-management skills for aiding you in developing lifetime behaviors such as regular physical activity. The Surgeon General's recent report has an entire chapter devoted to the factors which help you to adhere to physical activity. We agree with the need for such a discussion and in this edition we emphasize the factors that aid you in adhering to lifetime activity. The section concludes with a concept on planning for healthy lifestyles.

Features

Over the years we have listened to teachers and students who use our books. Suggestions from you help us add to the features of the book that have proved to be so successful over time. Some of the key features that we think you will appreciate include:

- **Full-color Format.** The use of full color is intended not only to make the book attractive but to make the materials educationally sound. Full color allows us to highlight muscles used in each exercise, to present figures and pictures in a way that is easy to understand, and to help you locate materials (color tabs connecting concepts to labs, color pages for exercise illustrations, color bands for figures and tables).

- **Concepts.** We use concepts statements to introduce each major topic of the book. The concept statement and the evidence to support the statement are referred to as a concept rather than a chapter.
- **Health Goals.** Each concept includes health goals based on *Healthy People 2000*. **NEW** to this edition are updates of progress toward the nation's health goals.
- **Glossary.** A glossary of terms is listed at the beginning of each concept, then each term appears in boldface when it occurs in the text for the first time. This gives the reader an opportunity to refer back to the definitions if necessary.
- **Fact Statement Format.** Each major topic within each concept is made as a fact statement. This fact statement is followed by an explanation, discussion, and practical applications. Presenting information in this way allows us to present more information in less space and cuts through verbiage often found in texts of this type. This feature has been highly rated by users over the years.
- **Suggested Readings and References.** Suggested readings are listed at the end of each concept to aid those who are interested in learning more about a topic. In addition, an extended list of references is included so that you can know the source of materials presented in the text. We have gone to great lengths to get the most recent scientific information. It is for this reason that this book is widely used as a reference book as well as a text.
- **Laboratory Experiences and Questionnaires.** Most concepts are accompanied by laboratory exercises. Lab sheets provide spaces for recording personal data. Some labs require you to perform activities while others are questionnaires which help you learn more about yourself. Two planning labs are especially important (planning for active living and planing for healthy lifestyles). Color tabs (same color and location on the page) help you easily locate corresponding concepts and labs.
- **Lab Resource Materials.** At the end of each concept, lab resource materials are presented. These are materials that you will need to perform the lab experiences and complete the lab sheets at the end of the book. This allows you to easily locate the materials and to read about the various activities at the same time as you read each concept. These materials are available for future reference when the lab sheets have been used.
- **Appendices.** Metric conversion charts and charts of nutrient values are included for your use.
- **Inclusive Personalized Coverage.** No matter who you are, becoming physically active on a regular basis and adopting other healthy lifestyles will pay dividends. In this book we have been very careful to show how we are all *included* among those who can benefit. We are each individuals and for this reason we must be careful to personalize our lifestyles to suit individual needs. To help you personalize the information, we have provided fitness standards for different age groups and for men and women. We have noted instances when age, gender, and/or ethnic differences might affect disease risks of various kinds. Our intent is to point out our similarities while at the same time providing information that will be inclusive and personalized.
- **Criterion Referenced Fitness Standards.** For nearly thirty years we have provided criterion-referenced standards for use in rating your health-related fitness. We have based fitness ratings on levels of fitness deemed to be associated with improved health and wellness. Only recently have others come to recognize the wisdom of this system. Criterion-referenced standards allow you to decide how much fitness you need for your own good health and wellness. Your success is judged by self-comparisons and comparisons to health standards rather than the fitness of another person. Consult concept 4 for more information.

Concepts of Physical Fitness is intended to help you make important decisions about a wide variety of fitness issues. We feel that this book will empower you to take responsibility for personal fitness and wellness by adopting and maintaining healthy lifestyles, particularly regular physical activity designed to promote health-related physical fitness. We hope that you will find the book interesting and useful, and that you will want to share its message with your family and friends.

A Note to Instructors

Over the years, *Concepts of Physcial Fitness* has changed to make it easier to use for both students and instuctors. With each edition we have made changes recommended by users. The larger trim size introduced with the 5th edition, and the full color introduced in the 7th edition, were especially well received. Users continue to appreciate the outline format and tearout labs, and these are retained in the 9th edition.

We hope you agree that we continue to "lead the way" by including the most up-to-date facts that are documented by current references. You will note that the references are located at the end of the book. This allows us to reduce duplication so that we can avoid lengthening the book, which in turn keeps the price down. Many of you have expressed your thanks for our efforts to keep the price of the book low while still providing essential factual information.

Concepts of Physical Fitness is more than just a text; it is a full educational package. Many ancillary materials are available as part of the total educational package. The components of this package are:

- **Instructor s Manual (IM).** This revised manual includes: course objectives, suggestions for organization and scheduling lectures and labs, attention to using our electronic Lecture Presentation CD, grading suggestions, lecture outlines (complete with visual aids), chapter objectives, key points, discussion questions, ideas for outside activities, audiovisual resources, sources of equipment, blackline masters for use in making overhead transparencies, and an expanded test item file.

- **MicroTest III.** *MicroTest III* allows you to prepare custom exams using our prepared test bank along with your own test items. To improve the quality of our test items, we retained the services of a leading test expert, Dr. Weimo Zhu, to review and assist in writing the very best test items possible. MicroTest is available in IBM DOS, Windows, and Macintosh versions.
- **Color Transparencies.** Two sets of transparencies are now available (on request). The first set of 50 color images includes anatomical, physiological, fitness, and wellness images specifically for use with *Concepts of Physical Fitness*. A second set of general fitness and wellness transparencies supplements the *Concepts* set.
- **Videos.** Videos continue to be available to instructors. The first tape focuses on physical fitness. This newly released video presents the fitness philosophy, an overview of the administration of fitness tests found within the text, and describes the concept approach. The second video focuses on wellness. It includes basic wellness definitions as well as a general wellness philosophy. Both tapes are perfect classroom tools for use in motivating students at an early stage in the course. They can be used in class prior to the presentation of those tests, or can serve as resource material for the instructor.
- **Computer Programs.** In addition to Testpak, several computer programs continue to be available in both IBM and Macintosh formats. The computer assessment programs evaluate students in the areas of physical activity, target heart rate, heart disease risk, nutrition, and stress. Students enter information and receive instant feedback on their current status as well as ways to maintain or improve their levels of fitness.
- **Teacher s Resource Notebook (Binder).** A special notebook (binder) will be given free to each adopter of the text. This handy binder comes complete with tabbed dividers to contain such items as the Instructor's Manual, Transparencies, etc.

Acknowledgments

In the years since the first *Concepts* book was published, many people have helped to make it successful. There is great risk in attempting to identify all of those who have helped us through the years because there is the very real possibility that we will forget to name someone who has made an important contribution to the book's success. Nevertheless, we want to extend a thanks to the many people who have helped. To those of you who we no doubt missed (including all of the users who have written us with suggestions over the years), we apologize. We do want to make these acknowledgments because without the help of those named, the *Concepts* books would not have experienced the success that they have.

First, we would like to acknowledge a few people who have made special contributions over the years. **Linus Dowell, Carl Landiss,** and **Homer Tolson,** all of Texas A&M University, were involved in the development of the first *Concepts* book and their contributions were also important as we helped start the fitness movement back in the 1960s. Other pioneers were **Jimmy Jones** of Henderson State University who started one of the first *Concepts* classes in 1970 and has led the way in teaching fitness in the years that followed; **Charles Erickson,** who started a quality program at Missouri Western; and **Al Leister,** a leader in the east at Mercer County Community College in New Jersey. **David Laurie** and **Barbara Gench** (now at Texas Women's University) at Kansas State University, as well as others on that faculty, were instrumental in developing a prototype *Concepts* program which research has shown to be successful. A special thanks is extended to **Greg Welk** who has contributed so much to the development of the most recent editions of the book, including his coauthorship of the Instructor's Manual, CD-ROM presentation disk, and other ancillary materials. **Mark Ahn, Keri Chesney, Chris MacCrate, Guy Mullin, Stephen Hustedde, Greg Nigh,** and **Doreen Mauro,** along with other employees of the Consortium for Instructional Innovation and the Micro Computer Resource Facility at Arizona State University, and **Betty Craft** and **Ken Rudich** and other employees of the Distance Learning Technology Program at Arizona State University deserve special recognition. All of the above-named people were instrumental in the development of the *Concepts* books over the years.

Second, we wish to extend thanks to the following people who provided comments on the current editions of our *Concepts* book: **Debra A. Beal,** Northern Essex Community College; **Roger Bishop,** Wartburg College; **David S. Brewster,** Indiana State University; **Ronnie Carda,** University of Wisconsin–Madison; **Curt W. Cattau,** Concordia University; **Cindy Ekstedt Connelley,** Catawba College; **J. Ellen Eason,** Towson State University; **Bridgit A. Finley,** Oklahoma City Community College; **Diane Sanders Flickner,** Bethel College; **Judy Fox,** Indiana Wesleyan University; **Earlene Hannah,** Hendrix College; **Carole J. Hanson,** University of Northern Iowa; **David Horton,** Liberty University; **John Merriman,** Valdosta State College; **Beverly F. Mitchell,** Kennesaw State College; **George Perkins,** Northwestern State University; **James J. Sheehan,** Fitchburg State College; **Mary Slaughter,** University of Illinois; **Paul H. Todd,** Polk Community College; **Susan M. M. Todd,** Vancouver Community College–Langara Campus; **Kenneth E. Weatherman,** Floyd College; **Newton Wilkes, Bridget Cobb, John Dippel,** and **Todd Kleinfelter** of Northwestern State University of Louisiana and **John R. Webster,** Central Connecticut State University. A special thanks is extended to **Patty Williams, Ann Woodard, Laurel Smith,** and **Bill Carr** (Polk Community College) for their helpful suggestions. Without their help, the book could not have been the success that it has proven to be over the years. We thank you all.

Third, we want to acknowledge the following people who have aided us in the preparation of past editions: **James Angel, Jeanne Ashley, Stanley Brown, Ronnie Carda, Robert Clayton, Melvin Ezell Jr., Brigit Finley, Pay Floyd, Carole Hanson, James Harvey, John Hayes, David Horton, Sister Janice Iverson, Tony Jadin, Richard Krejei, Ron Lawman, James Marett, Pat McSwegin, Betty McVaigh, John Merriman, Beverly Mitchell, Sandra Morgan, Robert Pugh, Larry Reagan, Mary Rice, Roberta Stokes, Paul Todd, Susan Todd, Marjorie Avery Willard, Karen Cookson, Dawn Strout, Earlene Hannah, Ken Weatherman, J. Ellen Eason, William Podoll, John Webster, James Sheehan, David Brewster, Kelly Adam, Lisa Hibbard, Roger Bishop, Mary Slaughter, Jack Clayton Stovall, Karen Watkins, Ruth Cohoon, Mark Bailey, Nena Amundson, Bruce Wilson, Sarah Collie, Carl Beal, George Perkins, Stan Rettew, Ragene Gwin, Judy Fox, Diane Flickner, Cindy Connelley, Curt Cattau, Don Torok,** and **Dennis Wilson.** They all helped us build the foundation for success of the current editions.

Finally, we want to acknowledge others who have contributed, including **Virginia Atkins, Charles Cicciarella, Donna Landers, Susan Miller, Robert Pangrazi, Karen Ward, Carl Waterman,** and **Weimo Zhu.** Among other important contributors are former graduate students who have contributed ideas, made corrections, and contributed in other untold ways to the success of these books. We wish to acknowledge **Jeff Boone, Laura Borsdorf, Lisa Chase, Tom Cuddihy, Darren Dale, Bo Fernhall, Connie Fye, Louie Garcia, Steve Feyrer-Melk, Ken Fox, Ron Hager, Brian Nielsen, Debbie Ostlund, Kirk Rose, Jack Rutherford, Scott Slava, Dave Thomas, Min Qi Wang, Jim Whitehead,** and **Ashley Woodcock.**

The challenge of **Healthy People 2000** *is to use the combined strength of scientific knowledge, professional skill, individual commitment, community support, and political will to enable people to achieve their potential to live full, active lives. It means preventing premature death and preventing disability, preserving a physical environment that supports human life, cultivating family and community support, enhancing each individual's inherent abilities to respond and to act, and assuring that all Americans achieve and maintain a maximum level of functioning.*

Public Health Service
Healthy People 2000

The **Healthy People 2000** *goals . . . emphasize the quality of life—not just its quantity—as measured through use of quality-adjusted life expectancy (years of healthy life).*

J. Michael McGinnis
Public Health Service
Healthy People 2000 at Mid Decade

We must get serious about improving the health of the nation by affirming our commitment to healthy physical activity on all levels: personal, family, community, organizational, and national. Because physical activity is so directly related to preventing disease and premature death and to maintaining a high quality life, we must accord it the same level of attention that we give other important public health practices that affect the entire nation. Physical activity thus joins the front ranks of essential health objectives, such as sound nutrition, the use of seat belts, and the prevention of adverse health effects of tobacco.

Audrey F. Manley
Surgeon General (Acting)

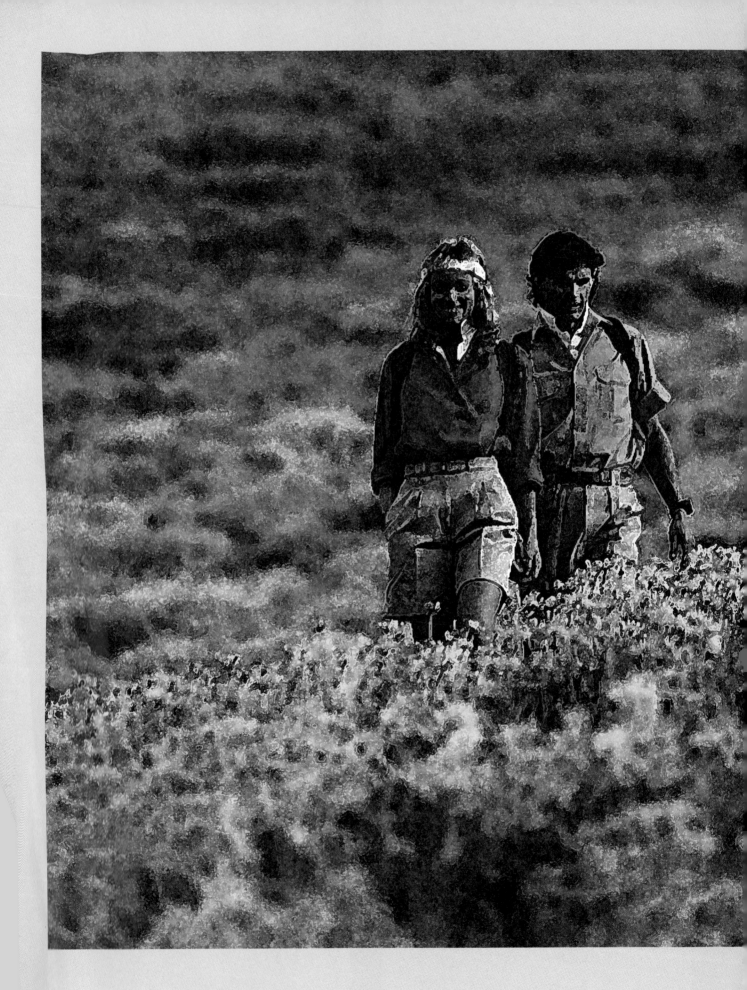

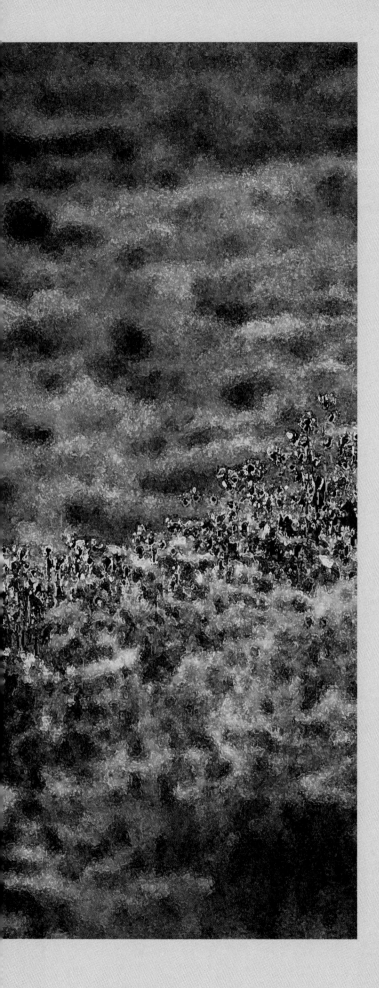

SECTION

I

Physical Activity, Fitness, and Wellness

CONCEPT
·1·

Introduction to Physical Activity, Fitness, and Wellness

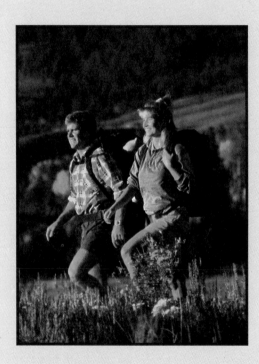

Concept 1

Good physical fitness, regular exercise, and optimal wellness are important for all people.

A Statement About National Health Goals

At the beginning of each concept in this book is a section containing abbreviated statements of national health goals from the document *Healthy People 2000: National Health Promotion and Disease Prevention Objectives.* These statements, established by expert groups representing more than 300 national organizations, are intended as realistic national health goals to be achieved by the year 2000. In 1995 a mid-decade review was conducted and it was determined that progress was being made in more than half of the priority goal areas. Throughout the book we have indicated areas in which improvements have been made and areas in which progress has been lacking. Although the goals are intended to improve the health of those in the United States, they seem important for all people in North America and in other cultures throughout the world. This book is written with the achievement of these important health goals in mind.

Introduction

The recently published *Surgeon General's Report on Physical Activity and Health* (1996) traces the link between physical activity and good health to the 5th century B.C. The exercise to health relationship was traced through Greek cultures to modern times. The early notion that activity is beneficial to health is now well-documented. Evidence is available to support the idea that lack of regular physical activity results in poor physical fitness. Those who are not physically fit and who are sedentary often suffer from hypokinetic diseases and other conditions discussed in this book.

As western civilization becomes more automated, physical exertion becomes less necessary as a part of the normal work of many adults. However, the need for regular exercise has not decreased; if anything, it has increased. Regular physical activity is, however, only one of many lifestyle patterns that can enhance health and wellness. Recent scientific evidence, as summarized in the Surgeon General's report and other recent documents, suggests that a healthy lifestyle, more than any other single factor, is responsible for optimal wellness. The implication is that each of us can learn to alter our lifestyles to foster lifetime fitness, health, and wellness.

Health Goals for the Year 2000

- Increase the span of healthy life. (↑)
- Increase the proportion of people who do regular physical activity for cardiovascular fitness. (↑)
- Increase the proportion of people who do regular physical activity for strength, muscular endurance, and flexibility. (<>)
- Decrease the proportion of people who do no leisure-time physical activity. (↓)

Reduce the prevalence of overfatness and increase physical activity among those who have excess body fatness. (↓)

Note: (↑) indicates progress toward goal, (↓) indicates regression from goal, and (<>) indicates either no change or lack of new data since 1990.

General Terms

Throughout the book, key terms are in bold type the first time they appear in the text. You may wish to check the definition of each term as you read.

- **Bone Integrity** Soundness of the bones associated with high density and absence of symptoms of deterioration.

- **Exercise** Formally exercise is defined as physical activity done for the purpose of getting physically fit. Physical activity is generally considered to be a broader term used to describe all forms of large muscle movements including sports, dance, games, work, lifestyle activities, and exercise for fitness. In this book, exercise and physical activity will often be used interchangeably to make reading less repetitive and more interesting.

- **Health** Health is optimal well-being that contributes to quality of life. It is more than freedom from disease and illness, though freedom from disease is important to good health. Optimal health includes high-level mental, social, emotional, spiritual, and physical fitness within the limits of one's heredity and personal disabilities.

- **Hypokinetic Diseases or Conditions** Hypo means under or too little, and kinetic means movement or activity. Thus, hypokinetic means "too little activity." A hypokinetic disease or condition is one associated with lack of physical activity or too little regular exercise. Examples of such conditions include heart disease, low back pain, adult-onset diabetes, and obesity.

- **Illness** Illness is the ill feeling and/or symptoms associated with a disease or circumstances that upset homeostasis.

- **Lifestyles** Lifestyles are patterns of behavior or ways an individual typically lives.

- **Physical Fitness** Physical fitness is the body's ability to function efficiently and effectively. It consists of health-related physical fitness and skill-related physical fitness, which have at least eleven different components, each of which contributes to total quality of life. Physical fitness is associated with a person's ability to work effectively, to enjoy leisure time, to be healthy, to resist hypokinetic diseases, and to meet emergency situations. It is related to but different from health, wellness, and the psychological, sociological, emotional, and spiritual components of fitness. Although the development of physical fitness is the result of many things, optimal physical fitness is not possible without regular exercise.

- **Wellness** Wellness is the integration of all parts of health and fitness (mental, social, emotional, spiritual, and physical) that expands one's potential to live and work effectively and to make a significant contribution to society. Wellness reflects how one feels (a sense of well-being) about life as well as one's ability to function effectively. Wellness, as opposed to illness (a negative), is sometimes described as the positive component of good health.

Health-Related Fitness Terms

- **Body Composition** The relative percentage of muscle, fat, bone, and other tissues of which the body is composed. A fit person has a relatively low, but not too low, percentage of body fat (body fatness).

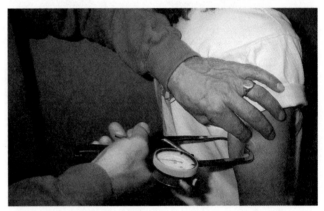

Body composition (fatness)

- **Cardiovascular Fitness** The ability of the heart, blood vessels, blood, and respiratory system to supply fuel, especially oxygen, to the muscles and the ability of the muscles to utilize fuel to allow sustained exercise. A fit person can persist in physical activity for relatively long periods without undue stress.

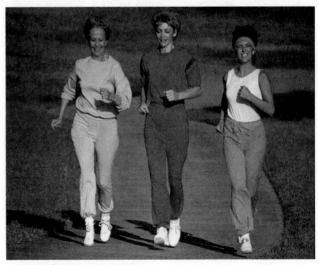

Cardiovascular fitness

Flexibility The range of motion available in a joint. It is affected by muscle length, joint structure, and other factors. A fit person can move the body joints through a full range of motion in work and in play.

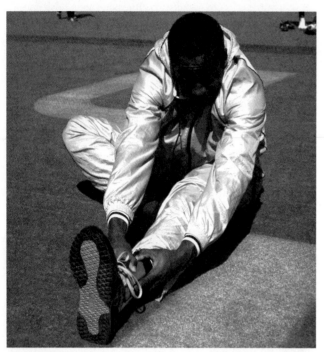

Flexibility

Muscular Endurance The ability of the muscles to repeatedly exert themselves. A fit person can repeat movements for a long period without undue fatigue.

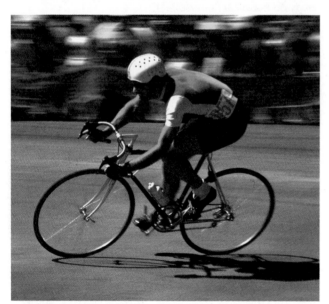

Muscular endurance

Strength The ability to exert an external force or to lift a heavy weight. A fit person can do work or play that involves exerting force, such as lifting or controlling one's own body weight.

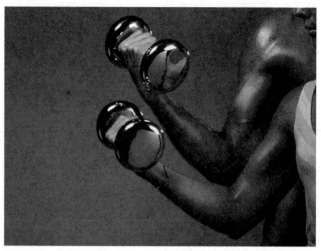

Strength

Skill-Related Fitness Terms

Agility The ability to rapidly and accurately change the direction of the movement of the entire body in space. Skiing and wrestling are examples of activities that require exceptional agility.

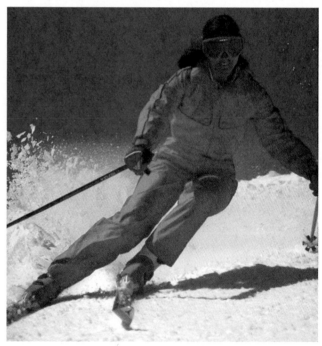

Agility

Balance The maintenance of equilibrium while stationary or while moving. Water skiing, performing on the balance beam, or working as a riveter on a high-rise building are activities that require exceptional balance.

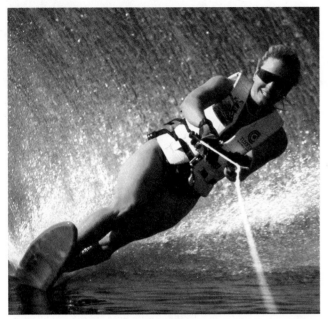

Balance

Coordination The ability to use the senses with the body parts to perform motor tasks smoothly and accurately. Juggling, hitting a golf ball, batting a baseball, or kicking a ball are examples of activities requiring good coordination.

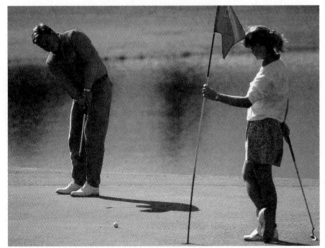

Coordination

Power The ability to transfer energy into force at a fast rate. Throwing the discus and putting the shot are activities that require considerable power.

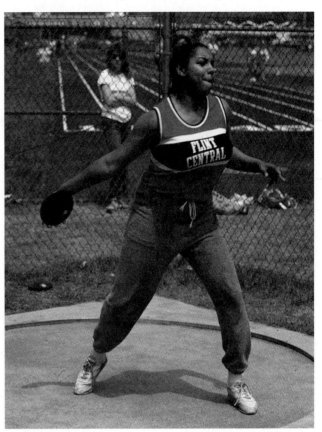

Power

Reaction Time The time elapsed between stimulation and the beginning of reaction to that stimulation. Driving a racing car and starting a sprint race require good reaction time.

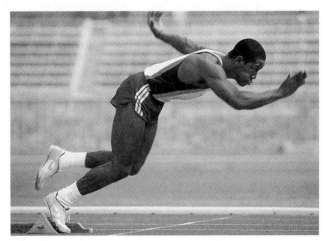

Reaction time

Speed The ability to perform a movement in a short period of time. A runner on a track team or a wide receiver on a football team needs good foot and leg speed.

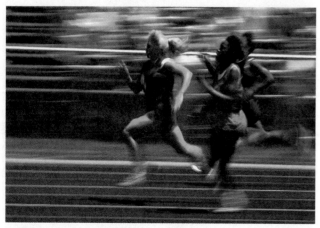

Speed

The Facts

Good **health** is of primary importance to adults in our society.

When polled about important social values, 99 percent of adults in the U.S. identified "being in good health" as one of their major concerns. The three concerns expressed most often were good health, good family life, and good self-image. The one percent who did not identify good health as an important concern had no opinion on any social issues. Among those polled, none felt that good health was unimportant.

Optimal health is more than freedom from disease.

During this century the life expectancy for the average person has increased by 60 percent. A child born in 1900 could expect to live only 47 years. A child born today can expect to live to the age of 75.8. Much of the increase in life span can be attributed to modern medical science. Many diseases that killed thousands in earlier times can now be easily treated. Pneumonia, which can be treated with antibiotics, is a good example.

As treatment for killer diseases became available, the emphasis shifted to disease prevention. Curing disease was still of concern, but the development of vaccines and other preventions for disease became central to the efforts of public health and medical experts. Many lives have been saved and much pain and suffering has been avoided as a result of the development of vaccines for diseases such as smallpox and polio.

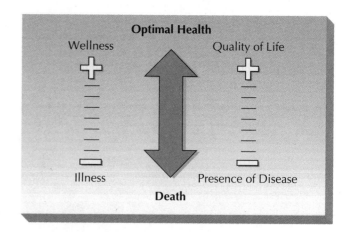

Figure 1.1

Wellness is an important part of optimal health.

As a result of the advances in illness treatment and prevention, an effort can now be made to focus on **wellness.** Wellness, or a sense of well-being, includes one's ability to live and work effectively and to make a significant contribution to society. It reflects how one feels about life as well as one's ability to function effectively. Wellness represents a quality of living component that is essential for optimal health.

As illustrated in figure 1.1, good health is partly associated with freedom from illness and disease. Disease treatment and prevention efforts are important to good health. However, as noted previously, a sense of well-being or wellness as reflected in quality living is critical to optimal health. Health promotion programs often go beyond disease treatment and prevention in that they contribute to optimal **physical fitness** and spiritual and emotional health, as well as other components that enhance the quality of life.

Increasing the span of healthy life is a principal health goal.

Consistent with the notion that optimal health includes a wellness dimension that is more than freedom from disease, the Public Health Service has adopted as its principal goal the increase in *healthy* span of life. In this regard we have been effective in meeting national health goals as the life expectancy for the average person has increased from 73.7 to 75.8 years since the national health goals were developed. Unfortunately, the average person can expect to have only about 64 years of healthy life (see figure 1.2). The remaining 11.8 years are characterized as dysfunctional or lacking in the wellness component. For these people quality of life is diminished.

Lack of wellness is not, however, a problem exclusive to older people. Many young people fail to achieve

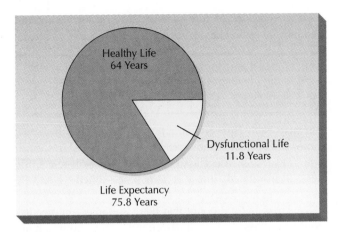

Figure 1.2

Years of healthy life as a proportion of life expectancy (U.S. population)

Source: Data from *National Vital Statistics System* and *National Health Interview Survey*. Centers for Disease Control and Prevention, Atlanta, GA.

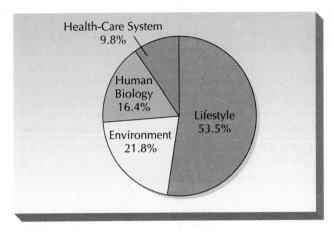

Figure 1.3

Percentage contribution of four sources to early death

Source: Data From K. E. Powell, et al., "The Status of the 1990 Objectives for Physical Fitness and Exercise" in *Public Health Reports*, 19: 101, 1989. U.S. Public Health Service.

wellness because of **illness** and/or less than quality living. Increasing the quality of life for people of all ages is as important as increasing the number of years lived. In addition to adding years to life, the goal is to add life to our years.

> Lifestyle change, more than any other factor, is considered to be the best way of preventing illness and early death in our society.

When people in Western society die before the age of 65, it is considered to be early or premature death. The four major factors contributing to early death are noted in figure 1.3. Human biology, which includes hereditary predisposition to disease, accounts for only a small share of the causes of early death. Improvements in the environment and in the health-care system could substantially decrease early death, but by far the best way to decrease this problem is the promotion of healthy lifestyles.

> Healthy lifestyles are critical to wellness.

Just as unhealthy lifestyles are the principal causes of modern-day illnesses such as heart disease, cancer, and diabetes, healthy **lifestyles** can result in an improved feeling of wellness that is critical to optimal health. In recognizing the importance of "years of healthy life," the Public Health Service also recognizes what it calls "measures of well-being." This well-being or wellness is associated with social, mental, spiritual, and physical functioning. Being physically active and eating well are two examples of healthy lifestyles that can improve well-being and add years of quality living. Many of the healthy lifestyles associated with good physical fitness and optimal wellness will be discussed in detail later in this book.

> Regular physical activity is a healthy lifestyle that helps prevent **hypokinetic diseases** and conditions.

An increase in physical activity designed to improve physical fitness is a central goal in the plan designed to enhance the healthy life span of people in the U.S. by the year 2000. Physical activity and physical fitness have been shown to reduce the risk of such hypokinetic illnesses as heart disease, hypertension, adult-onset diabetes, osteoporosis, obesity, mental-health problems, some forms of cancer, and chronic musculoskeletal problems such as back pain.

> Good physical fitness and regular physical activity are important to wellness.

Wellness is quality of life. Regular physical activity and good physical fitness have been shown to enhance quality of life in many ways. Physical fitness and **exercise** can help you look good, feel good, and enjoy life. Exercise helps keep body fat levels in normal ranges and is responsible for muscle development that can improve one's perception of self. Fitness and exercise have been associated with various mental and physical health benefits that help an individual feel good and function effectively. Physical activity provides an enjoyable way to spend one's leisure time. Each of the wellness benefits of physical activity and physical fitness will be discussed in greater detail in the concepts that follow.

> If optimal health is to be achieved, personal control of lifestyles is necessary.

A recent poll indicates that 91 percent of adults would like to change their lifestyles to make their lives more enjoyable and to change factors associated with wellness, such as reducing stress and tension. Unfortunately, many people feel that they do not have personal control over good health and wellness. For example, one survey suggests that most of the lifestyle changes deemed important by millions in our society will remain in the realm of fantasies, just beyond realization.

Experts have shown that people who feel that health is beyond personal control express such ideas as "Bad things (illness) can't happen to me and good things (wellness) are beyond my reach." Evidence is presented in this book to show that many of the most serious health problems in our society can happen to anyone, and that the risk of suffering from these problems can be greatly reduced by making lifestyle changes that are possible for all people. Adopting healthy lifestyles not only helps in disease prevention but also can promote wellness—the quality of life component of optimal health.

The Facts About Physical Fitness Components

Physical fitness consists of many components, each of which is specific in nature.

Physical fitness is a combination of several aspects rather than a single characteristic. A fit person possesses at least adequate levels of each of the health-related fitness components, and each of the skill-related fitness components. People who possess one aspect of physical fitness do not necessarily possess all of the other aspects.

Some relationships exist among different fitness characteristics, but each of the components of physical fitness is separate and different from the others. For example, people who possess exceptional strength do not necessarily have good cardiovascular fitness, and those who have good coordination do not necessarily possess good flexibility.

Body composition, cardiovascular fitness, flexibility, muscular endurance, and strength are the health-related components of physical fitness.

Because each fitness characteristic has a direct relationship to good health and lessens the risk of hypokinetic disease, each is considered a part of health-related physical fitness. Some experts consider **bone integrity** to be an additional part of health-related fitness.

Possessing a moderate amount of each component of health-related fitness is essential to disease prevention and health promotion. To some extent, having exceptionally high levels of health-related fitness is similar to having high level skill-related fitness. For example, moderate amounts of strength are necessary to prevent back and posture problems, whereas high levels of strength contribute most to improved performance in activities such as football and jobs involving heavy lifting.

Agility, balance, coordination, power, reaction time, and speed are often considered to be the main components of skill-related physical fitness.

Because each fitness characteristic is related to certain motor skills, such as those required in sports and in specific types of jobs, each is classified as a part of skill-related fitness. Skill-related fitness is sometimes called "sports fitness" or "motor fitness."

There is little doubt that there are other abilities that could be classified as skill-related fitness components. Also, each part of skill-related fitness is multidimensional. For example, coordination could be hand-eye coordination such as batting a ball, foot-eye coordination such as kicking a ball, or any of many other possibilities. The six parts of skill-related fitness identified here are those that are commonly associated with successful sports and work performance. It should be noted that each could be measured in ways other than those presented in this book. Measurements are provided to help the reader understand the nature of total physical fitness and to help the reader make important decisions about lifetime physical activity.

Other Facts About Fitness and Physical Activity

Heredity influences physical fitness, total fitness, and optimal health.

There is good evidence that a person's potential to develop exceptionally high levels of physical fitness, especially skill-related physical fitness, is based on heredity. Just as physical fitness is influenced by heredity, so are other parts of total fitness and health. Predispositions to various diseases and health problems can be inherited.

Healthy lifestyles are important to optimal health and quality of life.

Doing physical activity is one of many healthy lifestyles that contribute to optimal health and quality of life. Unlike heredity, lifestyles can be changed to improve fitness and health.

North Americans have become more active in recent years.

Adults in the United States have become more active in recent years. Since the Gallup Poll on exercise was begun in 1961, there has been a consistent increase in physical activity among adults. In 1961 only 24 percent of adults said they

Adults who do 30 minutes of exercise 5 days a week.

Currently = 24%

Goal = 36%

Adults who do cardiovascular fitness activity 3 days a week for at least 20 minutes a day.

Currently = 12%

Goal = 20%

People aged 6 and older who do regular strength, muscular endurance, and flexibility exercise.

Current = not known

Goal = 40%

People aged 6 and older who do no leisure-time physical activity.

Current = 24%

Goal = 15%

Figure 1.4

Physical activity and fitness goals for the year 2000

Source: Data from the Public Health Service. *Healthy People 2000: National Health Promotion and Disease Prevention Objectives*, Washington, D.C.: U.S. GPO, 1991 and from J. M. McGinnis and P. R. Lee "Healthy People 2000 at Mid Decade," in *Journal of the American Medical Association*, 273, 1123.

were physically active during their free time. Currently, more than half say they are active. Surveys in Canada show similar increases in adult physical activity. This indicates that the "fitness movement" is more than a fad. Regular exercise is becoming a part of the lifestyle of an increasing number of people. Since 1990 the number of people who are active enough to achieve fitness, health, and wellness benefits has increased from 22 percent to 24 percent, showing progress toward our national goal. This has led to increasing the goal for the year 2000 from 30 percent to 36 percent (see figure 1.4).

Too many North Americans are not as active as they should be.

Though more adults are active than in the past, many who say they are active participate only occasionally. Research results indicate that most adults do not exercise enough to improve fitness and that many are totally inactive. Unfortunately, attempts to decrease the number of people who are totally inactive have been ineffective. In fact, more adults are now totally sedentary than in 1990, when national health goals were established.

Some segments of the population are more fit and active than others.

In spite of the concerns of some about the fitness of our youth, children are the most active and fit segment of the population. Evidence indicates that teens are less active than children, and adults are less active than teens. Today,

children have been shown to be as fit as children 30 years ago, with one exception: they are fatter than children of previous generations. There is concern that teens are less active than in past years. This fact is important because the teen years are a time when proper exercise and healthy lifestyles can result in exceptional fitness gains.

Among the adult population, young, middle-class males are most likely to be active. Women have become more active in recent years but are still less active than men. Older adults experience the same general benefits of regular physical activity that younger people do, but nearly twice as many are likely to be sedentary. People with disabilities and those with low incomes are also considerably less active than other adults.

Good physical fitness and regular physical activity contribute to optimal health and wellness.

Good fitness resulting from regular exercise reduces the risk of hypokinetic disease and contributes to wellness as evidenced by an improved quality of life. The health benefits of exercise and fitness will be outlined in greater detail later.

Industry has recognized the importance of exercise programs to employee fitness and productivity.

Realizing that many jobs are not as active as they were prior to automation, industries have taken steps to provide on-the-job exercise and fitness programs for their employees. More than one-half of all companies with 750 or more employees now have an exercise program. A national goal is to increase this number to 80 percent. Since 1990 significant progress has been made in achieving this goal. Company officials endorse the fitness-in-industry movement because medical costs are skyrocketing; hypokinetic diseases, such as back pain, account for a billion-dollar annual loss in production; and absenteeism can be reduced considerably by offering employees an exercise and fitness program. Evidence indicates that such programs are cost-effective as well as popular among employees. The increase in worksite wellness programs has been cited as one reason for progress in other important national health goals. One company official notes, "It's the best fringe benefit we've offered."

Many people are ignorant of the facts about physical activity and physical fitness.

Unfortunately, many adults in the U.S. hold misconceptions about health, fitness, and exercise. For example, more than 50 percent of inactive adults feel that such sports as baseball and bowling provide enough exercise to develop good health and physical fitness. Although the facts indicate otherwise, those who do not exercise regularly believe that they get all the exercise they need. Interestingly, those who report that they participate in regular exercise are also the ones who are likely to feel that they do not get enough exercise for their own good.

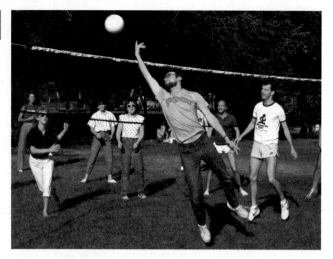
Exercise provides an opportunity for social involvement.

The most popular forms of exercise among adults require very little skill or equipment and are easily accessible.

The Surgeon General's Report on Physical Activity and Health indicates that the most popular participation activities among adults are walking, gardening or yard work, stretching exercises, bicycling, strength exercises, stair climbing, jogging, aerobic dancing, and swimming. Other national surveys consistently show similar results. All these can be done in or near the home for little or no cost. None requires a high degree of physical skill in order for a person to be successful or to enjoy the benefits associated with regular involvement. These activities are not often those that people value for their children, nor those in which they themselves were involved in as children. And although football, baseball, basketball, gymnastics, and boxing are the activities adults most enjoy watching, they usually are not the ones in which they participate.

Regular exercise and good fitness can save money.

Studies show that sedentary living costs taxpayers huge amounts of money each year. It is projected that society could save $1,900 annually for each sedentary person who began regular exercise. The extra costs to taxpayers are the result of increased health insurance premiums, life insurance premiums, sick leave coverage, and disability insurance premiums.

Physical activity can be important for many reasons, but it is not a cure-all, and if done improperly, it can be dangerous.

The many benefits of exercise are well-documented in this book. However, certain types of exercise are contraindicated for some people. Doing too much too soon can be dangerous for those who have not been involved in exercise on a regular basis. Those who exercise irregularly, such as the "weekend athlete" who exercises vigorously only on weekends or other special occasions, may be asking for trouble. Even avid exercisers can become over-involved with their commitment to physical activity and develop an activity neurosis. This condition can develop if an individual becomes irrationally concerned about his or her need for involvement in exercise.

There is no single best form of physical activity for all people.

Different people participate in different types of exercise for different reasons. This is as it should be. Each person has his or her own unique movement personality—no two people move in exactly the same way. Because movement personalities differ, there is a wide variety of leisure activities from which individuals can select. The choice of exercise and physical activities should be made only after carrying out the following steps:

- Assess your current health and physical fitness status to determine your individual needs.
- Examine your current interests. (Exercise should be enjoyable.)
- Acquire a knowledge and an understanding of the values of different activities.
- Determine which activities will best meet your needs and interests.
- Acquire skill and knowledge in the selected activities.

Physical activity is for virtually everyone.

Exercise, whether it be sports or some other form of physical activity, should not be limited to those with good athletic ability. Regardless of age, sex, or athletic ability (if there is no serious medical limitation), there is some form of activity that everyone will find enjoyable and in which everyone can succeed.

Facts About Why People Do Not Exercise

The number one reason people give for not exercising is, "I don't have the time."

"I'm too busy!" This reason has been shown repeatedly to be the leading reason why people do not do regular exercise. Invariably, these people indicate that they know they should do more exercise and that they plan to in the future when "things are less hectic." For example, young people say that they will soon be established in a career and then they will have the time to exercise. Older people say that they wish they had taken the time to be active when they were younger.

Another major reason people do not exercise is, "It's too inconvenient."

Many who avoid exercise do so because it is inconvenient. They are exercise procrastinators. Specific reasons for

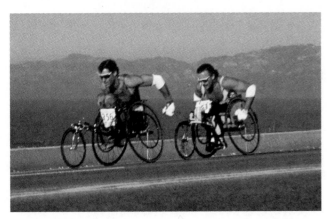

Exercise is for everyone.

procrastinating include: "It makes me sweaty"; "It messes up my hair"; and "I just can't find the energy." (It is interesting, though, that those who do exercise regularly report improvements in their appearance and a feeling of increased energy.)

Large numbers of adults are not active because they "just don't enjoy exercise."

The reasons some people say they do not enjoy exercise include: "People might laugh at me"; "Sports make me nervous"; and "I am not good at physical activities." These people often lack confidence in their own abilities. In some cases, this is because of their past experiences in physical education or in athletics. With properly selected activities, even those who have never enjoyed exercise can get "hooked."

Poor health is a reason some people avoid exercise.

Some people avoid exercise because of health reasons. Though it is true that there are good medical reasons for not exercising, many people with such problems can benefit from exercise if it is properly designed for them.

Lack of facilities and bad weather are reasons some people do not exercise regularly.

Regular exercise is much more convenient if facilities are easy to reach and the weather is good. Still, recreational opportunities have increased considerably in recent years. Furthermore, some of the most popular activities for building fitness require very little equipment, can be done in or near the home, and are inexpensive.

Some people do not perform regular physical activity because they think they are too old.

As people grow older, many begin to feel that exercise is something they cannot do. For most people this is simply not true! Studies conducted over a period of years indicate that properly planned exercise for older adults is not only

safe but also has many health benefits, including longer life, fewer illnesses, increased working capacity, and an improved sense of well-being.

Facts About Why People Do Exercise

The number one reason people exercise regularly is "for health and physical fitness."

Nearly all adults recognize the importance of exercise for good health and fitness. More than one national survey has shown that health and fitness is the single most important reason why people engage in regular exercise. Unfortunately, many adults say that a "doctor's order to exercise" would be the most likely reason to get them to begin a regular program. For some, however, waiting for a doctor's order may be too late.

Physical appearance is a common reason cited for doing regular exercise.

An important reason for exercising is to improve physical appearance. In our society, looking good is highly valued, thus physical attractiveness is another major reason why people participate in regular exercise. Of major importance to many adults is weight or fat control.

While the evidence suggests that exercise can be effective in helping you look your best, there is a danger of unrealistic expectations on the part of many people. Most would like to make a change in their appearance that is not likely to happen as a result of exercise alone.

Enjoyment is a major reason for exercising regularly.

A majority of adults say that enjoyment would be of paramount importance in deciding to exercise. This is not surprising, given statements from joggers that they began exercising for fitness but continue for such reasons as the "peak experience," the "runner's high," and "spinning free." In fact, movement can be an end in itself. Satisfaction can be derived from the mere involvement in the movement activity. The sense of fun, the feeling of well-being, and the general enjoyment associated with physical activity is well-documented.

Relaxation and release from tension are reasons given for doing regular exercise.

Relaxation and release from tension rank high as reasons why people do regular exercise. Exercise, such as walking, jogging, or cycling, is a way of getting some quiet time away from the stress of the job. For years, it has been recognized that exercise in the form of sports and games provides a catharsis, or outlet, for the frustrations of normal daily activities. Evidence indicates that regular exercise can help reduce depression and anxiety, both common symptoms in Western culture.

Physical activity can provide a way of meeting a challenge and developing a sense of personal accomplishment.

A sense of personal accomplishment associated with performing various physical activities is frequently a reason people exercise. In some cases, it is merely learning a new skill, such as racquetball or tennis; in other cases, it is running a mile or doing a certain number of sit-ups that provides this feeling of accomplishment. The challenge of doing something never done before is apparently a very powerful experience. Physical activities provide opportunities not readily available in other aspects of life.

An important reason many people exercise is the social experience of involvement.

Physical activity often provides the opportunity to be with other people. It is this social experience that many appreciate most about exercise. Frequent answers to the question, "Why do you exercise?" include: "It is a good way to spend time with other members of the family"; "It is a good way to spend time with close friends"; and "Being part of the team is a satisfying feeling." Physical activity settings can also provide an opportunity for making new friends.

The competitive experience is an important reason people participate in sports and physical activities.

"The thrill of victory" and "sports competition" are two reasons often given by people who participate in physical activities. For many, the competitive experiences can be very satisfying.

A positive balance of feelings enhances your chances of being active.

People who have more postive feelings about physical activity than negatives one are said to have a positive balance of feelings. A positive balance of feelings increases the chances that a person will be active. On the other hand, a person who has more negative feelings than positive ones is more likely to be inactive. You can use the charts in the lab resource materials to assess your "balance of feelings."

Suggested Readings

Bouchard, C. "Heredity and Health-Related Fitness." *Physical Activity and Fitness Research Digest* 1(1993): 1.
Bruess, C., and G. Richardson. *Decisions for Health*. 4th ed. Dubuque, IA: Wm. C. Brown Publishers, 1995.
Corbin, C. B. and Pangrazi, R. P. "What You Need to Know About the Surgeon General's Report on Physical Activity and Health," *Physical Activity and Fitness Research Digest*, 2(1996):1.
McGinnis, J. M. "The Public Health Burden of a Sedentary Lifestyle." *Medicine and Science in Sports and Exercise* 24 (1992): S196 (Supplement).
McGinnis, J. M., and P. R. Lee. "Healthy People 2000 at Mid Decade." *Journal of the American Medical Association* 273 (1995): 1123.
Paffenbarger, R., et al. "Physical Activity and Physical Fitness as Determinants of Health and Longevity." In Bouchard, C., et al., *Exercise, Fitness, and Health*. Champaign, IL: Human Kinetics Publishers, 1990.
Public Health Service. Healthy People 2000: National Health Promotion and Disease Prevention Objectives. Washington, D.C.: U.S. Government Printing Office, 1991.
Shephard, R. J. *Physical Activity and Health-Related Fitness*. Champaign, IL: Human Kinetics Publishers, 1993.
Surgeon General's Office. Surgeon General's Report on Physical Activity and Health. Washington D.C.: U.S. Government Printing Office, (1996).

LAB RESOURCE MATERIALS

Physical Activity Questionnaire: Scoring Directions.

1. For items 1 through 7 give 5 points for strongly agree, 4 for agree, 3 for undecided, 2 for disagree, and 1 for strongly disagree.

2. For items 8 through 14 give 1 point for strongly agree, 2 for agree, 3 for undecided, 2 for disagree, and 1 for strongly disagree.

3. Write the number scores in Chart 1.1 and in the spaces below.

Health and fitness	Item 1 _____ + Item 8 _____ = _____	Fun/enjoyment	Item 1 _____ + Item 8 _____ = _____
Relaxation/tension	Item 1 _____ + Item 8 _____ = _____	Challenge/achiev.	Item 1 _____ + Item 8 _____ = _____
Social	Item 1 _____ + Item 8 _____ = _____	Appearance	Item 1 _____ + Item 8 _____ = _____
Competition	Item 1 _____ + Item 8 _____ = _____		

4. Calculate a "balance to feelings" score. Give yourself one point for each score totaling 4 or 5 (above). Give yourself a −1 for each score totaling 1 or 2. Give yourself a 0 for each score of 3. You have a positive score if you have more plus scores than minus scores. You have a negative score if you have more minus scores than plus scores (see Chart 1.2 for ratings).

Chart 1.1 Physical Activity Questionnaire

The term "physical activity" in the following statements refers to all kinds of activities, including sports, formal exercises, and informal activities, such as jogging and cycling. Check your answers first, then read the directions for scoring at the end of the questionnaire.

	Strongly Agree	Agree	Undecided	Disagree	Strongly Disagree	Score
1. I should exercise regularly for my own good health and physical fitness.	☐	☐	☐	☐	☐	_____
2. One of the main reasons I do regular physical activity is because it is fun.	☐	☐	☐	☐	☐	_____
3. I enjoy taking part in physical activity because it helps me to relax and get away from the pressures of daily living.	☐	☐	☐	☐	☐	_____
4. The challenge of physical training is one reason why I participate in physical activity.	☐	☐	☐	☐	☐	_____
5. One of the things I like about physical activity is the participation with other people.	☐	☐	☐	☐	☐	_____
6. Regular exercise helps me look my best.	☐	☐	☐	☐	☐	_____
7. Competition is a good way to keep a game from being fun.	☐	☐	☐	☐	☐	_____
8. Doing regular physical activity can be as harmful to health as it is helpful.	☐	☐	☐	☐	☐	_____
9. Doing exercise and playing sports is boring.	☐	☐	☐	☐	☐	_____
10. Participating in physical activities makes me tense and nervous.	☐	☐	☐	☐	☐	_____
11. Most sports and physical activities are too difficult for me to enjoy.	☐	☐	☐	☐	☐	_____
12. I do not enjoy physical activities that require the participation of other people.	☐	☐	☐	☐	☐	_____
13. Doing regular physical activity does little to make me more physically attractive.	☐	☐	☐	☐	☐	_____
14. Competing against others in physical activities makes them enjoyable.	☐	☐	☐	☐	☐	_____

Chart 1.2 Physical Activity Questionnaire *Rating Scale*

Classification	Each of Seven Scores	Balance of Feeling Score
Excellent	9–10	Excellent = more than +4
Good	7–8	Good = +2 to +3
Fair	6	Fair = +1
Poor	4–5	Poor = 0
Very poor	3 or less	Very poor = negative scores

Chart 1.3 Physical Fitness Stunts

Item	Fitness Aspect	Pass	
1. *One-foot balance.* Stand on one foot; press up so that the weight is on the ball of the foot with the heel off the floor. Hold the hands and the other leg straight out in front for ten seconds.	Balance	Yes ☐	
2. *Standing long jump.* Stand with the toes behind a line; using no run or hop step, jump as far as possible. To pass, men must jump their height plus six inches. Women must jump their height only.	Power	Yes ☐	
3. *Paper ball pickup.* Place two wadded paper balls on the floor five feet away. Run, pick up the first ball, and return both feet behind the starting line. Repeat with the second ball. Finish in five seconds.	Agility	Yes ☐	
4. *Paper drop.* Have a partner hold a sheet of notebook paper so that the side edge is between your thumb and index finger, about the width of your hand from the top of the page. When your partner drops the paper, catch it before it slips through the thumb and finger. Do not move your hand lower to catch the paper.	Reaction time	Yes ☐	
5. *Double heel click.* With the feet apart, jump up and tap the heels together twice before you hit the ground. You must land with your feet at least three inches apart.	Speed	Yes ☐	

16   Physical Activity, Fitness, and Wellness

Chart 1.3 continued

Item	Fitness Aspect	Pass
6. *Paper ball bounce*. Wad up a sheet of notebook paper into a ball. Bounce the ball back and forth between the right and left hands. Keep the hands open and palms up. Bounce the ball three times with each hand (six times total), alternating hands for each bounce.	Coordination	Yes ☐
7. *Run in place*. Run in place for one and a half minutes (120 steps per minute). Rest for one minute and count the heart rate for thirty seconds. A heart rate of 60 or lower passes. A step is counted each time the right foot hits the floor.	Cardiovascular fitness	Yes ☐
8. *Backsaver toe touch*. Sit on the floor with one foot against a wall. Bend the other knee. Bend forward at the hips. After three warm-up trials, reach forward and touch your closed fists to the wall. Bend forward slowly; do not bounce. Repeat with the other leg straight. Pass if fists touch the wall with each leg straight. Note: This is a test-stunt, not an exercise.	Flexibility	Yes ☐
9. *The pinch*. Have a partner pinch a fold of fat on the back of your upper arm (body fatness), halfway between the tip of the elbow and the tip of the shoulder. Men: No greater than ¾ of an inch. Women: No greater than one inch.	Body composition	Yes ☐
10. *Push-up*. Lie face down on the floor. Place the hands under the shoulders. Keeping the legs and body straight, press off the floor until the arms are fully extended. Women repeat once; men, three times.	Strength	Yes ☐
11. *Side leg raise*. Lie on the floor on your side. Lift your leg up and to the side of the body until your feet are 24 to 36 inches apart. Keep the knee and pelvis facing forward. Do not rotate so that the knees face the ceiling. Perform 10 with each leg.	Muscular endurance and strength	Yes ☐

CONCEPT
·2·

The Health Benefits of Physical Activity and Fitness

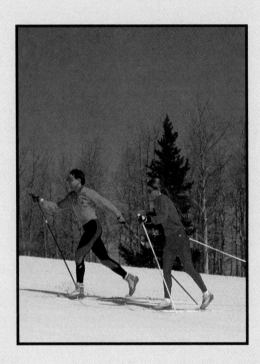

Concept 2

Physical activity and good physical fitness can contribute to optimal health and wellness.

Introduction

At no time in our history has so much evidence been accumulated to demonstrate the health and wellness benefits of physical activity and fitness. In 1990 the National Health Goals (Healthy People 2000) highlighted physical activity in its first chapter. This indicated the importance that public health officials placed on physical activity in improving health and quality of life. In 1992 the American Heart Association elevated sedentary living to status as a "primary risk factor" for heart disease indicating that activity was of primary rather than secondary importance in preventing heart disease. In 1995 a group of experts from the Centers for Disease Control and Prevention and the American College of Sports Medicine issued a recommendation for physical activity and public health that established the strong link between regular physical activity and good health and wellness. The recent *Surgeon General's Report on Physical Activity and Health* is the latest and most powerful of the documents summarizing the benefits of regular physical activity and good fitness. This extensive document provides definitive evidence of the value of physical activity and fitness to sound health and wellness. Each of these documents is cited to support the facts in this concept.

Health Goals for the Year 2000

- Increase the span of life. (↑)
- Decrease years of dysfunctional life. (<>)
- Reduce coronary heart disease deaths. (↑)
- Reduce cholesterol levels among adults. (↑)
- Reduce the incidence of overweight among adults. (↓)
- Reduce the proportion of adults with high blood pressure. (↑)
- Reduce stroke deaths. (↑)
- Reduce the incidence of and deaths from diabetes. (<>)
- Reduce the incidence of chronic back conditions. (<>)
- Reverse the rise in cancer deaths. (↑)
- Reduce the prevalence of stress-related disorders. (↑)
- Reduce the suicide rate. (↑)
- Reduce hip fractures among older people. (<>)

Note: (↑) indicates progress toward goal, (↓) indicates regression from goal, and (<>) indicates either no change or lack of new data since 1990.

Terms

- **Acquired Aging** The acquisition of characteristics commonly associated with aging but that are, in fact, caused by immobility or sedentary living.
- **Angina Pectoris** Chest or arm pain resulting from reduced oxygen supply to the heart muscle.
- **Arteriosclerosis** Hardening of the arteries due to conditions that cause the arterial walls to become thick, hard, and nonelastic.
- **Atherosclerosis** The deposition of materials along the arterial walls; a type of arteriosclerosis.

Chronic Disease A disease or illness that is associated with lifestyle or environmental factors as opposed to infectious diseases (hypokinetic diseases are considered to be chronic diseases).

Congestive Heart Failure The inability of the heart muscle to pump the blood at a life-sustaining rate.

Coronary Circulation Circulation of blood to the heart muscle associated with the blood-carrying capacity of a specific vessel or development of collateral vessels (extra blood vessels).

Coronary Heart Disease (CHD) Diseases of the heart muscle and the blood vessels that supply it with oxygen, including heart attack.

Coronary Occlusion The blocking of the coronary blood vessels.

Disease/Illness Prevention Altering lifestyles and environmental factors with the intent of preventing or reducing the risk of various illnesses and diseases.

Disease/Illness Treatment Altering lifestyles and use of medical procedures to aid in rehabilitation or reduction in symptoms or debilitation from a disease or illness.

Emotional Storm A traumatic emotional experience that is likely to affect the human organism physiologically.

Fibrin The substance that in combination with blood cells forms a blood clot.

Health and Wellness Promotion Altering lifestyles and environmental factors with the intent of improving quality of life.

High-Density Lipoprotein (HDL) A blood substance that picks up cholesterol and helps remove it from the body; often called "good cholesterol."

Hyperkinetic Condition A disease/illness or health condition caused by or contributed to by too much exercise.

Hypertension High blood pressure.

Hypokinetic Diseases or Conditions *Hypo* means "under" or "too little," and *kinetic* means movement or activity. Thus, hypokinetic means "too little activity." A hypokinetic disease or condition is associated with lack of physical activity or too little regular exercise. Examples of such conditions include heart disease, low back pain, adult-onset diabetes, and obesity.

Lipids All fats and fatty substances.

Lipoprotein Fat-carrying protein in the blood.

Low-Density Lipoprotein (LDL) A core of cholesterol surrounded by protein; the core is often called "bad cholesterol."

Parasympathetic Nervous System Branch of the autonomic nervous system that slows the heart rate.

Peripheral Vascular Disease Lack of oxygen supply to the working muscles and tissues of the arms and legs resulting from decreased blood supply.

Stroke (Cerebrovascular Accident or CVA) condition in which the brain, or part of the brain receives insufficient oxygen as a result of diminished blood supply; sometimes called apoplexy.

Sympathetic Nervous System Branch of the autonomic nervous system that prepares the body for activity by speeding up the heart rate.

Time-Dependent Aging The loss of function resulting from growing older.

Facts About Physical Activity, Fitness, and Disease Prevention/Treatment

There are three major ways in which regular physical activity and good fitness contribute to optimal health and wellness.

The methods by which physical activity and fitness contribute to optimal health and wellness are illustrated in figure 2.1. First, they can aid in **disease/illness prevention.** There is considerable evidence that the risk of hypokinetic diseases and conditions can be greatly reduced among those who do regular exercise and achieve good physical fitness.

Leading public health officials have suggested that "Physical activity is related to the health of all Americans. It has the ability to reduce directly the risk for several major **chronic diseases,** as well as to catalyze positive changes with respect to other risk factors for these diseases. Physical activity may produce the shortcut we in public health have been seeking for the control of chronic diseases, much like immunization has facilitated progress against infectious diseases" (McGinnis 1992).

Second, exercise and fitness can be a significant contributor to **disease/illness treatment.** Even with the best disease-prevention practices, some people will become ill. Regular exercise and good fitness has been shown to be effective in alleviating symptoms and rehabilitation after illness for such hypokinetic conditions as diabetes, heart attack, back pain, and others.

Finally, physical activity and fitness are methods of **health and wellness promotion.** They contribute to quality living associated with wellness, the positive component of good health. In the process they aid in meeting many of the nation's health goals for the year 2000.

Too many adults suffer from **hypokinetic diseases.**

In 1961, Kraus and Raab coined the term "hypokinetic disease." They pointed out that recent advances in medicine had been quite effective in eliminating infectious diseases but that degenerative diseases, characterized by sedentary or "take-it-easy" living, had increased in recent decades. In fact, heart disease is the leading cause of death in North America. High blood pressure, stroke, and coronary artery disease including heart attack afflict millions each year. The second leading

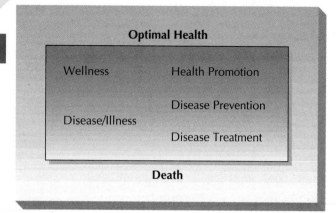

Figure 2.1
Contributors to optimal health and wellness

medical complaint (headache is number one) is low back pain, and as many as one-half of all adults are considered to be obese. Studies now show that the symptoms of hypokinetic disease begin in youth. This suggests that the incidence of hypokinetic disease in our culture will not be reduced without considerable lifestyle change in people of all ages (see figure 2.2).

> The link between regular physical activity and good health is now well documented.

People who exercise regularly can reduce their risk of death, regardless of the cause. Active people increase their life expectancy by two years compared to those who are inactive. The *Surgeon General's Report* indicates that sedentary people experience a 20 percent to two fold increase in early death compared to active people. One leading public health official indicates that increasing physical activity among the adult population would do wonders for the health of the nation because there are so many sedentary people who could benefit from active lifestyles. "In fact, the national pattern of physical inactivity, in combination with the dietary patterns . . . ranks with tobacco use among the leading preventable contributors to death for Americans—well ahead of the contributions of infectious diseases" (McGinnis 1992). "Physical Activity and Public Health," a recommendation from the Centers for Disease Control and Prevention and the American College of Sports Medicine concludes, "If Americans who lead sedentary lives would adopt a more active lifestyle, there would be enormous benefit to the public's health and to individual well-being" (Pate, et al., 1995).

The Facts About Physical Activity and Cardiovascular Diseases

> There are many types of cardiovascular diseases.

Hypertension (high blood pressure), **coronary occlusion** (heart attack), **atherosclerosis, arteriosclerosis, angina pec-**

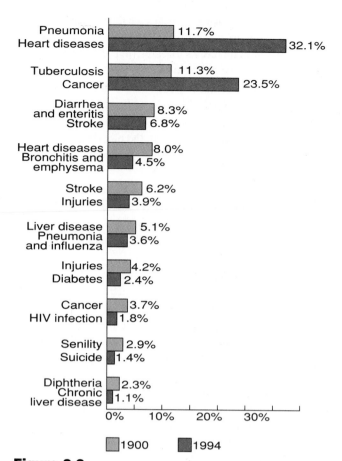

Figure 2.2
Major causes of death in the United States.

Source: Data from the Centers for Disease Control and Prevention, National Center for Health Statistics.

Note: The sum of data for the ten causes may not equal the total due to rounding.

toris (chest or arm pain), **stroke, peripheral vascular disease,** and **congestive heart failure** are among the more prevalent forms of heart disease. Evidence indicates that inactivity relates in some way to each of these types of disease.

> The various forms of cardiovascular disease (CVD) are the leading killers in automated societies.

As noted in figure 2.2, cardiovascular diseases are the leading cause of death in the United States. Similar death rates are apparent in Canada, Great Britain, Australia, and other automated societies.

> A wealth of statistical evidence indicates that active people are less likely to have coronary heart disease than sedentary people.

Much of the research relating inactivity to heart disease has come from occupational studies that show a high incidence of heart disease in people involved only in sedentary work. Even with the limitations inherent in these types of studies, the findings of more and more occupational studies present convincing evidence that the inactive individual has an increased risk of coronary heart disease. A study summarizing all of the important occupational studies shows a 90 percent reduced risk of coronary heart disease for those in active versus inactive occupations.

Studies also indicate that people who are physically active in their leisure time have reduced risk of coronary heart disease if they expend a significant number of calories per week in strenuous sports and other activities. In fact, it was concluded that improving activity levels was among the best ways to reduce the risk of heart disease among adults.

> Recent research suggests that regular exercise can be a primary factor in reducing the risk of heart disease and early death from the heart disease.

The American Heart Association, after carefully examining the research literature, said ". . . the body of research is now of sufficient strength to identify a sedentary lifestyle as a risk factor comparable to high blood pressure, high blood cholesterol, and cigarette smoke" (Cooper 1992). After reviewing hundreds of studies on exercise and heart disease, the Surgeon General's Report on Physical Activity and Health concluded that "physical activity is causally linked to atherosclerosis and coronary heart disease."

> Recent decreases in the incidence of heart disease in the United States may be, in part, due to recent increases in activity levels of adults.

Though heart disease is still present in epidemic proportions (one in three males will have a heart attack by age sixty), many experts feel that the increase in regular exercise by previously sedentary Americans is one reason for the modest decreases in heart disease in recent decades. Though more attention has been given to heart disease as a killer among men, it is also the leading cause of death among women.

The Facts About Physical Activity and the Healthy Heart

> There is evidence that regular physical activity will increase the ability of the heart muscle to pump blood as well as oxygen.

A fit heart muscle can handle extra demands placed on it. Through regular exercise, the heart muscle gets stronger, contracts more forcefully, and therefore pumps more blood with each beat, resulting in a slower heart rate and greater heart efficiency. Of importance is the fact that the heart is just like any other muscle—it must be exercised regularly if it is to stay fit. The fit heart has open, clear arteries free of atherosclerosis. (See figure 2.3.)

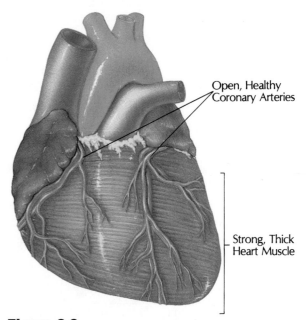

Figure 2.3
The fit heart muscle

The Facts About Physical Activity and Atherosclerosis

> Atherosclerosis is implicated in many cardiovascular diseases.

Atherosclerosis is a condition that contributes to heart attack, stroke, hypertension, angina pectoris, and peripheral vascular diseases. Deposits on the walls of arteries restrict blood flow and oxygen supply to the tissues. Atherosclerosis of the coronary arteries, the vessels that supply the heart muscle with oxygen, is particularly harmful. If these arteries become narrowed, the blood supply to the heart muscle is diminished and angina pectoris may occur. Atherosclerosis increases the risk of heart attack because a clot is more likely to obstruct a narrowed artery than a healthy, open one.

> Atherosclerosis, which begins early in life, is the result of a systematic build-up of deposits in an arterial wall.

Current theory suggests that atherosclerosis begins when damage occurs to the cells of the inner wall of the artery (intima). Substances associated with blood clotting are attracted to the damaged area. These substances seem to cause the migration of smooth muscle cells, commonly found only in the middle wall of the artery (media), to the intima. In the later stages, fats (including cholesterol) and other substances are thought to be deposited, forming plaques or protrusions (see figure 2.4) that diminish the internal diameter of the artery. Research indicates that the first signs of atherosclerosis begin in early childhood.

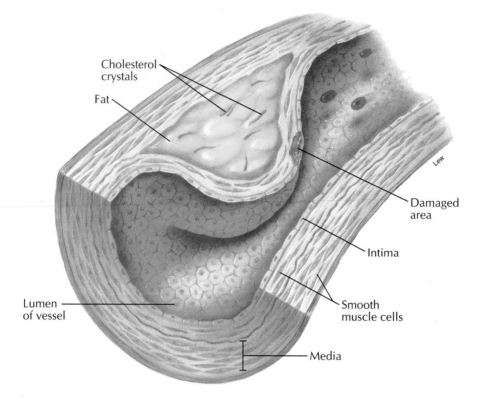

Cholesterol crystals

Fat

Damaged area

Intima

Lumen of vessel

Smooth muscle cells

Media

Figure 2.4
Atherosclerosis

There is evidence that regular physical activity can help prevent atherosclerosis.

All of the ways in which regular exercise helps prevent atherosclerosis are not yet known. However, three of the most plausible theories are discussed below.

Lipid Deposit Theory

There are several kinds of **lipids** in the bloodstream, including **lipoproteins,** phospholipids, triglycerides, and cholesterol. Cholesterol is the most well-known, but it is not the only culprit. Many blood fats are manufactured by the body itself, while others are ingested in high fat foods, particularly saturated fats (fats that are solid at room temperature). As noted earlier, blood lipids are thought to contribute to the development of atherosclerotic deposits on the inner walls of the artery. One substance, called **low-density lipoprotein (LDL),** is considered to be a major culprit in the development of atherosclerosis. LDL is basically a core of cholesterol surrounded by protein and another substance that makes it water soluble. The theory is that regular exercise can reduce blood lipid levels, including LDL-C (the cholesterol core of LDL). People with high total cholesterol and LDL-C levels have been shown to have a higher than normal risk of heart disease (see table 2.1). New evidence indicates that a substance called apolipoprotein B (Apo B or phenotype B) combines with LDL to increase risk. A low Apo B level is desirable.

Protective Protein Theory

Whereas LDLs carry a core of cholesterol that is involved in the development of atherosclerosis, **high-density lipoprotein (HDL)** picks up cholesterol (**HDL-C**) and carries it to the liver, where it is eliminated from the body. For this reason it is often called the "protective protein." High levels of HDL are considered to be desirable. When you have a blood test it is wise to determine the amount of HDL-C compared to the total amount of cholesterol (TC) in your blood. A low TC/HDL-C ratio is a good indicator of the protection you are receiving from HDL (see table 2.1). The theory is that people who do regular exercise have high HDL amounts, as evidenced by TC/HDL-C ratios, and therefore less heart disease. Just as Apo B together with LDL increases risk, another substance called apolipoprotein A-I (Apo A-I), attaches itself to HDL to help lower LDL levels. A high Apo A-I level is desirable.

Blood Coagulant (Fibrin and Platelet) Theory

Fibrin is a sticky, threadlike substance in the blood that is important to the clotting process. Platelets are another type of cell involved in blood coagulation. The blood coagulant theory suggests that fibrin and platelets may be involved in the development of atherosclerosis. Specifically, blood coagulants may deposit at the site of an injury on the wall of an artery, contributing to the process of plaque build-up or atherosclerosis. Exercise has been shown to reduce fibrin levels

Table 2.1
Cholesterol Goals (mg/100 ml)

	Total Cholesterol	LDL-C	HDL-C	TC/HDL-C
Goal	200 or less	130 or less	55+	3.5 or less
Borderline	201–239	130–159	36–55	3.6–5.0
High risk	240+	160+	35 or less	5.0+

Source: Data from B. Liebman, "Rating Your Risk" in *Nutrition Action*, 19:8, 1992 and Fifth Committee on Detection, Evaluation, and Treatment of High Blood Pressure in *Archives of Internal Medicine*, 153, 154, 1993.

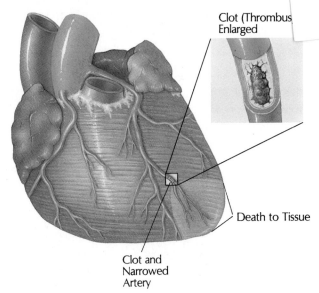

Figure 2.5
Heart attack

in the blood. The breakdown of fibrin resulting from regular physical activity seems to reduce platelet adhesiveness and the concentration of platelets in the blood. This in turn is thought to reduce the risk of atherosclerosis development.

The Facts About Physical Activity and Heart Attack

Heart attack is the most prevalent and serious of all cardiovascular diseases.

A heart attack occurs when a coronary artery is blocked (see figure 2.5). A clot or thrombus is the most common cause. When a coronary occlusion or heart attack occurs, blood flow and oxygen to the heart muscle are cut off. If the coronary artery that is blocked supplies a major portion of the heart muscle, death will occur within minutes. Occlusions of lesser arteries may result in angina pectoris or a nonfatal heart attack.

Regular physical activity reduces the risk of heart attack (coronary occlusion).

People who perform regular sports and physical activity have half the risk of a first heart attack compared to those who are sedentary. Possible reasons are less atherosclerosis, greater diameter of arteries, and less chance of a clot forming.

There is evidence that regular exercise can improve **coronary circulation** and thus reduce the chances of a heart attack or dying from one.

Within the heart, there are many tiny branches extending from the major coronary arteries. All of these vessels supply

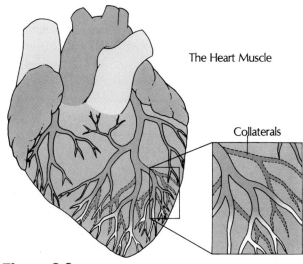

Figure 2.6
Coronary collateral circulation

blood to the heart muscle. Healthy arteries can supply blood to any region of the heart as it is needed. Active people are likely to have greater blood-carrying capacity in these vessels, probably because the vessels are larger and more elastic. Also, the active person may have a more profuse distribution of arteries within the heart muscle (see figure 2.6) which results in greater blood flow. A few studies show that physical activity may promote the growth of "extra" or collateral blood vessels that are thought to open up to provide the heart muscle with the necessary blood and oxygen when the oxygen supply is diminished as in a heart attack. The most recent evidence has yet to fully support this idea.

Improved coronary circulation may provide protection against a heart attack because a larger artery would require more atherosclerosis to occlude it. In addition, the development of collateral blood vessels supplying the heart may diminish the effects of a heart attack if one does occur. These "extra" (or collateral) blood vessels may take over the function of regular blood vessels during a heart attack.

> The heart of the inactive person is less able to resist stress and is more susceptible to an **emotional storm** that may precipitate a heart attack.

The heart is rendered inefficient by one or more of the following circumstances: high heart rate, high blood pressure, and excessive stimulation. All of these conditions require the heart to use more oxygen than is normally necessary and decrease its ability to adapt to stressful situations.

The "loafer's heart" is one that beats rapidly because it is dominated by the **sympathetic nervous system,** which speeds up the heart rate. Thus, the heart continuously beats rapidly, even at rest, and never has a true rest period. Further, high blood pressure makes the heart work harder and contributes to its inefficiency.

Research indicates four things concerning exercise and the loafer's heart.

- Regular exercise leads to dominance of the **parasympathetic nervous system** rather than to sympathetic dominance; thus the heart rate is reduced and the heart works efficiently.
- Regular exercise helps the heart rate return to normal faster after emotional stress.
- Regular exercise strengthens the loafer's heart, making the heart better able to weather emotional storms.
- Regular exercise decreases sympathetic dominance and its associated hormonal effects on the heart, thus lessening the chances of altered heart contractility and the likelihood of the circulatory problems that accompany this state.
- Regular exercise reduces the risk of sudden death from ventricular fibrillation (arrhythmic heartbeat).

> Regular exercise is one effective means of rehabilitation for a person who has **coronary heart disease** or who has had a heart attack.

Not only does regular exercise seem to reduce the risk of developing coronary heart disease, but there is also evidence that those who already have the condition may reduce the symptoms of the disease through regular exercise. For those who have had heart attacks, regular and progressive exercise can be an effective prescription when carried out under the supervision of a physician. Remember, however, that exercise is not the treatment of preference for all heart attack victims. In some cases, it may be contraindicated.

Physical Activity and Other Cardiovascular Diseases

> Regular physical activity and accompanying good physical fitness are associated with a reduced risk of high blood pressure (hypertension).

Approximately 30 percent of adults have borderline or high-risk hypertension. More men than women are likely to be hypertensive, as are more blacks than whites. Native Americans have a higher than normal incidence of hypertension, and the incidence for all groups increases as people grow older. A recent research summary indicates that the effects of physical activity on blood pressure are more dramatic than previously thought and are independent of age, body fatness, and other factors. Inactive, less fit individuals have a 30 to 50 percent greater chance of being hypertensive than active, fit people. Regular exercise can also be one effective method of reducing blood pressure for those with hypertension. Physical inactivity in middle age has now been associated with risk of high blood pressure later in life.

The most plausible reason why physical activity seems to reduce the chances of high blood pressure is a reduction in resistance to blood flow in the blood vessels probably resulting from dilation of the vessels. Goals for blood pressure are indicated in table 2.2.

> Regular exercise can help reduce the risk of stroke.

Stroke is a major killer of adults. Those with high blood pressure and atherosclerosis are susceptible to stroke. Since regular exercise and good fitness are important to the prevention of both high blood pressure and atherosclerosis, exercise and fitness are considered helpful in the prevention of stroke.

> Regular exercise is helpful in the prevention of peripheral vascular diseases.

There is evidence that people who exercise regularly have better blood flow to the working muscles and other tissues than inactive, unfit people. Since peripheral vascular disease is associated with poor circulation to the extremities, regular exercise can be considered one method of preventing this condition.

Table 2.2
Blood Pressure Goals

	Blood Pressure (mm/hg) Systolic	Diastolic
Goal	130 or less	85 or less
Near Goal	131–139	86–89
Borderline	140–159	90–99
Moderate Hypertension	160–180	100–109
Severe Hypertension	180+	110+

The Facts About Physical Activity, Health-Related Fitness, and Other Hypokinetic Conditions

> Some forms of cancer can now be considered as hypokinetic diseases.

As illustrated in figure 2.2, cancer is the second leading cause of death in the United States. Cancer is a number of different diseases of which several are considered hypokinetic. Adequate data are now available to document the relationship of inactivity to colon cancer. Inactive people have a 50 to 250 percent greater risk of getting colon cancer than active people. Consistent findings also suggest that rectal cancer is also associated with inactivity. The relationship between fitness, exercise, and other forms of cancer is not yet fully understood. However, preliminary evidence suggests that fit people who regularly exercise have increased protection against reproductive system and breast cancers. One possible reason for the reduced risk of colon/rectal cancer (the second most common cause of cancer deaths among males) is the reduced intestinal transit time among regular exercisers. Among women, nonathletes have been found to have a greater risk of breast cancer than athletes, though this finding needs further verification. For those who have cancer, there is evidence that exercise can help them lead more fulfilling and productive lives.

> Active people who possess good muscle fitness are less likely to have back and other musculoskeletal problems than inactive, unfit people.

Because few people die from it, back pain does not receive the attention given to such medical problems as heart disease and cancer. But back pain is considered to be the second leading medical complaint in the United States, second only to headaches. Only common colds and flu cause more days lost from work than this ailment. At some point in

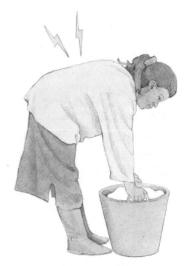

Figure 2.7
Back pain is a hypokinetic condition, but it may also be caused by incorrect lifting techniques.

their lives, approximately 80 percent of all adults will experience back pain that limits their ability to function normally. Recent National Safety Council data indicated that the back was the most frequently injured of all body parts and the injury rate was double that of any other part of the body.

Many years ago, medical doctors began to associate back problems with the lack of physical fitness. It is now known that the great majority of back ailments are the result of poor muscle strength and endurance, and poor flexibility. Tests on patients with back problems show weakness and lack of flexibility in key muscle groups.

Though lack of fitness is probably the leading reason for back pain in Western society, there are many other factors that increase the risk of back ailments, including poor posture, improper lifting (see figure 2.7) and work habits, heredity, and disease states, such as scoliosis and arthritis.

> Obesity, as well as lesser degrees of fatness, is not a disease state in itself but is a hypokinetic condition associated with a multitude of far-reaching complications.

Obesity is associated with serious organic impairments, shortened life, psychological maladjustments, poor relationships with peers (especially among children), awkward physical movement, and lack of achievement in athletic activities. Obesity can be both a cause and an effect of physical unfitness. Those who are overfat have a higher risk of respiratory infections; are prone to developing high blood pressure, atherosclerosis, and disorders of the circulatory and respiratory systems; and have a greater than normal risk of some forms of cancer. The symptoms of adult-onset diabetes are associated with excessive fatness. (Fortunately, fat loss to normal levels is usually followed by remission of adult-onset diabetic symptoms). Because exercise, together with sound nutritional management, is an effective means of lowering body fat, it can be helpful in reducing the risk of those conditions associated with fatness and obesity.

> Diabetes is often considered a hypokinetic condition because of the important role exercise plays in managing the disease.

Diabetes is the sixth leading cause of death among people over forty. It accounts for at least 10 percent of all short term hospital stays and has a major impact on health-care costs in western society. By itself, exercise is not an effective treatment for Type I (insulin-dependent) diabetes. However, with proper medical supervision, exercise is encouraged for maintaining physical fitness for most diabetics. Those who perform regular physical activity are less likely to suffer from Type II (noninsulin dependent, adult-onset) diabetes than sedentary people. For those with Type II diabetes, regular exercise can help reduce body fatness and improve insulin sensitivity and glucose tolerance, all of which contribute to controlling the disease. Together with sound nutritional habits and proper medication, exercise can be useful in the management of diabetes.

> Regular physical activity is important to bone growth and development.

Studies indicate that excessive bed rest can result in deterioration of the bones. When the long bones do not bear weight, they lose calcium and become porous and fragile. Even excessive sitting can result in bone deterioration, regardless of age. Bones are strengthened not only by bearing weight, but by the pull of active muscles. Regular exercise is as necessary for healthy bone development as it is for healthy muscle development.

The maximum amount of bone you will ever develop is called peak bone mass. Peak bone mass is usually achieved in the teen years. Lack of load-bearing exercise and poor nutrition during this time results in a low peak bone mass. As we grow older, bone mass decreases. If it decreases to exceptionally low levels, osteoporosis occurs. Those who develop greater peak bone mass when young can lose bone density without becoming osteoporotic. Those particularly susceptible to osteoporosis are post menopausal women not taking an estrogen supplement, those who do not consume adequate calcium, and those who do not do regular weight-bearing exercise. Weight training has been shown to be an effective method of retaining bone mass as you grow older.

> Common mental health disorders can be considered hypokinetic conditions.

Some mental health conditions are prevalent in modern society. According to the Surgeon General's Report on Physical Activity and Health, nearly one of every two adult Americans will report having a mental health disorder at some point in life. A few that are associated with inactive lifestyles are noted here.

Insomnia is a condition that afflicts many people in our culture and one that is often stress related. Results from a survey of American adults indicate that 52 percent feel regular exercise helps them to sleep better.

Depression is another stress-related condition experienced by many adults. Thirty-three percent of inactive adults report that they often feel depressed. For some, depression is a serious disorder that exercise alone will not cure; however, recent research does indicate that exercise, combined with other forms of therapy, can be effective in its treatment. For those with minor depression, exercise may also be helpful. One-third of very active people in one study felt that regular exercise helped them to better cope with life's pressures.

Even more common than depression and insomnia is the condition called Type A behavior. "Type A personalities" are stress-prone individuals with a greater than normal incidence of diseases. A Type A person is tense, overcompetitive, and worried about meeting time schedules. Regular exercise can be of special benefit to the Type A person, though noncompetitive exercise would probably be best.

> Hypokinetic diseases and conditions have many causes.

Regular exercise and good physical fitness are only two preventative factors associated with the conditions described in this concept as hypokinetic diseases. Other healthy lifestyle factors cannot be overlooked in the prevention of these diseases.

Physical Activity, Physical Fitness, and Nonhypokinetic Diseases

> Regular physical activity can have positive effects on some nonhypokinetic conditions.

- Infections. Infectious diseases are not generally considered to be hypokinetic conditions. However, regular exercise that fosters physical fitness and good health may help you resist diseases resulting from lowered general resistance. On the other hand, when the body is fighting an infection, too much exercise can result in a lowered state of resistance.
- Arthritis. Many, if not most, arthritics are in a deconditioned state resulting from a lack of activity. The traditional advice that exercise is to be avoided by arthritics is now being modified in view of the findings that carefully prescribed exercise can improve general fitness and, in some cases, reduce the symptoms of the disease.

- Chronic Pain. There are many sources of pain that persist for long periods of time without relief; some are difficult to understand. Nevertheless, large numbers of adults are victims of chronic pain. Both aerobic exercise and resistance training are currently being prescribed as means of treating this problem.
- Premenstrual Syndrome (PMS). PMS, a mixture of physical and emotional symptoms that occurs prior to menstruation, has many causes. However, current evidence suggests that changes in lifestyle, including involvement in regular exercise, may be effective in relieving PMS symptoms.

Physical Activity, Physical Fitness, and Aging

In many ways, **acquired aging** is similar to a hypokinetic condition.

Forced inactivity in young adults can cause losses in function (acquired aging) very much like those that are generally considered to occur with aging (**time-dependent aging**). Studies suggest that acquired aging is a product of a sedentary lifestyle. In Africa, Asia, and South America, where older adults (age sixty-five and older) maintain an active lifestyle, individuals do not acquire many of the characteristics commonly associated with aging in North America.

Facts About Health and Wellness Promotion

Good health-related physical fitness and regular physical activity are important to health promotion and feeling well.

Optimal health is more than freedom from disease. Regular exercise and good fitness not only help prevent illness and disease but also promote quality of life and feeling well. Good health-related fitness can help you feel good, look good, and enjoy life. Some of the health and wellness benefits of regular exercise are outlined in table 2.3.

Good physical fitness can help an individual enjoy his or her leisure time.

A person who is not too fat, has no back problems, does not have to worry about high blood pressure, and has reasonable skills in lifetime sports is more likely to get involved and stay regularly involved in leisure-time activities than one who does not have these characteristics. It is said that enjoying your leisure time may not add years to your life, but can add life to your years.

Good physical fitness can help an individual work effectively and efficiently.

A person who can resist fatigue, muscle soreness, back problems, and other symptoms associated with poor health-related fitness is capable of working productively and having energy left over at the end of the day. Surveys of employees who have the opportunity to improve fitness through involvement in employee fitness programs indicate that 75 percent have an improved sense of well-being. Employers indicate that absenteeism decreased by up to 50 percent among program participants. People with good skill-related fitness may be more effective and efficient in performing specific motor skills required for certain jobs.

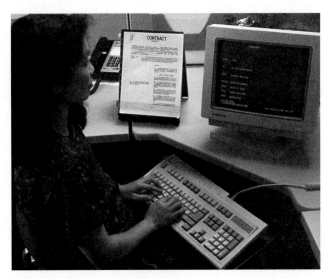

Fitness improves work efficiency.

Good physical fitness is essential to effective living.

Although the need for each component of physical fitness is specific to each individual, every person requires enough fitness to perform normal daily activities without undue fatigue. Whether it be walking, performing household chores, or merely feeling good and enjoying the simple things in life without pain or fear of injury, good fitness is important to all people.

Good physical fitness may help you function safely and assist you in meeting unexpected emergencies.

Emergencies are never expected, but when they do arise, they often demand performance that requires good fitness. For example, flood victims may need to fill sandbags for hours without rest, and accident victims may be required to walk or run long distances for help. Also, good fitness is required for such simple tasks as safely changing a spare tire or loading a moving van without injury.

Table 2.3
Health and Wellness Benefits of Regular Exercise

Major Benefit	Related Benefits	Major Benefit	Related Benefits
Improved cardiovascular fitness and health	• Stronger heart muscle • Lower heart rate • Better electric stability of heart • Decreased sympathetic control of heart • Increased O_2 to brain • Reduced blood fat, including low-density lipids (LDL) • Increased protective high-density lipids (HDL) • Delayed development of atherosclerosis • Increased work capacity • Improved peripheral circulation • Improved coronary circulation • Resistance to "emotional storm" • Reduced risk of heart attack • Reduced risk of stroke • Reduced risk of hypertension • Greater chance of surviving a heart attack • Increased oxygen-carrying capacity of the blood	Diabetes	• Decreased chance of adult-onset diabetes • Improved quality of life for Type I diabetics
		Reduction in mental tension	• Relief of depression • Improved sleep habits • Fewer stress symptoms • Ability to enjoy leisure • Possible work improvement
		Opportunity for social interactions	• Improved quality of life
		Resistance to fatigue	• Ability to enjoy leisure • Improved quality of life • Improved ability to meet some stressors
		Opportunity for successful experience	• Improved self-concept • Opportunity to recognize and accept personal limitations • Improved sense of well-being • Enjoy life—fun
Greater lean body mass and less body fat	• Greater work efficiency • Less susceptibility to disease • Improved appearance • Less incidence of self-concept problems related to obesity	Improved appearance	• Better figure/physique • Better posture • Fat control
Improved strength and muscular endurance	• Greater work efficiency • Less chance of muscle injury • Reduced risk of low back problems • Improved performance in sports • Quicker recovery after hard work • Improved ability to meet emergencies	Reduced effect of acquired aging	• Improved ability to function in daily life • Better short-term memory • Fewer illnesses • Greater mobility • Greater independence • Greater ability to operate automobile
Bone development	• Greater peak bone density • Less chance of osteoporosis	Improved flexibility	• Greater work efficiency • Less chance of muscle injury • Less chance of joint injury • Decreased chance of low back problems • Improved sports performance
Cancer	• Reduced risk of colon cancer • Possible reduced risk of rectal, reproductive and breast cancers	Other health benefits	• Extended life • Decrease in dysfunctional years

Physical fitness is the basis for dynamic and creative activity.

Though the following quotation by former President John F. Kennedy is now more than thirty years old, it clearly points out the importance of physical fitness.

"The relationship between the soundness of the body and the activity of the mind is subtle and complex. Much is not yet understood, but we know what the Greeks knew: that intelligence and skill can only function at the peak of their capacity when the body is healthy and strong, and that hardy spirits and tough minds usually inhabit sound bodies. Physical fitness is the basis of all activities in our society; if our bodies grow soft and inactive, if we fail to encourage physical development and prowess, we will undermine our capacity for thought, for work, and for the use of those skills vital to an expanding and complex America."

Table 2.4
Hypokinetic Disease Risk Factors

Factors That Cannot Be Altered

1. **Age**—As you grow older, your risk of contracting hypokinetic diseases increases. For example, the risk of heart disease is approximately three times as great after sixty as before. The risk of back pain and ulcer disease is considerably greater after forty.

2. **Heredity**—People who have a family history of hypokinetic disease are more likely to develop a hypokinetic condition. Heart disease, hypertension, ulcers, back problems, obesity, high blood lipid levels, and other problems have been shown to be more prevalent among those who have a family history of these conditions. Black Americans are 45 percent more likely to have high blood pressure than whites; therefore, they suffer strokes at an earlier age with more severe consequences than whites.

3. **Sex**—Men have a higher incidence of many hypokinetic conditions than women. Although the number of women with heart disease is increasing, women still have only about half the incidence of the disease as men; however, the incidence increases sharply in women after menopause.

Factors That Can Be Altered

4. **Body Fatness**—Having too much body fat is considered by many to be a hypokinetic condition because it may limit your ability to function efficiently and effectively. Even those who do not classify overfatness as a hypokinetic condition agree that it does increase the risk of other hypokinetic conditions. For example, loss of fat can result in relief from symptoms of adult-onset diabetes, can reduce problems associated with certain types of back pain, and can reduce the risks of surgery.

5. **Diet**—There is a clear association between hypokinetic disease and certain types of diets. The excessive intake of saturated fats, such as animal fats, is linked to atherosclerosis and other forms of heart disease. Excessive salt in the diet is associated with high blood pressure.

6. **Diseases**—People who have one hypokinetic disease are more likely to develop a second or even a third condition. For example, if you have diabetes, atherosclerosis, or high blood pressure, your risk of having a heart attack or stroke increases dramatically. People with poor posture have a high risk of experiencing back pain, and those with too much body fat have a greater than normal risk of diabetes. Although you may not be entirely able to alter the extent to which you develop certain diseases and conditions, reducing your risk and following your doctor's advice can improve your odds significantly.

7. **Regular Physical Activity**—As noted throughout this book, regular exercise can help reduce the risk of hypokinetic disease.

8. **Smoking**—Smokers have a much higher risk of developing and dying from heart disease than nonsmokers. The risk of heart attack is twice as great among young smokers as among young nonsmokers. (Most striking is the difference in risk between older women smokers and nonsmokers.) Smokers have five times the risk of heart attack as nonsmokers. Smoking is also associated with the increased risk of high blood pressure, cancer, and several other medical conditions. Apparently, the more you smoke, the greater the risk. To stop smoking even after many years can significantly reduce the hypokinetic disease risk.

9. **Stress**—There is evidence that people who are subject to excessive stress are predisposed to various hypokinetic diseases including heart disease and back pain. Statistics indicate that hypokinetic conditions are common among those in certain high-stress jobs and those having type A personality profiles.

The Facts About Risk Factors

> There are many different positive lifestyles that can reduce the risk of disease.

Many of the factors that contribute to optimal health and quality of life are also considered risk factors. Changing these risk factors can dramatically reduce the risk of hypokinetic diseases such as heart disease, obesity, back pain, and cancer, as well as other diseases such as infections and sexually transmitted diseases. Lack of exercise, poor nutrition, smoking, and inability to cope with stress are all risk factors associated with various diseases (see table 2.4).

> Not all risk factors can be altered by lifestyle changes.

Some factors that can contribute to the increased risk of disease are not under your personal control. Three uncontrollable risk factors are: age, heredity, and sex. These factors that cannot be altered by lifestyle changes are presented in table 2.4.

> Altering risk factors can help reduce the risk of more than one adverse condition at the same time.

By altering the risk factors that are controllable, you can reduce the risk of several hypokinetic conditions. For example, controlling body fatness reduces the risk of diabetes, hypertension, and back problems. Altering your diet can reduce the chances of developing high levels of blood lipids, and thus reduce the risk of atherosclerosis.

Reducing risk alters the probability of disease, but does not assure disease immunity.

Some risk factors are more likely to contribute to heart disease than others. These are considered to be primary risk factors. Inactivity, high blood pressure (hypertension), particularly high systolic pressure, high blood fat levels (cholesterol and other fats), and smoking are considered to be primary risk factors. Others, such as age, and stress, are considered secondary risk factors.

The Facts About Hyperkinetic Conditions

Hypokinetic means too little exercise. Conversely, hyperkinetic means too much exercise. Just as reasonable amounts of exercise can help reduce the risk of hypokinetic health problems, it has become apparent that excessive exercise can lead to **hyperkinetic conditions** that have negative effects on health and wellness. Several of the more common hyperkinetic conditions are described next.

Musculoskeletal Overuse Injuries

Evidence suggests that periodic rest is necessary to allow the body to recover from the stress of continuous and vigorous training. For example, runners who train seven days a week have more muscle and joint injuries than those who take off at least one day a week or reduce training levels several days a week. The most common overuse injuries are joint injuries to the foot, ankle, and knee; stress fractures in the lower extremities; and muscle/connective tissue injuries such as shin splints, strained hamstring muscles, and calf pain. These injuries are apparent among any type of exerciser who overdoes it. For example, dance aerobics instructors have been shown to be particularly likely to have overuse injuries. Tennis and baseball players often have similar problems, but their problems occur in different parts of the body (the arm and shoulder). The best way to prevent this type of hyperkinetic condition is periodic rest. Pain, the body's warning signal, is a good clue that the body needs rest.

Activity Neurosis

Activity neurosis is a compulsion to exercise. People with activity neurosis become irrationally concerned about their exercise regimen. They may exercise more than one time a day and rarely take a day off. The activity neurotic feels the need to exercise even when ill or injured. Musculoskeletal overuse injuries are especially common among activity neurotics. The excessive desire to exercise can also be the source of poor performance in other aspects of life, as well as a source of stress. Competitive athletes with this condition may have reduced performance, and among females, amenorrhea (no menstrual flow).

Anorexia Nervosa

Anorexia nervosa is an eating disorder associated with an obsessive desire to be lean. There is increasing evidence that many anorexics use compulsive exercise, as well as undereating, to keep body fat at low levels. For this reason anorexia nervosa can often be considered a hyperkinetic condition.

Body Neurosis

Body neurosis is an obsessive concern for having an attractive body. Among females, it is associated with an extreme desire to be lean. In some cases it can lead to anorexia. Among males, this condition is associated with an extreme desire to be muscular. Recent research indicates that increasing numbers of males are interested in leanness and a number of females are now compulsive about muscle mass gains. Those with body neurosis are often compulsive exercisers, though they are also more likely to be subject to nutritional quackery (use of quack dietary supplements) and in some cases resort to the use of anabolic steroids.

Suggested Readings

Blair, S., et al. "Bone Gain in Young Adult Women." *Journal of the American Medical Association* 268(1992):2403.

Cooper, E. "Statement on Physical Activity and Heart Disease." American Heart Association News Release. July 1, 1992, pp. 1–2.

Cooper, K. *Controlling Cholesterol.* New York: Bantam Books, 1988.

Corbin, C. B., and R. P. Pangrazi. "The Health Benefits of Exercise." *Research Digest for Physical Activity and Fitness* 1(1993):1.

Corbin, C. B. and Pangrazi, R. P. "What You Need to Know About the Surgeon General's Report on Physical Activity and Health," *Physical Activity and Fitness Research Digest,* 2(1996):1.

Haskell, W. L. "Physical Activity in the Prevention and Management of Coronary Heart Disease." *Physical Activity and Fitness Research Digest* 2(1995):1.

International Society of Sport Psychology. "Physical Activity and Psychological Benefits: Position Statement." 20(1992):179.

McGinnis, J. M. "The Public Health Burden of a Sedentary Lifestyle." *Medicine and Science in Sports and Exercise* 24(1992):S196.

McGinnis, J. M., and P. R. Lee. "Healthy People 2000 at Mid Decade." *Journal of the American Medical Association* 273(1995):1123.

Pate, R. R., et al. "Physical Activity and Public Health." *Journal of the American Medical Association* 273(1995):402.

Plowman, S. A. "Physical Fitness and Healthy Low Back Function." *Physical Activity and Fitness Research Digest* 1(1993):1.

Public Health Service. *Healthy People 2000: National Health Promotion and Disease Prevention Objectives.* Washington, DC: U.S. Government Printing Office, 1991.

Public Health Service. *Surgeon General's Report on Physical Activity and Health.* Washington, DC: U.S. Government Printing Office, 1996.

Shaw, J. M., and C. Snow-Harter. "Osteoporosis and Physical Activity." *Physical Activity and Fitness Research Digest.* Washington, DC: President's Council on Physical Fitness and Sports, 1995.

Heart Disease Risk Factor Questionnaire

Circle the appropriate answer to each question.

Risk Points

	1	2	3	4	Score
Unalterable Factors					
1. How old are you?	30 or less	31–40	41–54	55+	_____
2. Do you have a history of heart disease in your family?	none	grandparent with heart disease	parent with heart disease	more than one with heart disease	_____
3. What is your sex?	female		male		
			Total Unalterable Risk Score		_____
Alterable Factors		↑↓			
4. What is your percent of body fat?	F=20%↓ M=15%↓	25%↓ 20%↓	30%↓ 25%↓	35%↑ 30%↑	_____
5. Do you have a high-fat diet?	no	slightly high in fat	above normal in fat	eat a lot of meat, fried and fatty foods	_____
6. What is your blood pressure? (systolic or upper score)	120↓	121–140	141–160	160↑	_____
7. Do you have other diseases?	no	ulcer	*diabetes	both	_____
8. Do you exercise regularly?	4–5 days a week	3 days a week	less than 3 days a week	no	_____
9. Do you smoke?	no	cigar or pipe	less than ½ pack a day	more than ½ pack a day	_____
10. Are you under much stress?	less than normal	normal	slightly above normal	quite high	_____
			Total Alterable Risk Score		_____
			Grand Total Risk Score		_____

*Diabetes is a risk factor that is often not alterable.

From CAD Risk Assessor, William J. Stone, Reprinted by permission of the author.

Chart 1 Heart Disease Risk Rating Scale			
Rating	**Unalterable Score**	**Alterable Score**	**Total Score**
Very High	9 or More	21 or More	31 or More
High	7–8	15–20	26–30
Average	5–6	11–14	16–25
Low	4 or Less	10 or Less	15 or Less

CONCEPT ·3·

Preparing for Physical Activity

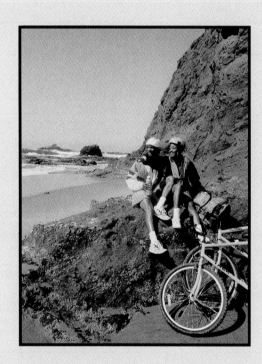

Concept 3

Proper preparation can help make physical activity enjoyable, effective, and safe.

Introduction

Since 1990, when physical activity goals were established, there has been an increase in the number of adults who do enough exercise for fitness, health, and wellness. Unfortunately, many others who started exercising dropped out after a few days, weeks, or months. As noted previously, part of the problem is that people lack information concerning the correct way to exercise.

For those just beginning a physical activity program, adequate preparation may be the key to persistence. It is hoped that a person armed with good information about preparing for exercise will become involved and stay involved with that exercise for a lifetime. To be effective, physical activity must be something that is a part of a person's normal lifestyle. Some facts that will help you prepare for exercise and make it part of your normal routine are presented in this concept.

Health Goals for the Year 2000

- Increase the proportion of people who do adequate physical activity for fitness, health, and wellness.(↑)
- Decrease the proportion of people who do no leisure-time physical activity.(↓)

Note: (↑) indicates progress toward goal, (↓) indicates regression from goal, and (<>) indicates either no change or lack of new data since 1990.

Terms

- **Adults with Increased Risk** People classified as having increased risk possess two of the following risk factors identified by medical groups: diabetes, high blood pressure, regular use of tobacco, sedentary lifestyle, high cholesterol, family history of heart attack in parent, men above age 45, and women above age 55.
- **Apparently Healthy Adults** Adults who have less than two of the commonly identified heart disease risk factors and who have no known disease or disease symptoms.
- **Clinical Exercise Test** A test typically administered on a treadmill in which exercise is gradually increased in intensity while the heart is being monitored by an EKG. Symptoms, such as an abnormal EKG, not present at rest may be present in an exercise test.
- **Cool-Down Exercise** Light to moderate tapering-off activity after vigorous exercise; often consisting of the same exercises used in the warm-up.
- **Dehydration** Excessive loss of water from the body, usually through perspiration, urination, or evaporation.

- **PAR-Q** This is an acronym for Physical Activity Readiness Questionnaire. It is designed to help you determine if you are medically suited to begin an exercise program.
- **Warm-Up Exercise** Light to moderate activity done prior to the workout. Its purpose is to reduce the risk of injury and soreness and possibly to improve performance in a physical activity.
- **Wind-Chill Factor** An index that uses air temperature and wind speed to determine the chilling effect of the environment on humans.

The Facts to Consider Before Beginning Physical Activity

> Before beginning a regular physical activity program, it is important to establish your medical readiness to participate.

The British Columbia (Canada) Ministry of Health conducted extensive research to devise a procedure that would help people know when it was advisable to seek medical consultation prior to beginning or altering an exercise program. The goal was to prevent unnecessary medical examinations, while at the same time helping people to be reasonably assured that regular exercise was appropriate. The research resulted in the development of the **PAR-Q** questionnaire. The PAR-Q, revised in 1994, consists of seven simple questions you can ask yourself to determine if medical consultation is necessary prior to exercise involvement.

The American College of Sports Medicine (ACSM) has divided people into three general categories for making determinations as to whether a medical exam or a **clinical exercise test** is necessary before beginning an exercise program. The categories include **apparently healthy adults,** those with **increased risk,** and those with known disease. Healthy young adults (men under 40 and women under age 50) who have no known health problems and answer "no" to all seven PAR-Q questions are generally cleared for participation in both moderate and vigorous exercise designed to improve fitness, health, and wellness. For older men and women (men over 40 and women over 50) and those with increased risk but no symptoms of disease, moderate exercise programs do not necessarily need to be preceded by an exam and clinical exercise test. The ACSM does recommend a medical exam and a clinical exercise test for older adults and those with increased risk who plan to begin vigorous exercise programs, for those with symptoms of disease regardless of age, and for those with known heart disease. When resuming physical activity after an injury or illness, consultation with a physician is always wise no matter what your age or medical condition.

There is no way to be absolutely sure that you are medically sound to begin a physical activity program. Even a thorough exam by a physician cannot guarantee that a person does not have some limitations that may cause a problem during exercise. The ACSM guidelines are designed to minimize the risk while preventing unnecessary medical cost. However, if there is any doubt about your readiness for activity, a medical exam is the surest way to make certain that you are ready to participate.

Those who plan to do intensive training (particularly for sports) may want to answer some additional questions concerning whether a medical exam is necessary before beginning (see Lab 3.1).

> It is important to dress properly for physical activity.

The clothing you wear for exercise should be specifically for that exercise. It should be comfortable and not too tight or binding at the joints. Though appearance is important to everyone, comfort in exercise is more important than looks. Clothing should not restrict movement in any way. Preferably, the clothing that comes in direct contact with the body should be porous to allow for sweat evaporation. Some women, especially those who need extra support, should consider using an exercise bra, and men will need an athletic supporter. A warm-up suit over other exercise apparel is recommended because it can be removed during exercise if desired. Many exercise suits are nonporous and therefore are not desirable for exercise.

Socks that fit properly should be worn during exercise. Socks that are too short can cause ingrown toenails, and loose-fitting socks can cause blisters. Sockless feet can result in blisters, abrasions, shoe odor, and excess wear on shoes.

> Proper exercise footwear is important.

Most manufacturers now produce athletic shoes in six categories: running/jogging, walking, tennis, court, aerobic/fitness, and cross trainers. Many produce even more specialized shoes within each category. For example, many have separate court shoes for basketball and volleyball. For those who are highly dedicated to a specific activity, a specialized pair of shoes should be purchased. For those who do not specialize in one activity, the cross trainer is a good choice.

The essential characteristics of all athletic shoes are described below:

- Support. The heel counter and the heel stabilizer provide stability and control foot movement. The heel tab protects the Achilles tendon from trauma. A wide heel in running shoes provides stability and protects against ankle turns. For court games such as basketball, a high-top shoe is recommended for additional ankle support.
- Cushioning. It is generally agreed that good cushioning is important, especially in the heel and midsole. However, excessive cushioning is not recommended. Too much cushioning may increase risk of injury by inhibiting the reflexes that help the body protect itself against the impact of the foot with the ground.

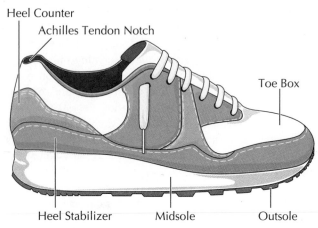

Heel Counter

Achilles Tendon Notch

Toe Box

Heel Stabilizer   Midsole   Outsole

Proper exercise shoes are important.

- Performance. A lightweight shoe requires less energy output over lengthy exercise periods. Good traction for a given sport is also important. For lengthy performances, a shoe that is at least partially made from a material that can breathe, such as nylon mesh, helps sweat evaporation and inhibits shoe weight gain.
- Fit. The toe box should be roomy enough so that you can wiggle your toes. Regardless of the type of shoe worn, exercise shoes should generally be one-half size larger than your regular shoes. If you wear two pairs of socks while exercising, you should wear two pairs when trying on the shoes. It is important to try on the shoes and move around in them before making a purchase. Make sure they feel good to you.

Probably the biggest mistake made in purchasing footwear is failure to replace shoes when they are worn out. The condition of the sole of the shoe is far less important than the breakdown of the heel (rundown to the inside or outside), or disproportionate wear that results in unusual movement patterns. It is better to replace shoes too soon than to risk injury from worn-out shoes.

Facts to Consider During Daily Physical Activity

There are three key components of the daily exercise program: **warm-up exercise,** the workout, and the **cool-down exercise.**

The key component of a fitness program is the daily workout. Experts agree, however, that the workout should be preceded by a warm-up and followed by a cool-down.

The warm-up prior to exercise is recommended to prepare the muscles and heart for the workout.

There are two good reasons for warming up prior to exercise. The first is to prepare the heart muscle for exercise. The second is to stretch the skeletal muscles.

A warm-up designed to prepare the heart muscle for moderate to vigorous exercise should include two to five minutes of walking, jogging, or mild exercise. Research shows that for some people, starting vigorous exercise abruptly is not wise. Apparently in some exercises, the increased blood flow to the heart and other muscles does not begin immediately when the exercise starts, at least not for all people. Adults who do this type of warm-up do not experience electrocardiogram abnormalities that are apparent in some people who do not warm-up.

The skeletal muscle warm-up should include static stretching of the major muscle groups involved in the exercise that is to follow. It should be emphasized that even though warming up prior to an activity may help reduce the chance of muscle injury, it is not a substitute for a regular program of exercise designed to improve flexibility.

A warm-up that is suitable for walking, jogging, running, cycling, and even basketball is included here as an example. This warm-up can be used for other activities provided stretching exercises for the major muscle groups involved in the activities are added. The cardiovascular warm-up is suitable for most activities, but other mild exercise (such as a slow, two to five minute swim for swimmers or a slow, two to five minute ride on a bicycle for cyclists) can be substituted.

The stretching portion of the warm-up can be done before or after the cardiovascular portion.

Some experts believe that the cardiovascular portion of the warm-up should precede the stretching portion because warm muscles are less apt to be injured by the stretch. Warm muscles also stretch farther. If you choose to stretch before the warm-up, make certain it is a gentle, static stretch. This is not the time for a flexibility workout in which you try to increase your normal range of motion. Rather, it should be for the purpose of limbering-up or loosening. It is acceptable to begin your warm-up with stretching as long as static stretches are used.

A cool-down after exercise is important.

Proper exercise planning is very important. One part of this planning is the organization of each exercise session. Each session should include a warm-up, a workout, and a cool-down. The warm-up has already been discussed. The workout, or actual exercise, is discussed in greater detail in other concepts. The cool-down is done immediately after the workout and should consist of exercise similar to the warm-up to permit a gradual decrease in the heart rate and gentle stretches of the muscles used in the workout.

There is still some controversy about the best time to stretch and about the benefits of warming up and cooling down. However, given current evidence, both a warm-up and a cool-down seem wise. Like the warm-up, there are two principal components of a cool-down: static muscle stretching and an activity for the cardiovascular system. Although not all experts agree, some believe that static muscle stretching *after* the workout is more important than stretching before because it may help relieve spasms in fatigued muscles. Stretching done as part of the cool-down may be more effective for lengthening the muscles than stretching done at other times because the stretching is done when the muscle temperature is elevated and therefore is more likely to produce optimal flexibility improvements.

A cardiovascular portion of the cool-down is also important. During exercise, the heart pumps a large amount of blood to the working muscles to supply the oxygen necessary to keep moving. The muscles squeeze the veins (see figure 3.1), which forces the blood back to the heart. Valves in the veins prevent the blood from flowing backward. As long as exercise continues, the blood is moved by the muscles back to the heart, where it is once again pumped to the body. If exercise is stopped abruptly, the blood is left in the area of the working muscles and has no way to get back to the heart. In the case of the runner, the blood pools in the legs. Because the heart has less blood to pump, blood pressure may drop. This can result in dizziness, and can even cause a person to pass out. The best way to prevent this problem is to taper off or slow down gradually after exercise. A cardiovascular cool-down should include approximately two minutes of walking, slow jogging, or any nonvigorous activity that uses the muscles involved in the workout.

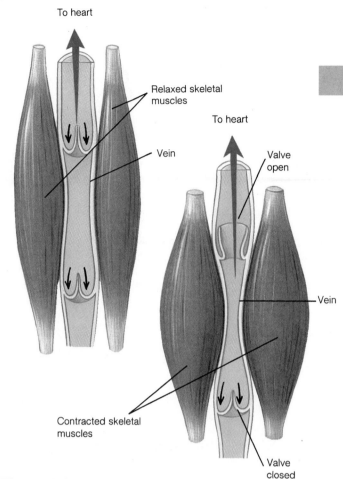

Figure 3.1
The pumping action of the muscles

A Sample Warm-up and Cool-down for an Aerobic Workout

The exercises shown here can be used before a moderate aerobic workout as a warm-up, or after a workout as a cool-down. Perform these exercises slowly. Do not bounce or jerk against the muscle. Hold each stretch for at least ten seconds. Perform each exercise at least once and up to three times. In concept 7, other stretching exercises are presented that can be used in a warm-up or cool-down.

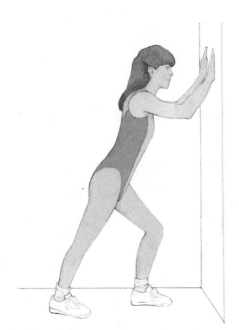

Face a wall with your feet two or three feet away. Step forward on left foot to allow both hands to touch the wall. (1) Keep the heel of your right foot on the ground, toe turned in slightly, knee straight, and buttocks tucked in. Lean forward by bending your front knee and arms and allowing your head to move nearer the wall. Hold. (2) Bend right knee, keeping heel on floor. Hold. Repeat with the other leg. (See figure 3.2.)

Figure 3.2
Calf stretcher for (1) gastrocnemius and (2) soleus

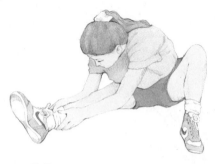

Figure 3.3
Back-saver toe touch (for hamstrings)

Sit on the floor. Extend one leg and bend the other knee, placing the foot flat on the floor. Bend at the hip and reach forward with both hands. Grasp one foot, ankle, or calf, depending upon how far you can reach. Pull forward with your arms trying to touch your head to your knee. Keep your knee relatively straight. Hold. Repeat with the opposite leg. (See figure 3.3.)

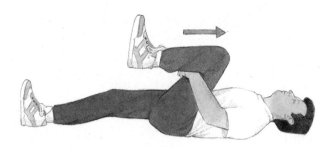

Figure 3.4
Leg hug (for the hip and back extensors)

Lie on your back. Bend one leg and grasp your thigh under the knee. Hug it to your chest. Keep the other leg straight and on the floor. Hold. Repeat with the opposite leg. (See figure 3.4.)

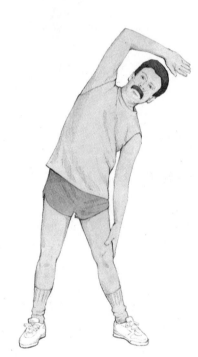

Figure 3.5
Side stretch

With the feet apart approximately shoulder width, lean to one side. Reach down with the arm on that side and reach up over your head with the opposite arm. Let your body weight stretch the muscles as you lean sideward. Do not twist or arch the back. Hold. Repeat to the other side. (See figure 3.5.)

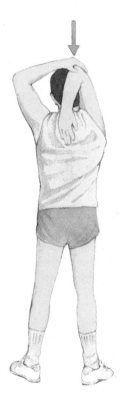

Figure 3.6
Zipper (for triceps and lower "pecs")

Lift right arm and reach behind head and down the spine (as if pulling up a zipper). With the left hand, push down on right elbow and hold. Reverse arm position and repeat. (See figure 3.6.)

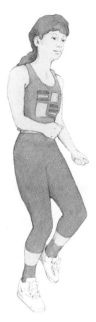

Figure 3.7
The cardiovascular warm-up

Before you perform a vigorous workout, walk or jog slowly for two minutes. After exercise, do the same. (See figure 3.7.)

Facts About the Exercise Environment

Exercise in exceptionally hot or humid weather can be dangerous.

The normal human body temperature is 98.6 degrees. During vigorous exercise, or when the surrounding temperature is above this level, the body temperature begins to rise. If the body get too hot, various heat problems can occur including heat cramps, heat exhaustion, and heat stroke (see table 3.1).

The body has its own methods of avoiding heat problems. The principal method of cooling is evaporation. During exercise, or even inactivity in hot weather, you perspire

Table 3.1
Types of Heat-Related Problems

Problem	Symptoms	Severity
Heat cramps	Muscle cramps, especially in muscles most used in exercise	Least severe
Heat exhaustion	Muscle cramps, weakness, dizziness; headache, nausea, clammy skin, paleness	Moderate severity
Heat stroke	Hot, flushed skin; dry skin (lack of sweating); dizziness; fast pulse; unconsciousness; high temperature	Extremely severe

or sweat. Evaporation of the sweat results in cooling that helps keep the body temperature within normal limits. If the weather is both hot and humid, evaporation is a less effective means of cooling the body. Excessive sweating or lack of fluid replacement (drinking water) can result in **dehydration.** A person who is dehydrated stops sweating so evaporation can no longer be used to cool the body. The body diverts blood to the blood vessels in an attempt to cool the body by exchanging heat directly with the environment. This can result in the most dangerous type of heat problem—heat stroke (see table 3.1).

When exercising in hot and humid environments, special precautions should be taken to prevent heat-related problems.

- Limit or avoid exercise in hot or humid environments. The apparent temperature is a combined value determined by both temperature and humidity. When the apparent temperature is below 90 degrees (32.2 degrees Celsius), exercise is safe for most people. Caution should be used when exercising at apparent temperatures ranging from 90 degrees to 100 degrees (37.7 degrees Celsius). Above 100 degrees, apparent temperature is the danger zone, and exercise should be done with extreme care, be limited, or be canceled. (See table 3.2.)
- Replace fluids regularly. Drink water at regular intervals *during* exercise. Drink water before and after exercise. For exercise lasting more than one or two hours, simple carbohydrates (glucose, fructose, or sucrose) in concentrations less than 5 percent are considered beneficial to performance and body cooling. Salt (sodium) in drinks is generally considered unnecessary.
- Gradually expose yourself to exercise in hot and humid environments. The body gets better at handling heat and humidity with repeated exposure. Too much at once is especially dangerous.
- Dress properly for exercise in the heat and humidity. Wear white or light colors that reflect rather than absorb heat. Porous clothing allows the passage of air to cool the body. Rubber, plastic, or other nonporous clothing is especially dangerous. A hat or porous cap can help when exercising in direct sunlight.
- Rest at regular intervals, preferably in the shade.
- Watch for signs of heat stress. If signs are present, stop immediately.

If overheating occurs, take immediate steps to cool the body.

- Get out of the heat—stop exercise.
- Remove excess clothing.

Table 3.2
Exercise in the Heat (Apparent Temperatures).

To read the table, find the air temperature on the top, then find the humidity on the left. Find the apparent temperature where the columns meet.

Relative Humidity (%)	Air Temperature (Degrees F)										
	70	75	80	85	90	95	100	105	110	115	120
100	72	80	91	108	132						
95	71	79	89	105	128						
90	71	79	88	102	122						
85	71	78	87	99	117	141					
80	71	78	86	97	113	136					
75	70	77	86	95	109	130					
70	70	77	85	93	106	124	144				
65	70	76	83	91	102	119	138				
60	70	76	82	90	100	114	132	149			
55	69	75	81	89	98	110	126	142			
50	69	75	81	88	96	107	120	135	150		
45	68	74	80	87	95	104	115	129	143		
40	68	74	79	86	93	101	110	123	137	151	
35	67	73	79	85	91	98	107	118	130	143	
30	67	73	78	84	90	96	104	113	123	135	148
25	66	72	77	83	88	94	101	109	117	127	139
20	66	72	77	82	87	93	99	105	112	120	130
15	65	71	76	81	86	91	97	102	108	115	123
10	65	70	75	80	85	90	95	100	105	111	116
5	64	69	74	79	84	88	93	97	102	107	111
0	64	69	73	78	83	87	91	95	99	103	107

= Safe Zone
= Caution Zone
= Danger Zone

"Apparent Temperatures"

Source: Data from the National Oceanic and Atmospheric Administration.

- Drink cool water.
- Immerse the body in cool water.
- If symptoms of heat stroke are present, seek immediate help.
- Statically stretch cramped muscles.

Exercise in exceptionally cold and windy weather can be dangerous.

Exercise in the cold is not considered to be as dangerous as exercise in the heat because you can always add clothing to keep warm. However, extreme cold can be dangerous to the exerciser because of a drop in body temperature or frostbite. A combination of wind and cold temperatures (**wind-chill factor**) poses the greatest danger.

When exercising in cold and windy environments, special precautions should be taken.

- Limit or cancel exercise if the wind-chill factor reaches the danger zone. (See table 3.3.)

- Dress properly for exercise in the wind and cold. Wear light clothing in several layers rather than one heavy garment. The layer of clothing closest to the body should be absorbent. A porous wind-breaker will keep wind from cooling the body and will allow the release of body heat. Since the hands, feet, nose, and ears are most susceptible to frostbite, these body parts should be covered. Wear a hat or cap, mask, and mittens. Mittens are warmer than gloves.
- Try to keep from getting wet in cold weather.

High altitude may limit performance and require adaptation of normal exercise.

The ability to do vigorous physical tasks is diminished as altitude increases. Breathing rate and heart rates increase at high altitude for similar types of activities done at sea level. With proper acclimation (gradual exposure), the body adjusts to the lower oxygen pressure found at high altitude, and performance improves. Nevertheless, performance ability at high altitudes, especially for activities requiring cardiovascular fitness, is usually less than would be expected at sea level. At extremely high altitudes, the ability to perform vigorous physical activity may be impossible without an extra oxygen supply. When moving to a high altitude from sea level, vigorous exercise should be done with caution. Acclimation to high altitudes requires a minimum of two weeks and may not be complete for several months.

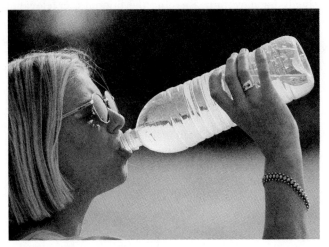
It is important to replace water during exercise.

Vigorous exercise may need to be limited or avoided if air pollution is high.

Various pollutants such as ozone, carbon monoxide, pollens, and particulates can cause poor physical performance, and in some cases health problems. Ozone, a pollutant produced primarily by the sun's reaction to car exhaust, can cause symptoms including headache, coughing, and eye irritation. Similar symptoms result from exposure to carbon monoxide, a tasteless and odorless gas, caused by combustion of oil, gasoline, and cigarette smoke. Most news media in metropolitan areas now give ozone and carbon monoxide levels as a part of their weather reports. When levels of these pollutants reach moderate levels, exercise may need to be modified for some people. When levels are high, exercise may need to be postponed. Exercisers wishing to avoid ozone and carbon monoxide may want to exercise indoors early in the morning, or later in the evening. It is wise to avoid areas with a high concentration of automobiles.

Pollens from certain plants may cause allergic reactions for certain people. Some people are allergic to dust or other particulates in the air. Weather reports of pollens and particulates may help exercisers determine the best times for their activities and when to avoid vigorous activities.

Table 3.3
Wind-Chill Factor Chart

Wind-Chill Factor Chart										
Actual Temperature Reading (Degrees F)	Estimated Wind Speed (mph)									Zones
	Calm	5	10	15	20	25	30	35	40	
50	50	48	40	36	32	30	28	27	26	Relatively safe with proper clothing
40	40	37	28	22	18	16	13	11	10	
30	30	27	16	9	4	0	-2	-4	-6	
20	20	16	4	-5	-10	-15	-18	-20	-21	
10	10	6	-9	-18	-25	-29	-33	-35	-37	Danger to exposed skin
0	0	-5	-24	-32	-39	-44	-48	-51	-53	
-10	-10	-15	-33	-45	-40	-59	-63	-67	-69	
-20	-20	-26	-46	-58	-67	-74	-79	-82	-85	Unsafe— postpone exercise
-30	-30	-36	-58	-72	-82	-88	-94	-98	-100	
-40	-40	-47	-70	-85	-96	-104	-109	-113	-116	
*NOTE: Wind speeds above 40 mph do not seem to add to danger of cold										

Based on data from Taylor, K. Runner's World, 8(1973):28.

Source: Data from J. Karr Taylor in *Runner's World*, 8 (1973): 28.

Facts About Soreness and Injury

Understanding soreness can help you persist in exercise and avoid problems.

Some people avoid exercise because they remember earlier experiences such as team practices or training for special events that led to soreness 24 to 48 hours after the intense exercise. They feel that all exercise will make them sore and they want to avoid this unpleasant experience. It is true that intense exercise, especially to muscle groups that are not normally exercised, can cause what is called **delayed-onset muscle soreness** or **DOMS.** We now know that DOMS results from microscopic muscle tears, not a build-up of lactic acid as some people thought. In some cases DOMS is accompanied by swelling in addition to pain but in general the condition has no long-term consequences.

There are several steps that can be taken to avoid DOMS and to make exercise more enjoyable. Starting exercise gradually (not doing too much after being inactive) is perhaps the most important thing you can do. It is known that lengthening contractions (eccentric—see terms in concept 9) are more likely to cause DOMS than shortening muscle contractions (concentric contractions). For this reason walking or running downhill or downstairs should be phased into your program gradually. Of course a regular warm-up is also advised. Fortunately DOMS lasts only a day or so. Doing moderate exercise when you have soreness does not seem to put you at risk of muscle injury. DOMS is only temporary and not a regular occurrence for those who exercise regularly and consistently. Understanding this will keep it from being a deterrent to regular physical activity.

Being able to treat minor injuries will help reduce their negative effects.

Minor injuries such as muscle sprains and strains are not uncommon to those who are persistent in their exercise. If a serious injury should occur it is important to get immediate medical attention. However, for minor injuries, following the **RICE formula** will help you reduce the pain or the injury and will speed recovery. In this acronymn **R** stands for rest. Muscle sprains and strains heal best if rested and rest also helps you avoid further damage to the muscle. **I** stands for ice. The quick application of cold (ice or ice water) to a minor injury minimizes swelling and speeds recovery. Cold should be applied to as great a surface area as possible (soaking is best). If ice is used it should be wrapped to avoid direct contact with the skin. Apply cold for 20–30 minutes three times a day for several days. **C** stands for compression. Wrapping or compressing the injured area also helps minimize swelling and speeds recovery. Elastic bandages are good for applying compression. For a sprained ankle, wearing a high-top shoe (tied) until a bandage can be located provides good compression. Elastic socks may also be useful. Care should be taken to avoid wrapping an injury too tightly because this can result in loss of circulation to the area. **E** stands for elevation. Keeping the injured area elevated (above the level of the heart) is also effective in minimizing swelling. If pain or swelling persists or if there is any doubt about the seriousness of an injury seek medical help.

Muscle cramps can be relieved by statically stretching a muscle.

A muscle cramp is usually not considered to be an injury but they are painful and may seem like an injury. They are usually short in duration and can often be relieved with proper treatment. Muscle cramps are pains in the large muscles of the body that result when the muscle contracts vigorously for a continued period of time. Cramps can result from lack of fluid replacement (dehydration), from fatigue, and from a blow directly to a muscle. A true cramp is not the same as a muscle tear, sprain, or strain. A cramp can be relieved by statically stretching the cramped muscle. For example, the calf muscle, which often cramps among runners, football players, and other sports participants, can be relieved using the calf stretcher exercise which is part of the warm-up in this concept. Other stretching exercises from concept 8 can be used to relieve cramps to other muscles or muscle groups. If stretching causes persistent pain stop the stretching—you may have a muscle injury rather than a cramp. Of course replacing fluids regularly during exercise helps avoid cramps as does the development of flexibility (see concept 8).

Suggested Readings

American College of Sports Medicine. *ACSM's Guidelines for Exercise Testing and Prescription,* 5th ed. Baltimore, MD: Williams and Wilkins, 1995.

Brunick, T. "Choosing the Right Shoe." *Physician and Sportsmedicine* 18(1990):104.

Pate, R. R., et al. "Physical Activity and Public Health." *Journal of the American Medical Association* 273(1995):402.

Powers, S. K., and Howley, E. T. *Exercise Physiology.* (2nd ed.) Dubuque, IA: Brown & Benchmark Publishers, 1994.

Roberts, W. "Managing Heatstroke." *Physician and Sportsmedicine* 20(1992):17.

Shephard, R. J. "Readiness for Physical Activity." *Physical Activity and Fitness Research Digest* 1(1994):1.

Wichmann, S., and D. Martin. "Athletic Shoes: Finding the Right Fit." *Physician and Sportsmedicine* 21(1993):204.

Chart 3.1 Physical Activity Readiness Questionnaire (PAR-Q)
A Self-Administered Questionnaire for Adults

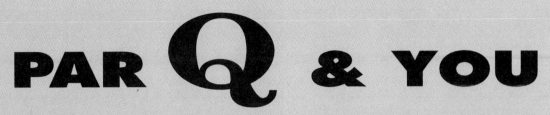

Regular physical activity is fun and healthy, and increasingly more people are starting to become more active every day. Being more active is very safe for most people. However, some people should check with their doctor before they start becoming much more physically active.

If you are planning to become much more physically active than you are now, start by answering the seven questions in the box below. If you are between the ages of 15 and 69, the PAR-Q will tell you if you should check with your doctor before you start. If you are over 69 years of age, and you are not used to being very active, check with your doctor.

Common sense is your best guide when you answer these questions. Please read the questions carefully and answer each one honestly: check YES or NO.

YES	NO	
☐	☐	1. Has your doctor ever said that you have a heart condition <u>and</u> that you should only do physical activity recommended by a doctor?
☐	☐	2. Do you feel pain in your chest when you do physical activity?
☐	☐	3. In the past month, have you had chest pain when you were not doing physical activity?
☐	☐	4. Do you lose your balance because of dizziness or do you ever lose consciousness?
☐	☐	5. Do you have a bone or joint problem that could be made worse by a change in your physical activity?
☐	☐	6. Is your doctor currently prescribing drugs (for example, water pills) for your blood pressure or heart condition?
☐	☐	7. Do you know of <u>any other reason</u> why you shoud not do physical activity?

If You Answered   Yes →

YES to one or more questions

Talk with your doctor by phone or in person BEFORE you start becoming much more physically active or BEFORE you have a fitness appraisal. Tell your doctor about the PAR-Q and which questions you answered YES.
- You may be able to do any activity you want—as long as you start slowly and build up gradually. Or, you may need to restrict your activities to those which are safe for you. Talk with your doctor about the kinds of activities you wish to participate in and follow his/her advice.
- Find out which community programs are safe and helpful for you.

No ↓

NO to all questions

If you answered NO honestly to <u>all</u> PAR-Q questions, you can be reasonably sure that you can:
- start becoming much more physically active—begin slowly and build up gradually. This is the safest and easiest way to go.
- take part in a fitness appraisal—this is an excellent way to determine your basic fitness so that you can plan the best way for you to live actively.

DELAY BECOMING MUCH MORE ACTIVE:
- if you are not feeling well because of a temporary illness such as a cold or a fever—wait until you feel better; or
- if you are or may be pregnant—talk to your doctor before you start becoming more active.

Please note: If your health changes so that you then answer YES to any of the above questions, tell your fitness or health professional. Ask whether you should change your physical activity plan.

<u>Informed Use of the PAR-Q</u>: The Canadian Society for Exercise Physiology, Health Canada, and their agents assume no liability for persons who undertake physical activity, and if in doubt after completing this questionnaire, consult your doctor prior to physical activity.

You are encouraged to copy the PAR-Q but only if you use the entire form

*Developed by the British Columbia Ministry of Health.

Produced by the British Columbia Ministry of Health and the Department of National Health & Welfare

Physical Activity Readiness
Questionnaire • PAR-Q
(revised 1994)

Note: It is important that you answer all questions honestly. The PAR-Q is a scientifically and medically researched preexercise selection device. It complements exercise programs, exercise testing procedures, and the liability considerations attendant with such programs and testing procedures. PAR-Q, like any other preexercise screening device, will misclassify a small percentage of prospective participants, but no preexercise screening method can entirely avoid this problem.

Chart 3.2 Physical Activity Questionnaire		
Answer the PAR-Q before using this chart. If you had one or more "yes" answers, follow the directions for the PAR-Q, concerning consultation with a physician. If you had all "no" answers on the PAR-Q, answer the additional questions below before beginning intensive training, particularly for sports.		
Yes	**No**	
☐	☐	1. Do you plan to participate on an organized team that will play intense competitive sports (i.e.,varsity team, professional team)?
☐	☐	2. If you plan to participate in a collision sport (even on a less organized basis), such as football, boxing, rugby, or ice hockey, have you been knocked unconscious more than one time?
☐	☐	3. Do you currently have symptoms from a previous muscle injury?
☐	☐	4. Do you currently have symptoms from a previous back injury, or do you experience back pain as a result of involvement in physical activity?
☐	☐	5. Do you have any other symptoms during physical activity that give you reason to be concerned about your health?
If your answer to any of these questions is "yes" then you should consult with your personal physician by telephone or in person to determine if you have a potential problem with vigorous involvement in physical activity.		

CONCEPT ·4·

How Much Physical Activity Is Enough?

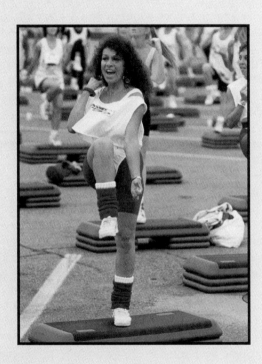

Concept 4

There is a minimal and an optimal amount of physical activity necessary for developing and maintaining each of the health-related aspects of physical fitness.

Introduction

Just as there is a correct dosage of medicine for treating an illness, there is a correct dosage of exercise for developing physical fitness. The minimum amount (dose) of exercise for developing physical fitness is called the threshold of training. The fitness target zone is the optimal amount of physical activity. New evidence indicates that the threshold for performance improvement differs from the threshold for achieving some health benefits of physical activity. Research also shows that the amount of exercise necessary for maintaining fitness may differ from the amount needed to develop it.

Health Goals for the Year 2000

- Increase the proportion of people who do *enough* physical activity for health and wellness. (↑)
- Decrease the proportion of people who do no leisure-time physical activity. (↓)

Note: (↑) indicates progress toward goal, (↓) indicates regression from goal, and (<>) indicates either no change or lack of new data since 1990.

Terms

- **FIT Formula**   A formula used to describe the frequency, intensity, and length of time for exercise to produce benefits. (When "FITT" is used, the second "T" refers to the type of physical activity you perform.)
- **Fitness Target Zone**   Amounts of exercise that produce optimal benefits.
- **Health Benefit**   A result of physical activity that provides protection from hypokinetic disease or early death.
- **Overload Principle**   A basic principle that specifies that you must perform exercise in greater than normal amounts (overload) to get an improvement in physical fitness or health benefits.
- **Performance Benefit**   A result of exercise that improves physical fitness and physical performance capabilities.
- **Physical Activity Pyramid**   This pyramid illustrates how different types of activities contribute to the development of physical fitness. Activities lower in the pyramid require more frequent participation whereas activities higher in the pyramid require less participation.
- **Principle of Progression**   A corollary of the overload principle that indicates the need to gradually increase overload to achieve optimal benefits.

- **Principle of Specificity** A corollary of the overload principle that indicates a need for a specific type of exercise to improve each fitness component or fitness of a specific part of the body.
- **Threshold of Training** The minimum amount of exercise that will produce benefits.

The Facts

The **overload principle** is the basis for improving physical fitness.

In order for a muscle (including the heart muscle) to get stronger, it must be "overloaded," or worked against a load greater than normal. To increase flexibility, a muscle must be stretched longer than is normal. To increase muscular endurance, muscles must be exposed to sustained exercise for a longer than normal period. If overload is less than normal for a specific component of fitness, the result will be a decrease in that particular component of fitness. A normal amount of exercise will maintain the current fitness level.

There is no substitute for overload in developing physical fitness.

Many people do not overload enough to develop good fitness. Often the programs found in health clubs and in exercises described in popular books and magazines do not provide for adequate overload. Some people try exercise machines or quack devices that violate the overload principle and are therefore ineffective.

The **principle of specificity** is an important law of exercise that should be observed if optimal fitness is to be obtained.

The "principle of specificity" simply states that to develop a certain characteristic of fitness, you must overload specifically for that particular fitness component. For example, strength-building exercises may do little for developing cardiovascular fitness, and flexibility exercises may do little for altering body composition.

Overload is specific to each component of fitness and is also specific to each body part. If you exercise the legs, you build fitness of the legs. If you exercise the arms, you build fitness of the arms. For this reason, it is not unusual to see some people with disproportionate fitness development. Some gymnasts, for example, have good upper body development but poor leg development, whereas some soccer players have well-developed legs but lack upper body development.

Specificity is important in designing your warm-up, workout, and cool-down programs for specific activities. Training is most effective when it closely resembles the activity for which you are preparing. For example, if your goal is to improve your skill in putting the shot, it is not enough to overload the arm muscles. You should perform a training activity requiring overload while doing a putting motion that closely resembles what you use in the actual sport.

The **principle of progression** is an important corollary of the overload principle.

The progression concept indicates that overload should not be increased too slowly or too rapidly if fitness is to result. Obviously, the concepts of threshold of training and fitness target zones are based on the "progression principle." Beginners can exercise progressively by starting near threshold levels and gradually increasing in frequency, intensity, and time (duration) within the target zone. Exercise above the target zone is counterproductive and can be dangerous. For example, the weekend athlete who exercises vigorously only on weekends does not exercise often enough, and so violates the principle of progression. Many people in the U.S., who consider themselves to be regular exercisers, violate the principle of progression by failing to exercise above threshold levels and in the exercise target zone. Clearly, it is possible to do too little or too much exercise to develop optimal fitness.

There is a **threshold of training** and a **fitness target zone** for each component of fitness.

The threshold of training is the minimum amount of exercise necessary to produce gains in fitness. What you normally do, or just a little more than your normal exercise, is not enough to cause improvements in fitness. Figure 4.1 shows the threshold of training and target zones for physical fitness improvement.

The fitness target zone begins at the threshold of training and stops at the point where the benefits of exercise become counterproductive, as shown in figure 4.1. This is the optimal level of exercise.

Some people incorrectly associate the concepts of threshold of training and fitness target zones with only cardiovascular fitness. As the principle of specificity suggests, each component of fitness has its own threshold and target zone. Details for each of the health-related aspects of fitness are presented later in this book.

The acronym FIT can help you remember the three important variables for determining threshold of training and fitness target zone levels.

For exercise to be effective, it must be done with enough **F**requency and **I**ntensity, and for a long enough **T**ime. The first letter from these three words spells **FIT** and can be considered as the formula for fitness.

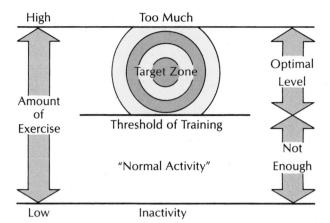

Figure 4.1
Exercise target zones

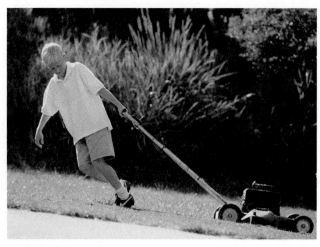

Doing lifestyle activities can benefit your health.

F Frequency (how often)—Exercise must be performed regularly to be effective. The number of days a person exercises per week is used to determine frequency. Exercise frequency depends on the specific component to be developed. However, most fitness components require at least three days and up to six days of activity per week.

I Intensity (how hard)—Exercise must be hard enough to require more exertion than normal to produce gains in health-related fitness. The method for determining appropriate intensity varies with each aspect of fitness. For example, flexibility requires stretching muscles beyond normal length, cardiovascular fitness requires elevating the heart rate above normal, and strength requires increasing the resistance more than normal.

T Time (how long)—Exercise must be done for a significant length of time to be effective. Generally, an exercise period must be at least fifteen minutes in length to be effective, while longer times are recommended for optimal fitness gains. As the length of time increases, intensities of exercise may be decreased. Time of exercise involvement is also referred to as exercise duration.

> The type of physical activity you do is often considered to be part of the FITT Formula.

Sometimes a second "T" is added to the FIT Formula (FITT) to indicate that the **T**ype of physical activity you perform is important. As the specificity principle indicates, different types of activity build different components of fitness. The **Physical Activity Pyramid** (see figure 4.2) is a good way to illustrate the different types of activities and how each contributes to the development of physical fitness. Like the Food Guide Pyramid (see concept 19) the Physical Activity Pyramid encourages more "portions" of activity (more frequent participation) in those activities lower in the pyramid and requires fewer "portions" from those higher in the pyramid.

Lifestyle physical activities are at the base of the pyramid. This type of activity is placed at the base of the pyramid because it is encouraged as a part of *everyday living* and can contribute significantly to good health, fitness, and wellness. Lifestyle activities include walking to or from work, climbing the stairs rather than taking an elevator, working in the yard, or doing any other type of exercise as part of your normal daily activities.

Aerobic activities include those which are of such an intensity that they can be performed for relatively long periods of time without stopping. Brisk fitness walking, jogging, biking, and aerobic dance are but a few of the common aerobic activities. This type of activity is included in the second level of the pyramid because it is encouraged *most days of the week* and is especially good for building cardiovascular fitness and helping to control body fatness.

Active sports are a type of activity that improve cardiovascular fitness and can help control body fatness if done for relatively long periods of time without stopping. They can also contribute to the development of other parts of fitness. Examples include basketball, tennis, golf, and bowling. Active sports done *more than a few days a week* can have many of the benefits of aerobic activities.

Flexibility (stretching) exercises are a type of exercise that are planned specifically to build flexibility. This type of exercise is necessary because activities lower in the pyramid often do not contribute to flexibility development. This type of exercise should be performed *at least three days per week* and for best results more often.

The strength and muscular endurance category includes exercises that are types of exercises that are planned specifically to build strength and muscular endurance. This type of exercise is necessary because activities lower in the pyramid often do not contribute to strength and muscular endurance development. This type of exercise should be performed *two to three days per week.*

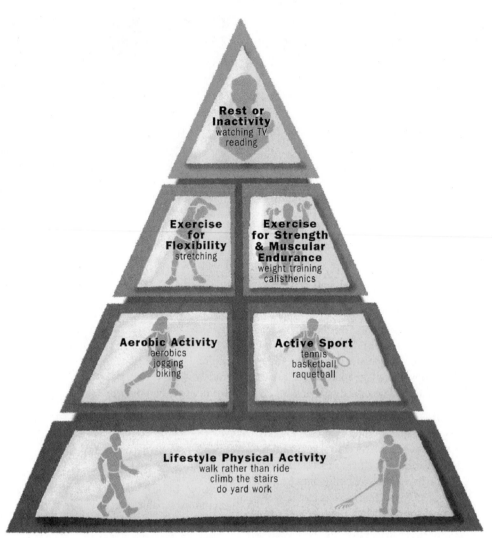

Figure 4.2
The Physical Activity Pyramid

Rest or inactivity can also be important to good health. Some time off just to relax is important to us all and of course proper amounts of rest and sleep help us recuperate. But, as you will learn later in this book, sedentary living (too much inactivity) results in low fitness as well as poor health and wellness. Rest and inactivity is placed at the top of the pyramid because it should be done *sparingly* compared to other types of activity in the pyramid.

In later concepts the Physical Activity Pyramid will be used to identify the types of activities that are appropriate for building different parts of fitness and contributing to overall health and wellness. For convenience the acronym FIT rather than FITT will be used in the remainder of this book.

> Threshold levels and target zones change as your fitness level changes.

As you become more fit by doing correct exercises, your threshold of training and fitness target zones may change.

Likewise, if you stop exercising for a period of time, they will also change. Your threshold of training and fitness target zones are based on your current physical fitness levels and your current exercise patterns. Recent research, for example, suggests that the exercise necessary to maintain fitness need not be as often as exercise designed to build fitness.

> It takes time for exercise to benefit health-related physical fitness.

Sometimes people just beginning an exercise program expect to see immediate results. They expect to see large losses in body fat in short periods of time, or great increases in muscle strength in just a few days. Evidence shows, however, that improvements in health-related physical fitness and the associated health benefits take several weeks to become apparent. Though some people report psychological benefits, such as "feeling better" and a "sense of personal accomplishment" almost immediately after beginning regular exercise, the physiological changes will take considerably longer to be realized. Proper preparation for exercise includes learning not to expect too much too soon, and not to do too much too soon. Attempts to overdo it and to try to get fit fast will probably be counterproductive, resulting in soreness and even injury. The key is to start slowly, stay with it, and enjoy the exercise. Benefits will come to those who persist.

> The threshold of training necessary for producing noticeable improvements in health-related physical fitness differs from the threshold necessary for producing some of the health benefits of exercise.

The FIT formula as presented in this concept outlines the amount of exercise necessary to achieve what is called a **performance benefit.** A performance benefit results in a significant improvement in a specific component of health-related fitness.There is good evidence that adequate amounts of fitness are necessary for good health and for improving performance in sports and physical activities.

New studies show that some of the **health benefits** of exercise occur at levels less than those necessary for producing performance benefits. For example, reduced risk of heart disease can result from exercise that is less intense than the threshold of training illustrated in figure 4.1. Gardening, walking, and other lifestyle activities of similar intensity have been shown to produce health benefits when done regularly and for a considerable duration. Whereas the performance and health benefits may occur within several weeks when exercise equals amounts prescribed by the FIT formula, the health benefits associated with less intense exercise are manifested only when regular exercise becomes a part of a permanent lifestyle. The lower threshold for sustained low-intensity exercise is illustrated in figure 4.3.

Exercise in the performance target zone illustrated in figure 4.3 is desirable. However, less intense physical activity should not be discounted as an important part of a healthy lifestyle.

Facts About Physical Fitness Testing

> Periodic physical fitness can aid in determining if a person is exercising enough and is fit enough for health, performance, and quality living.

At some point, it is wise to have an expert test your fitness. This helps you get an accurate assessment of your current fitness level. It is important, however, to learn to evaluate your own level of fitness. Learning to evaluate your own

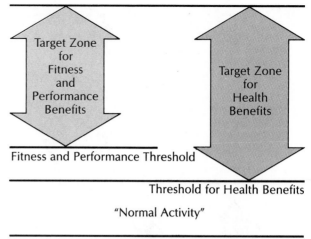

Figure 4.3
The threshold of training for health benefits of sustained lifestyle physical activity.

fitness allows you to have a personal record of your fitness on a regular basis, keeps you from being dependent on others, and aids you in staying fit for a lifetime.

> Comparison of physical fitness test results to health standards and improvement of your own fitness are more important than comparisons to other people.

In Western culture, we have a tendency to compare ourselves to others in almost all things we do. Rather than comparing your fitness scores to those of other people, you would be wise to concentrate on meeting good fitness standards and improving your personal fitness. Exceptionally high scores on fitness tests may improve performances in sports but probably are not necessary for good health. For example, a male having 10 to 15 percent body fat is considered to be more healthy than one having 25 to 30 percent body fat. However, having less than 10 percent of the body as fat is not necessarily more healthy than having 10 to 15 percent fat (though some people believe that low levels of fatness may enhance performance in some sports). As you will learn later in this book, having too little body fat can be harmful to good health.

Heredity also plays an important role in the amount of physical fitness a person can attain. More than a few people have become discouraged after completing an exercise program only to find that they have scored lower on fitness tests than friends who are less active. Though it is clear that regular exercise is critical to optimal physical fitness, each person also has a hereditary predisposition to fitness. Although achieving good scores on fitness tests is a desirable goal, it is important to understand that hereditary predispositions to fitness limit one's potential for achieving exceptionally high scores. Meeting standards for good health and improving personal fitness are more important than comparisons to other people.

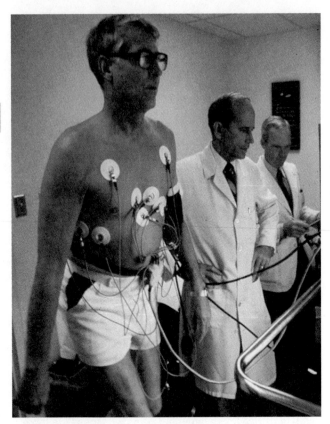

A fitness assessment by an expert can be useful.

Table 4.1
The Four Fitness Zones

High Performance Zone
The 'high performance zone' is a good indicator of adequate fitness, but it is not necessary to reach this level to experience good health benefits. Achievement of high performance scores has more to do with performance on various physical tasks than it does with good health.
Good Fitness Zone
If you reach the 'good fitness zone' you probably have enough of a specific fitness component to help reduce the risk of a specific hypokinetic condition, assuming that you maintain an active lifestyle. Even achievement in the good fitness zone may not result in optimal health benefits for inactive people.
Marginal Zone
'Marginal' scores indicate that some improvement is in order, but you are nearing minimal health standards set by experts.
Low Fit Zone
If you score 'low' in fitness, you are probably less fit than you should be for your own good health and wellness.

An assessment of all components of health-related fitness is important.

Because fitness has many different components, you will need to do many self-tests if you are going to get an accurate picture of your total fitness. It is recommended that each person do *several* tests of fitness for each component of health-related fitness. Multiple tests will give you a more complete and accurate picture of your total physical fitness.

An Important Note on Physical Fitness Testing

In this book we present many fitness tests. When possible, you should learn to give each test to yourself so that you can continue to reassess your fitness for a lifetime. Tests such as skin-fold measures are hard to administer to yourself, but you can learn to teach a friend or relative to measure you. You are encouraged to do as many tests as possible. For example, you may want to assess your cardiovascular fitness using all three tests described. You can use a summary of all tests to make accurate fitness assessments.

Finally, you should know how to use the Rating Scales in each concept to interpret your fitness results. Four rating

categories are provided for you to rate each part of health-related fitness. These are illustrated and described in table 4.1. Your first goal should be to be sure that you do not rate low on any health-related fitness part. Ultimately you should achieve the "good fitness zone" for all parts of fitness. You may, for personal reasons, wish to achieve the high performance zone for some fitness components. The fitness ratings used in this book help you determine "how much fitness is enough" for your good health and wellness, but do not require you to compare yourself to others or set unrealistic standards.

Suggested Readings

American College of Sports Medicine. *ACSM's Guidelines for Exercise Testing and Exercise Prescription.* 5th ed. Baltimore, MD: Williams and Wilkins, 1995.

Corbin, C. B., Pangrazi, R. P., and Welk, G. J. "Toward an Understanding of Appropriate Physical Activity Levels for Youth." *Physical Activity and Fitness Research Digest* 1(1994):1.

Corbin, C. B. and Pangrazi, R. P. "What You Need to Know About the Surgeon General's Report on Physical Activity and Health," *Physical Activity and Fitness Research Digest,* 2(1996):1.

Fletcher, G. F., et al. "American Heart Association Medical/Scientific Statement on Exercise." *Circulation.* 86(1992):340.

Paffenbarger, R., et al. "Physical Activity and Physical Fitness as Determinants of Health and Longevity." In Bouchard, C., et al., *Exercise, Fitness, and Health.* Champaign, IL: Human Kinetics Publishers, 1990.

Pate, R. R., et al. "Physical Activity and Public Health." *The Journal of the American Medical Association* 273(1995):402.

Sallis, J. F., and Patrick, K. "Physical activity guidelines for adolescents: consensus statement. *Pediatric Exercise Science,* 53(1994):302.

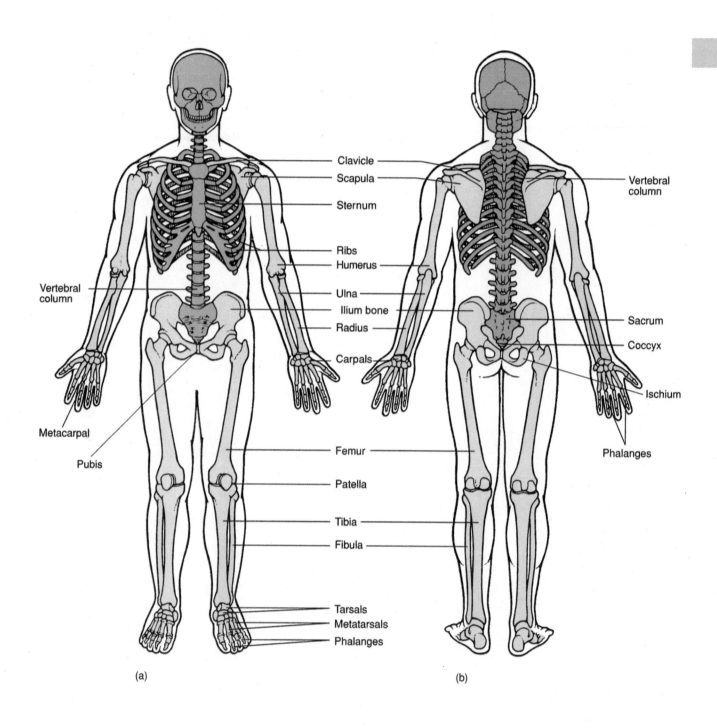

Clavicle
Scapula
Sternum

Ribs
Humerus
Ulna
Ilium bone
Radius
Carpals

Vertebral
column

Metacarpal

Pubis

Femur

Patella

Tibia

Fibula

Tarsals
Metatarsals
Phalanges

(a)

Vertebral
column

Sacrum
Coccyx

Ischium

Phalanges

(b)

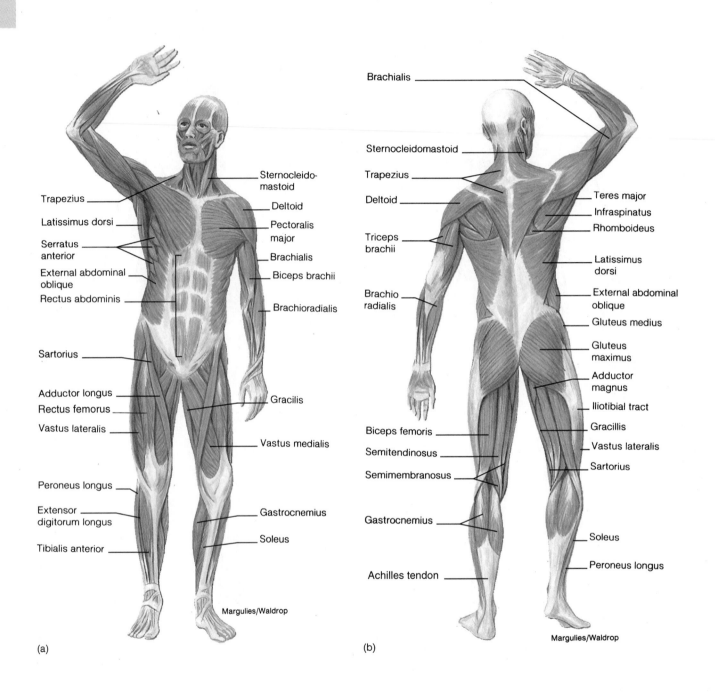

Trapezius

Latissimus dorsi

Serratus anterior

External abdominal oblique

Rectus abdominis

Sartorius

Adductor longus

Rectus femorus

Vastus lateralis

Peroneus longus

Extensor digitorum longus

Tibialis anterior

Sternocleido-mastoid

Deltoid

Pectoralis major

Brachialis

Biceps brachii

Brachioradialis

Gracilis

Vastus medialis

Gastrocnemius

Soleus

Margulies/Waldrop

(a)

Brachialis

Sternocleidomastoid

Trapezius

Deltoid

Triceps brachii

Brachio radialis

Biceps femoris

Semitendinosus

Semimembranosus

Gastrocnemius

Achilles tendon

Teres major

Infraspinatus

Rhomboideus

Latissimus dorsi

External abdominal oblique

Gluteus medius

Gluteus maximus

Adductor magnus

Iliotibial tract

Gracillis

Vastus lateralis

Sartorius

Soleus

Peroneus longus

Margulies/Waldrop

(b)

Major Blood Vessels

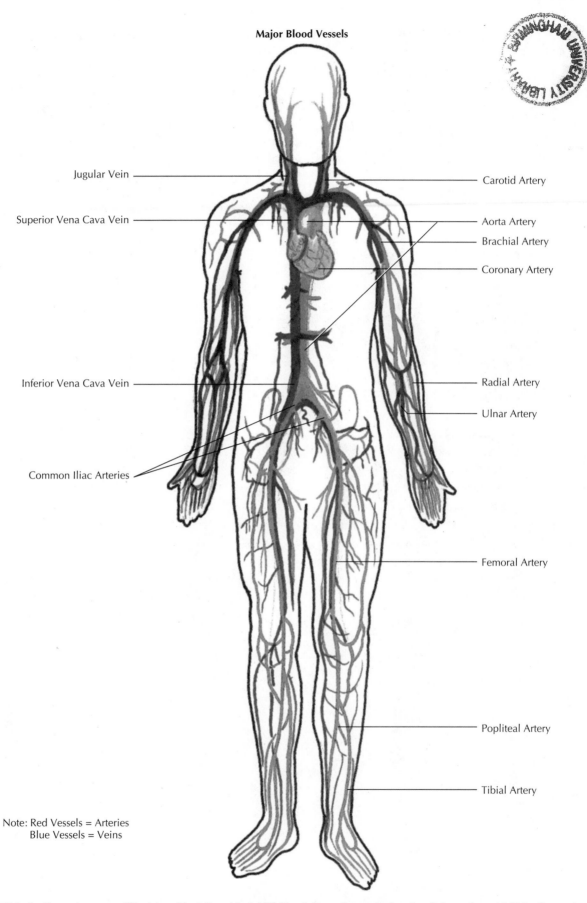

Jugular Vein

Superior Vena Cava Vein

Inferior Vena Cava Vein

Common Iliac Arteries

Carotid Artery

Aorta Artery

Brachial Artery

Coronary Artery

Radial Artery

Ulnar Artery

Femoral Artery

Popliteal Artery

Tibial Artery

Note: Red Vessels = Arteries
Blue Vessels = Veins

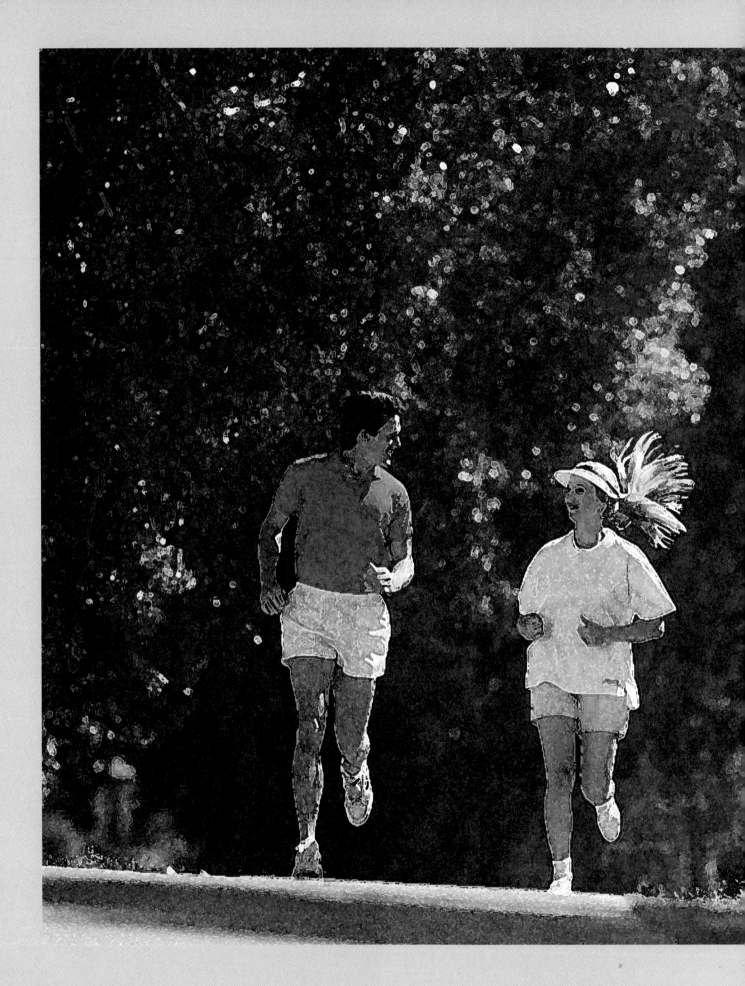

SECTION
·II·

Health-Related Physical Fitness

CONCEPT
·5·
Cardiovascular Fitness

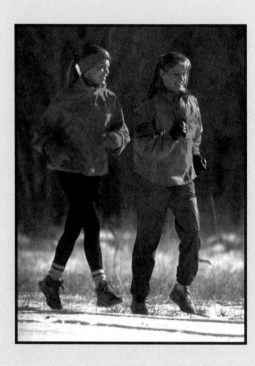

Cardiovascular fitness is probably the most important aspect of physical fitness because of its importance to good health and optimal physical performance.

Introduction

Cardiovascular fitness is frequently considered the most important aspect of physical fitness because those who possess it have a decreased risk of heart disease—the number one killer in our society. This is supported by the recent statements of the American Heart Association and the Surgeon General's Report on Physical Activity which indicate that sedentary living is a primary risk factor for heart disease and that increasing physical activity is a lifestyle change that has dramatic health and wellness benefits. In addition, cardiovascular fitness is important to the effective performance of virtually all types of work and play activities.

Health Goals for the Year 2000

- Reduce coronary heart disease deaths. (↑)
- Fewer stroke deaths. (↑)
- Better control of high blood pressure. (↑)
- Lower cholesterol levels. (↑)
- Increase the proportion of people who engage in activity that promotes cardiovascular fitness. (↑)

Note: (↑) indicates progress toward goal, (↓) indicates regression from goal, and (<>) indicates either no change or lack of new data since 1990.

Terms

- **Aerobic Capacity**   Another term used for maximal oxygen uptake ($\dot{V}O_2$ max).
- **Aerobic Physical Activity or Exercise**   Aerobic means "in the presence of oxygen." Aerobic activity is activity or exercise for which the body is able to supply adequate oxygen to sustain performance for long periods of time.
- **Anaerobic Capacity**   A measure of anaerobic fitness; the maximal work performed in a short burst of high-intensity exercise.
- **Anaerobic Exercise**   Anaerobic means "in the absence of oxygen." Anaerobic exercise is performed at an intensity so great that the body's demand for oxygen exceeds its ability to supply it.
- **Cardiovascular Fitness**   The ability of the heart, blood vessels, blood, and respiratory system to supply fuel, especially oxygen, to the muscles and the ability of the muscles to utilize fuel to allow sustained exercise.
- **Fast-Twitch (FT) Muscle Fibers**   The muscle fibers primarily used in anaerobic exercise or short, explosive exercise such as sprinting.
- **Health Benefit**   In this concept, health benefit refers to reduced risk of heart disease associated with exercise.
- **Hemoglobin**   Oxygen-carrying pigment of the red blood cells.

Lactic Acid   Substance that results from the process of supplying energy during anaerobic exercise; a cause of muscle fatigue.

Maximal Oxygen Uptake   A laboratory measure held to be the best measure of cardiovascular fitness. Commonly referred to as $\dot{V}O_2$ max or the volume ($\dot{V}$) of oxygen used when a person reaches his or her maximal (max) ability to supply it during exercise.

Performance Benefit   In this concept, performance benefit refers to an improved score on a cardiovascular fitness test or in performance of activities requiring cardiovascular fitness.

Ratings of Perceived Exertion (RPE)   The assessment of the intensity of exercise based on how the participant feels; a written questionnaire is used in the assessment.

Slow-Twitch (ST) Muscle Fibers   Muscle fibers primarily used in aerobic or sustained, continuous exercise; also referred to as fatigue-resistant fibers.

The Facts About Cardiovascular Fitness

Cardiovascular fitness is a term that has several synonyms.

Cardiovascular fitness is sometimes referred to as "cardiovascular endurance" because a person who possesses this type of fitness can persist in physical exercise for long periods of time without undue fatigue. It has been referred to as "cardio-respiratory fitness" because it requires delivery and utilization of oxygen, which is only possible if the circulatory and respiratory systems are capable of these functions.

The term "aerobic fitness" has also been used as a synonym for cardiovascular fitness because **aerobic capacity** is considered to be the best indicator of cardiovascular fitness and **aerobic physical activity or exercise** is the preferred method for achieving it. Regardless of the words used to describe it, cardiovascular fitness is complex because it requires fitness of several body systems (see figure 5.1).

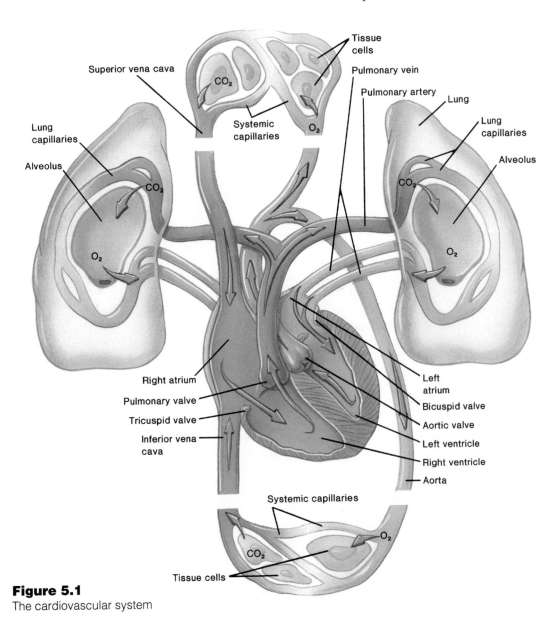

Figure 5.1
The cardiovascular system

Good cardiovascular fitness requires a fit heart muscle.

The heart is a muscle; to become stronger it must be exercised like any other muscle in the body. If the heart is exercised regularly, its strength increases; if not, it becomes weaker. Contrary to the belief that strenuous work harms the heart, research has found no evidence that regular, progressive exercise is bad for the normal heart. In fact, the heart muscle will increase in size and power when called upon to extend itself. The increase in size and power allows the heart to pump a greater volume of blood with fewer strokes per minute. For example, the average individual has a resting heart rate between seventy and eighty beats per minute, whereas it is not uncommon for a trained athlete's pulse to be in the low fifties or even in the forties.

The healthy heart is efficient in the work that it does. It can convert about half of its fuel into energy. An automobile engine in good running condition converts about one-fourth of its fuel into energy. By comparison, the heart is an efficient engine. The heart of a normal individual beats reflexively about 40 million times a year. During this time, over 4000 gallons, or 10 tons, of blood are circulated each day, and every night the heart's workload is equivalent to a person carrying a thirty-pound pack to the top of the 102-story Empire State Building.

Good cardiovascular fitness requires a fit vascular system.

As illustrated in figure 5.1, blood containing a high concentration of oxygen is pumped by the left ventricle through the aorta (a major artery), where it is carried to the tissues. Blood flows through a sequence of arteries to capillaries and to veins. Veins carry the blood containing lesser amounts of oxygen back to the right side of the heart, first to the atrium and then to the ventricle. The right ventricle pumps the blood to the lungs. In the lungs, the blood picks up oxygen and carbon dioxide is removed. From the lungs, the oxygenated blood travels back to the heart, first to the left atrium and then to the left ventricle. The process then repeats itself.

Healthy arteries are elastic, free of obstruction, and expand to permit the flow of blood. Muscle layers line the arteries and control the size of the arterial opening upon the impulse from nerve fibers. Unfit arteries may have a reduced internal diameter (atherosclerosis) because of deposits on the interior of their walls, or they may have hardened, nonelastic walls (arteriosclerosis).

Fit coronary arteries are especially important to good health. The blood in the four chambers of the heart does not directly nourish the heart. Rather, numerous small arteries within the heart muscle provide for coronary circulation (see figure 5.2). Poor coronary circulation precipitated by unhealthy arteries can be the cause of a heart attack (see figure 5.3).

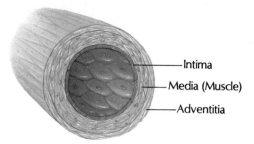

Figure 5.2
Healthy, elastic artery

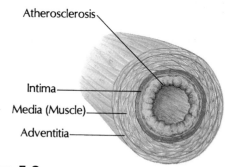

Figure 5.3
Unhealthy artery

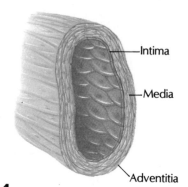

Figure 5.4
Healthy, nonelastic vein

Veins have thinner, less elastic walls than arteries as shown in figure 5.4. Also, veins contain small valves to prevent the backward flow of blood. Skeletal muscles assist the return of blood to the heart. The veins are intertwined in the muscle; therefore, when the muscle is contracted, the vein is squeezed, pushing the blood on its way back to the heart. A malfunction of the valves results in a failure to remove used blood at the proper rate. As a result, venous blood pools, especially in the legs, causing a condition known as varicose veins (see figure 3.1 on page 35).

Capillaries are the transfer stations where oxygen and fuel are released and waste products, such as CO_2, are removed from the tissues. The veins receive the blood from the capillaries for the return trip to the heart.

> Good cardiovascular fitness requires a fit respiratory system and fit blood.

The process of taking in oxygen (through the mouth and nose) and delivering it to the lungs, where it is picked up by the blood, is called external respiration. External respiration requires fit lungs as well as blood with adequate **hemoglobin** in the red blood cells (erythrocytes). Insufficient oxygen-carrying capacity of the blood is called anemia.

Delivering oxygen to the tissues from the blood is called internal respiration. Internal respiration requires an adequate number of healthy capillaries. In addition to delivering oxygen to the tissues, these systems remove CO_2. Good cardiovascular fitness requires fitness of both the external and internal respiratory systems.

> Cardiovascular fitness requires fit muscle tissue capable of using oxygen.

Once the oxygen is delivered, the muscle tissues must be able to use oxygen to sustain physical performance. Cardiovascular fitness activities rely mostly on **slow-twitch (ST) muscle fibers.** These fibers, when trained, undergo changes that make them especially able to use oxygen. Outstanding distance runners often have high numbers of slow-twitch fibers and sprinters often have high numbers of **fast-twitch (FT) muscle fibers.**

Facts About Physical Activity, Cardiovascular Fitness, and Heart Disease

> Regular physical activity reduces the risk of heart disease.

There is considerable evidence that regular physical activity reduces the incidence of heart disease. Also, it reduces the chances of early death from heart disease. In fact, the benefits of exercise in preventing heart disease have been shown to be independent of other risk factors. Inactivity is now considered a primary risk factor for heart disease. The amount of physical activity necessary to get these benefits is presented in the following section of this concept.

> People with low cardiovascular fitness have increased risk of heart disease.

The best evidence indicates that cardiovascular fitness is associated with heart disease. A classic research study at the Cooper Institute for Aerobics Research (Blair, et al., 1989) shows that low fit people are especially at risk. In addition it has now been demonstrated that improving your fitness (moving from low fitness to the good fitness zone) has a positive effect on health. Among those who are not low in fitness, further fitness increases bring additional health benefits but not equal in magnitude to the benefits received from getting out of the low fitness category.

Threshold and Target Zones for Reducing Heart Disease Risk and Improving Cardiovascular Fitness

> The frequency, intensity and time of your physical activity will vary depending on the benefits you hope to achieve.

The term "threshold of training" suggests that there is one level of physical activity that all people must do to achieve cardiovascular fitness as well as the **health benefits** of activity. We now know that the threshold differs for people depending on their current fitness and activity levels and the benefits they hope to achieve. New studies show that health benefits can be achieved by doing less activity than previously thought. However, those who desire **performance benefits** as indicated by a high level cardiovascular fitness, in addition to the health benefits of physical activity, will need to do activity at a higher threshold level than those who are interested primarily in the basic health benefits. Table 5.1 illustrates the threshold and target zones for performing physical activity designed to promote cardiovascular fitness and cardiovascular health. You should select activity amounts from this table based on the benefits you hope to achieve and your current fitness and activity levels.

> The type of physical activity you select is important to the benefits you will receive.

Lifestyle physical activity from the first level of the physical activity pyramid (see figure 5.5) can promote health benefits and make contributions to your cardiovascular fitness. Aerobic activities (see second level of the pyramid) are considered to be the most beneficial in promoting health benefits and are effective in promoting

Table 5.1
Threshold of Training and Target Zones for Aerobic Exercise

Performance and Health Benefit		Health Benefit
Frequency At least 3 and no more than 6 days a week. **Intensity** 50%* to 85% of working heart rate range, or 60%* to 90% of maximum heart rate, or exercise between 12 and 16 RPE. **Time** 20 to 60 minutes.	TARGET ZONE	Better 2000 to 3500 calories expended per week. Good 1000 to 2000 calories expended per week.
	THRESHOLD OF TRAINING	
Frequency 3 days a week. **Intensity** 50%* of its working heart rate range or 60% of maximal heart rate or exercise at 12 RPE. **Time** 20 minutes.		1000 calories expended per week in *regular* physical activity. or 1.35 calories per pound of body weight per day (3 calories per kg).

*Values of 40 to 50% are acceptable for those beginning exercise or with limitations.

performance increases needed for high-level performance. Though sports (see concept 15) can also be effective in contributing to the development of cardiovascular fitness, some are relatively ineffective and others can be very effective.

> As a minimum, adults should participate in regular physical activity equal to 30 minutes of brisk walking most, preferably all, days of the week.

The Surgeon General's Report on Physical Activity and Health, as well as a recent position statement by the Centers for Disease Control and Prevention and the American College of Sports Medicine, indicate that 30 minutes of physical activity equal to brisk walking most days a week is an important contributor to personal cardiovascular health and the cardiovascular health of the nation. Of course activity in addition to this minimum is endorsed (see table 5.1).

To achieve health benefits, physical activity can be accumulated in several 10 to 15 minute bouts that total 30 minutes daily. However, when possible, bouts of 30 minutes duration are recommended. Near daily activity is recommended because each activity session actually has short term benefits which do not occur if activity is not relatively frequent. This is sometimes referred to as the "last bout effect".

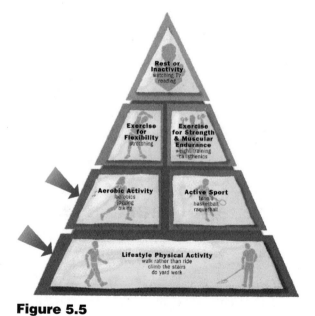

Figure 5.5
Select appropriate activities from the pyramid for cardiovascular fitness.

The threshold of training for producing many of the **health benefits** can be determined using a weekly calorie count. Scientific evidence suggests that people who regularly expend calories each week in lifestyle activities such as walking, stair climbing, and sports reduce death rates considerably compared to those who do not exercise. As few as 500 to 1000 calories expended in exercise per week can reduce death rate, but most experts suggest that to insure a health benefit from exercise, a person should expend no less than 1.35 calories per pound of body weight each day. This amounts to 1000 to 2000 calories per week for most people if exercise is done daily.

For optimal health benefits an expenditure of 2000 to 3500 calories per week is recommended, because people doing this much physical activity have 48 to 64 percent less risk of heart disease when compared to sedentary people. As the calories expended per week increase, the death rate decreases proportionally (see figure 5.6) up to 3500 calories. Because additional benefits do not occur for those expending more than 3500 calories per week, the target zone is 1000 to 3500 calories per week. For the health benefits to occur, calories must be expended on most days of the week and over long periods of time. In other words, moderate physical activity as described here must become regular lifetime physical activity if optimal health benefits are to be obtained. It should also be pointed out that some vigorous sports participation as part of the calories expended each week enhances the benefits of moderate regular calorie expenditure.

Meeting the minimum physical activity recommendation, as noted in the preceding fact statement (activity equal to 30 minutes of brisk walking most days of the week), equals approximately 1000 to 1400 Calories per week for most people. More information on the FIT formula for Calorie counting is illustrated in table 5.1.

As noted in the previous section, expending a significant number of calories each week can result in reduced risk of cardiovascular disease and improved health. To achieve these benefits it is only necessary to do relatively low-level exercise for extended periods of time. For example, a 150-pound person could walk for an hour and a half five days a week at three miles per hour to expend 2000 calories a week. Both cardiovascular health and performance benefits (improved fitness test results) could be obtained in much shorter periods of time if exercise is done more intensely. For busy people this method is often preferred. To achieve fitness by using shorter duration exercise, your heart rate must be elevated to target zone intensity. (Details are presented in table 5.1 and subsequent sections of this concept.) In addition to producing cardiovascular health benefits, ex-

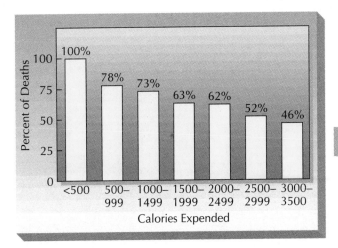

Figure 5.6
Deaths decrease as caloric expenditure increases.
The baseline death rate was established for inactive people [less than 550 calories].

Source: Data from R. Paffenbarger, et al., "Physical Activity and Physical Fitness as Determinants of Health and Longevity" in C. Bouchard, et al., *Exercise Fitness and Health,* 1990, Human Kinetics Publishers, Champaign, IL.

ercise that elevates the heart rate into the target zone has the added advantage of improved cardiovascular fitness test scores and improved performances in cardiovascular activities such as running, swimming, and cycling. Of course physical activity using the heart rate FIT formula can also be done by those who are not especially interested in getting benefits in a short period of time but who want a higher level of fitness and optimal health benefits. Those who exercise at a high heart rate for a long duration more than five days a week place themselves at risk of having musculoskeletal problems.

To determine the intensity of exercise for building cardiovascular fitness, it is important to know how to count your pulse. Each time the heart beats it pumps blood into the arteries. The surge of blood causes a pulse that can be felt by holding a finger against an artery. Major arteries that are easy to locate and are frequently used for pulse counts include the carotid on either side of the Adam's apple, and the radial just above the base of the thumb on the wrist (see figure 5.7). Heart (pulse) rate is important for determining the correct intensity of exercise for building cardiovascular fitness.

To count the pulse rate, simply place the fingertips (index and middle finger) over the artery at one of the previously mentioned locations. Move the fingers around until a strong pulse can be felt. Press gently so as not to cut off the blood flow through the artery. Counting the pulse with the thumb is *not* recommended because the thumb has a relatively strong pulse of its own and it could be confusing when counting another person's pulse.

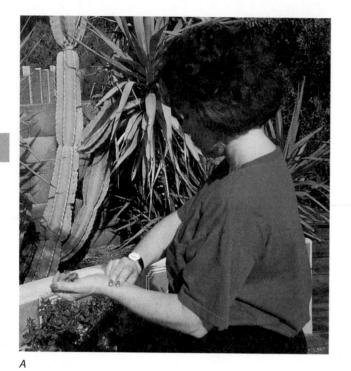

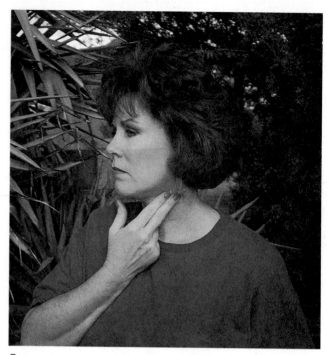

Figure 5.7
Counting your own pulse: *(A)* wrist (radial) and *(B)* neck (carotid)

Counting the pulse at the carotid artery is the most popular procedure, probably because the carotid pulse is easy to locate. Some researchers suggest that caution should be used when taking carotid pulse counts because pressing on this artery can cause a reflex that slows the heart rate. This could result in incorrect heart rate counts. More recent research indicates that carotid palpations, when done properly, can be used safely to count heart rate for most people.

The radial pulse is a bit harder to find than the carotid pulse because of the many tendons near the wrist. Moving the fingers around to several locations on the wrist just above the thumb will help you locate this pulse. For older adults or those with known medical problems, the radial pulse is recommended. Though less popular, the pulse can also be counted at the brachial artery. This is located on the inside of the upper arm just below the armpit.

Once the pulse is located, the heart rate can be determined in beats per minute. At rest, this is done simply by counting the number of beats in one minute. To determine exercise heart rate, it is best to count heart beats or pulses during exercise; however, during most activities this is difficult. Machines do exist that can count heartbeats during exercise, but they are not available to most people. The most practical method is to count the pulse immediately after exercise. During exercise, the heart rate increases; immediately after exercise, it begins to slow down or return to normal. In fact, the heart rate has already slowed considerably within one minute after exercise ceases. The key is to locate the pulse quickly and to count the rate for a short period of time. A full one-minute count after exercise does not give a good estimate of exercise heart rate, even if the pulse is quickly located, because the heart rate during the end of the count is much slower than it was during exercise. Keep moving while quickly locating the pulse, then stop and take a fifteen-second count. Multiply the number of pulses counted in a fifteen-second period by four to convert heart rate to beats per minute.

You can also count the pulse for ten seconds and multiply by six or count the pulse for six seconds and multiply by ten to estimate a one-minute heart rate. The latter method allows you to easily calculate heart rates by adding a zero to the six-second count. However, short duration pulse counts increase the chances of error because a miscount of one beat is multiplied by six or ten beats rather than by four beats.

The pulse rate should be counted after regular exercise, not after a sudden burst of activity. Some runners sprint the last few yards of their daily run and then count their pulse. Such a burst of exercise will elevate the heart rate considerably. This gives a false picture of the actual exercise heart rate. It would be wise for every person to learn to determine resting heart rate accurately and to estimate exercise heart rate by quickly and accurately making pulse counts after exercise.

In order to use heart rate properly in planning aerobic exercise for building cardiovascular fitness, it is important to know how to calculate heart rate threshold levels and target zones.

Two different procedures are commonly used to estimate threshold and target zone heart rates. The first involves calculating a percentage of your *working heart rate range,* also referred to by some as the maximum heart rate reserve. This method is considered by many to be the better of the two because it is more personal in that it uses your true resting heart rate in making the calculations. The second method, percentage of *maximal heart rate,* is easier to calculate but is less personalized. As noted in table 5.1, the percentage of heart rate intensity necessary to get you in the target zone differs depending upon which method of heart rate calculation you use. In the following paragraphs, both methods of determining threshold and target zone heart rates are described.

Percentage of Working Heart Rate Range

To calculate your working heart rate range (also called heart rate reserve), you must know your resting and maximal heart rates.

The resting heart rate is easily determined by counting the pulse for one minute while sitting or lying. Ideally, this should be done early in the morning when you are rested, rather than late in the day when you have been involved in many activities.

Maximal heart rate is harder to determine. It could be measured by an electrocardiogram while exercising to exhaustion; however, for most people it is safer and better to estimate *maximal heart rate* by using a formula. This is done by subtracting your age from 220. Maximal heart rates are near 200 in young people but decrease with age. The formula for calculating your maximal heart rate and an example of the calculations for a twenty-two-year-old individual are shown in table 5.2.

The *working heart rate* is determined by subtracting the resting heart rate from the maximal heart rate. The heart always works in the range between the resting (the lowest) and the maximal (the highest) rate of your pulse. The formula for calculating the working heart rate and an example for the twenty-two-year-old with a resting heart rate of sixty-eight beats per minute are also shown in table 5.2.

The *threshold of training,* or *minimum heart rate,* for building cardiovascular fitness, is determined by calculating 50 percent of the working heart rate and then adding it to the resting heart rate. The upper limit of the target zone is 85 percent of the working heart rate added to the resting heart rate. The formula for determining threshold and the upper limit of the target heart rate zone, and examples for the hypothetical exerciser, are shown in table 5.2. For best results, begin lower in the target zone and gradually increase exercise intensity.

Table 5.2

Formula and Example for Calculating Target Heart Rates Using Percentage of Working Heart Rate Range. (Example is for a twenty-two-year-old person with a resting heart rate of 68 bpm.)

Formula for Calculating Maximal Heart Rate	Example
220–Age (in years) = Maximal Heart Rate (beats per minute)	220 –22 = 198

Formula for Calculating Working Heart Rate	Example
Maximal Heart Rate–Resting Heart Rate = Working Heart Rate	198–68 = 130

Formula for Calculating Threshold of Training Heart Rate	Example
Working Heart Rate × 50%	130 × .50
	= 65
+ Resting Heart Rate = Threshold of Training Heart Rate	+ 68 = 133

Formula for Calculating the Upper Limit of the Target Heart Rate Zone	Example
Working Heart Rate × 85%	130 × .85
	= 110.5 (111)
+ Resting Heart Rate = Upper Limit for Target Heart Rate Zone	+ 68 = 179

The target zone for this twenty-two-year-old is 133–179 bpm.

Percentage of Maximal Heart Rate

To use this method, first estimate your maximal heart rate just as you did for the previous method, then determine the threshold heart rate by calculating 60 percent of the maximal heart rate. The upper limit of the target zone is determined by calculating 90 percent of the maximal heart rate. Table 5.3 gives an example for a hypothetical twenty-two-year-old person.

This procedure, using a percentage of maximal heart rate, is deemed an acceptable alternative to the procedure using a percentage of working heart rate range because it provides target heart rates similar to those using 50–85 percent of the working heart rate range (see examples).

You should learn to calculate your threshold and target heart rate values using one of the two methods. (The first method, percentage of working heart rate range, is a bit more difficult to calculate.) Regardless of which method you use, you should exercise vigorously enough to bring

Table 5.3

Formula and Example for Calculating Target Heart Rates Using the Percentage of Maximal Heart Rate Procedure. (Example is for a twenty-two-year-old person.)

Formula for Calculating Maximal Heart Rate	Example
220–Age (in years) = Maximal Heart Rate (beats per minute)	220–22 = 198
Formula for Threshold Heart Rate	**Example**
Maximal Heart Rate × 60%	198 × .60
Threshold of Training Heart Rate	= 118.8 (119)
Formula for Upper Limit Heart Rate	**Example**
Maximal Heart Rate × 90%	198 × .90
Upper Limit for Target Heart Rate Zone	= 178.2 (178)

The target zone for this person is 119–178 bpm.

your heart rate above threshold and into the target zone to get the cardiovascular performance benefits of exercise. For improvement to occur, gradually increase exercise intensity in the target heart rate zone.

It should be noted that there are several possible sources of error in calculating threshold and target heart rates. First, the method of calculating maximal heart rate is an estimate based on typical values for typical people. Second, errors in counting are possible. Finally, it is possible that the count you make *after* exercise may not actually reflect your heart rate *during* exercise. For this reason, it is important that you make several estimates of your threshold and target heart rates, especially when you are first starting a cardiovascular fitness program.

> Ratings of perceived exertion during exercise can be useful as a guide to intensity of cardiovascular exercise.

The American College of Sports Medicine suggests that experienced exercisers can use **Ratings of Perceived Exertion (RPE)** to determine if they are exercising in the target zone. This prevents the need to stop and count heart rate during exercise. A rating of 12 (somewhat hard) is equal to threshold, and a rating of 16 (hard) is equal to the upper limit of the target zone. With practice, most people can learn to recognize when they are in the target zone using ratings of perceived exertion. (See chart 5.7 in Lab Resource Material.)

> Your current fitness status and current activity patterns should influence the type and amount of activity you do to promote cardiovascular fitness and cardiovascular health benefits.

Making proper decisions about how much physical activity you should do is an art that is based on science. It is important that you listen to your body and do not try to do too much too soon. Part of the art of making good decisions about activity is using the principle of progression. The amount of activity performed by a beginner differs from that performed by a person who is more advanced. If you use heart rate counting to quantify your physical activity, the American College of Sports Medicine recommends you gradually increase your frequency, intensity and time of activity. Table 5.4 provides you with an example of a progressive program. Of course your current fitness and activity status will effect how quickly you progress. The type of activity you choose should be appropriate for the intensity of activity at each stage of the progression.

If you choose to count calories to determine appropriate activity levels you should also begin gradually. For example a beginner may choose 15 minute walks three days a week (about 300 Calories per week) and gradually build to 30 minutes most days of the week (1000 to 1400 Calories) or more.

The Facts About Measuring Cardiovascular Fitness

> Though cardiovascular fitness can be measured in several ways, **maximal oxygen uptake** is considered the best method of evaluation.

A person's maximal oxygen uptake ($\dot{V}O_2$ max), also commonly referred to as **aerobic capacity,** is determined in a laboratory by measuring how much oxygen a person can use in one minute of maximal exercise. Great endurance athletes can extract five or six liters of oxygen per minute from the environment during an all-out treadmill run or bicycle ride. An average person extracts only two or three liters in a one-minute exercise session. $\dot{V}O_2$ max is often adjusted to account for a person's body size because bigger people may have higher scores due to their larger size. Scores are often reported as milliliters of oxygen per kilogram of body weight ($ml/O_2/kg$). This score is calculated by dividing your $\dot{V}O_2$ max value by your weight in kilograms.

> Aerobic exercise is the most effective means of improving $\dot{V}O_2$ max.

As noted previously in this concept, good cardiovascular fitness requires a fit heart muscle, fit vascular and respiratory systems, fit blood, and fit muscles. Regular aerobic exercise improves these systems, which are essential for improved $\dot{V}O_2$ max.

Table 5.4
An Example of a Progression of Physical Activity for a Healthy Person (using heart rate)

Program Phase	Week	Exercise Frequency (session per week)	Exercise Intensity (% working HR range)	Exercise Duration (minutes)
Beginning	1	3	40–50	12
	2	3	50	14
	3	3	60	16
	4	3	60–70	18
	5	3	60–70	20
Improvement	6–9	3–4	70–80	21
	10–13	3–4	70–80	24
	14–16	3–4	70–80	24
	17–19	4–5	70–80	28
	20–23	4–5	70–80	30
	24–27	4–5	70–85	30
Maintenance	28+	3	70–85	30–45

From ACSM's Guidelines for Exercise Testing and Prescription, 5th edition. Copyright © Williams and Wilkins, 1995. Reprinted by permission.

$\dot{V}O_2$ max can be estimated using self-administered tests.

Several tests can be done with a minimum of equipment in or near your home. With proper instruction, you can learn to measure your own cardiovascular fitness using one of these methods. Commonly used tests are the step test, the twelve-minute run, the Astrand-Ryhming bicycle test, and the Rockport Walking Test. Since these tests are not as accurate as a laboratory test of $\dot{V}O_2$ max, the use of more than one test is recommended to help you get a valid assessment of your cardiovascular fitness.

The Facts About Aerobic and Anaerobic Exercise

Aerobic exercise can be sustained for considerably longer periods than anaerobic exercise.

Regardless of the type of exercise you perform, you derive energy from high-energy fuel that must be available in muscle fibers. The breakdown of this high-energy fuel in the muscle cells allows you to perform all types of exercise. Unfortunately, the energy resulting from the breakdown of this fuel is used up in a matter of seconds. Carbohydrates stored in the cells can be broken down to replenish the high-energy fuel supply to allow performance to continue

for an additional time (thirty to forty seconds for most people). The short-term, vigorous exercise performed in the absence of an adequate oxygen supply using these sources of energy is called **anaerobic exercise.**

Aerobic exercise, which means "in the presence of oxygen," is less vigorous and can be performed for much longer periods. Carbohydrates and fats available in the body can be used to rebuild the high-energy fuel necessary for doing regular exercises when oxygen is present.

Aerobic exercise produces cardiovascular fitness or aerobic capacity.

In accordance with the principle of specificity, regular aerobic exercise increases the body's ability to supply oxygen to the muscles as well as their ability to use it. Slow-twitch muscle fibers appear to benefit most from aerobic exercise.

Anaerobic exercise produces **anaerobic capacity.**

Anaerobic exercise produces **lactic acid** in the process of energy production. Muscle fatigue occurs when anaerobic energy supplies are depleted and lactic acid build-up occurs. Regular anaerobic exercise seems to allow the muscle to tolerate higher lactic acid levels before fatigue occurs. Also, anaerobic exercise improves anaerobic energy

Table 5.5
Threshold of Training and Target Zone for Anaerobic Exercise*

	Threshold of Training	Target Zone
Frequency	• 3 days a week.	• 3–4 days a week.
Intensity	• Short Interval—100% of maximum speed running, swimming, or other exercise of short duration (10–30 seconds).	• Short Intervals—100% of maximum speed running, swimming, or other exercise of short duration (10–30 seconds).
	• Long Intervals—90% of maximum speed running, swimming, or other exercise (30 seconds–2 minutes).	•Long Intervals—90–100% of maximum speed running, swimming, or other exercise (30 seconds–2 minutes).
Time	• Short Intervals—Exercise 10 seconds, rest 10 seconds, repeat 20 times.	•Short Intervals—Same as threshold but repeat up to 30 times.
	or	or
	• Exercise 20 seconds, rest 15 seconds. Repeat 10 times.	Same as threshold but repeat up to 20 times.
	or	or
	• Exercise 30 seconds, rest 1–2 minutes. Repeat 8 times.	Same as threshold but repeat up to 18 times.
	• Long Intervals—Exercise 1 minute, rest 3–5 minutes. Repeat 5 times.	•Long Intervals—Same as threshold but repeat up to 15 times.
	or	or
	Exercise 2 minutes, rest 5–15 minutes. Repeat 4 times.	Same as threshold but repeat up to 10 times.

*The threshold of training and target zone values depicted in this table are for healthy young adults. For older people, or those who have not been active recently, aerobic training is recommended. Those with known medical problems should consult a physician to determine appropriate exercise amounts. This is only a sample of several formats for meeting anaerobic target zones.

production capabilities, primarily in the fast-twitch fibers. These fibers appear to benefit most from anaerobic exercise. Anaerobic capacity is often measured in the laboratory using the Wingate Test, an all-out, thirty-second stationary bicycle ride at high resistance. The ability to perform a vigorous, short-term bout of exercise, and repeat it with a relatively short rest, will give you an indication of your anaerobic fitness.

Regular anaerobic exercise contributes to cardiovascular fitness development.

Though aerobic exercise is considered to be the preferred method of building cardiovascular fitness, anaerobic exercise can contribute to its development through increased heart rate and blood flow. Most experts agree that the primary contribution of anaerobic exercise to cardiovascular fitness is associated with improved delivery of oxygen in blood. Improvement of O_2 utilization within the cells seems to be specifically associated with aerobic exercise.

Improved anaerobic capacity can contribute to performance in activities considered to be aerobic.

Many physical activities commonly considered to be aerobic—such as tennis, basketball, and racquetball—have an anaerobic component. These activities require periodic vigorous bursts of exercise. Regular anaerobic training will help you resist fatigue in these activities. Even participants in activities such as long-distance running may benefit from some anaerobic training, especially if performance times or winning races is important. A fast start may be anaerobic, a sprint past an opponent may be anaerobic, and a kick at the end will no doubt be anaerobic. Anaerobic training can help prepare a person for these circumstances.

There is a threshold and target zone for performing anaerobic exercise.

The frequency, intensity, and time for anaerobic exercise threshold and target zone are presented in table 5.5.

Suggested Readings

American College of Sports Medicine. *ACSM's Guidelines for Exercise Testing and Exercise Prescription.* 5th ed. Baltimore, MD: Williams and Wilkins, 1995.

American College of Sports Medicine. "The Recommended Quantity and Quality of Exercise for Developing and Maintaining Cardiorespiratory and Muscular Fitness in Healthy Adults." *Medicine and Science in Sports and Exercise* 22(1990):2.

American Heart Association. "A Statement on Exercise: Benefits and Recommendations for Physical Activity Programs for All Americans," *Circulation,* 91(1995), 580.

Fletcher, G., et al. "American Heart Association: Statement on Exercise." *Circulation* 86(1992):2726.

Haskell, W. L. "Physical Activity in the Prevention and Management of Coronary Heart Disease." *Physical Activity and Fitness Research Digest* 2(1995):1.

Public Health Service. Surgeon General's Report on Physical Activity and Health. Washington, DC: U.S. Government Printing Office, 1996.

LAB RESOURCE MATERIALS

Chart 5.1 Twelve-Minute Run Test *Rating Chart* (scores in miles)			
Men (age)			
Classification	**17–26**	**27–39**	**40–49**	**50+**
High performance zone	1.80+	1.60+	1.50+	1.40+
Good fitness zone	1.55–1.79	1.45–1.59	1.40–1.49	1.25–1.39
Marginal zone	1.35–1.54	1.30–1.44	1.25–1.39	1.10–1.24
Low zone	<1.35	<1.30	<1.25	<1.10
Women (age)			
Classification	**17–26**	**27–39**	**40–49**	**50+**
High performance zone	1.45+	1.35+	1.25+	1.15+
Good fitness zone	1.25–1.44	1.20–1.34	1.15–1.24	1.05–1.14
Marginal zone	1.15–1.24	1.05–1.19	1.00–1.14	0.95–1.04
Low zone	<1.15	<1.05	<1.00	<.94

A chart showing the metric equivalents for this chart can be found in Appendix B.

Evaluating Cardiovascular Fitness

For an exercise program to be most effective, it should be based on personal needs. Some type of testing is necessary to determine your personal need for cardiovascular fitness. A treadmill test that includes continuous EKG monitoring or assessment of maximal oxygen uptake is the best test of cardiovascular fitness (see American College of Sports Medicine, 1995). However, there are some tests that do not require as much time and equipment and can give you a good estimate of cardiovascular fitness. The twelve-minute run, the step test, the Astrand-Ryhming bicycle test, and the Rockport Walking Test are some of these tests and are described here. Prior to performing any of these, be sure that

you are physically and medically ready. Prepare yourself by doing some regular exercise for three to six weeks before actually taking the tests. If possible, take more than one test and use the summary of your test results to make a final assessment of your cardiovascular fitness.

The Twelve-Minute Run Test

- Locate an area where a specific distance is already marked, such as a school track or football field; or measure a specific distance using a bicycle or automobile odometer.
- Use a stopwatch or wristwatch to accurately time a twelve-minute period.
- For best results, warm up prior to the test, then run at a steady pace for the entire twelve minutes (cool down after the tests).

- Determine the distance you can run in twelve minutes in fractions of a mile. Depending upon your age, locate your score and rating on the Twelve-Minute Run Test Rating Chart (chart 5.1).

The Step Test

- Warm up prior to exercise, and after finishing be sure to cool down.
- Step up and down on a twelve-inch bench for three minutes at a rate of twenty-four steps per minute. One step consists of four beats; that is, "up with the left foot, up with the right foot, down with the left foot, down with the right foot."
- Immediately after the exercise, sit down on the bench and relax. Don't talk.
- Locate your pulse or have another person locate it for you.
- Five seconds after the exercise ends, begin counting your pulse. Count the pulse for sixty seconds.
- Your score is your sixty-second heart rate. Locate your score and your rating on chart 5.2.

The Astrand-Ryhming Bicycle Test

- Ride a stationary bicycle ergometer for six minutes at a rate of fifty pedal cycles per minute (one push with each foot per cycle). Cool down after the test.
- Set the bicycle at a workload between 300 to 1200 kpm. For less fit or smaller people, a setting in the range of 300 to 600 is appropriate. Larger or fitter people will need to use a setting of 750 to 1200. The workload should be enough to elevate the heart rate to at least 125 bpm but no more than 170 bpm during the ride.
- During the sixth minute of the ride (if the heart rate is in the correct range—see previous step), count the heart rate for the entire sixth minute. The carotid or radial pulse may be used.
- Use the nomogram (chart 5.3) to determine your predicted oxygen uptake score. Connect the point that represents your heart rate with the point on the right-hand scale that represents the workload you used in riding the bike (use the scale for men and the scale for women). Read your score at the point where a straight line connecting the two points crosses the $\dot{V}O_2$ max line. For example, the sample score the woman represented by the dotted line is 2.55, or nearly 2.6. She had a heart rate of 150 and worked at a load of 600 kpm.
- Determine your score in terms of $\dot{V}O_2$ per kilogram of body weight by dividing your weight in kilograms

Chart 5.2 Step Test Rating Chart

Classification	60-Sec. Heart Rate
High performance zone	84 or less
Good fitness zone	85–95
Marginal zone	96–119
Low zone	120 and above

As you grow older you will want to continue to score well on this rating chart. Because your maximal heart rate decreases as you age, you should be able to score well if you exercise regularly.

Source: Data from F. W. Kasch and J. L. Boyer, *Adult Fitness: Principles and Practices,* 1968, Mayfield Publishing Company, Palo Alto, CA.

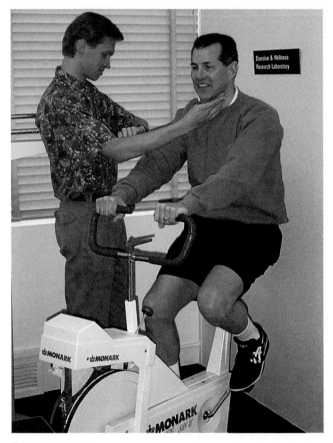

The bicycle test

into the score obtained from the nomogram. To compute your weight in kilograms, divide your weight in pounds by 2.2.
- To determine your cardiovascular fitness rating on the bicycle test, look up your $\dot{V}O_2$ per kilogram of body weight score on the nomogram and your rating in chart 5.4.

Chart 5.3 Nomogram

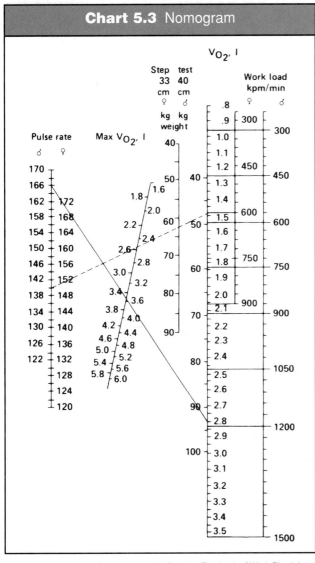

Source: Data from P. O. Astrand and K. Rodahl, *Textbook of Work Physiology*, 1986.

The Rockport Walking Test

- Warm up, then walk one mile as fast as you can. Record your time to the nearest second.
- Count your heart rate for 15 seconds immediately after the walk, then multiply by four to get a one-minute heart rate. Record your heart rate.
- Use your walking time and your post-exercise heart rate to determine your rating using chart 5.5 for males or 5.6 for females.

Chart 5.5 Walking Ratings for Males

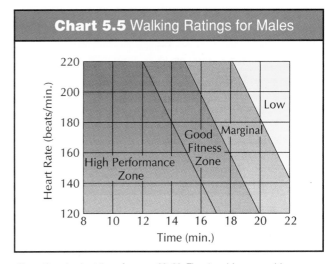

The ratings in chart 5 are for ages 20–29. They provide reasonable ratings for people of all ages.

Adapted from the *One Mile Walk Test,* with permission of the author, James M. Rippe, M.D.

Chart 5.4 Bicycle Test *Rating Scale* (ml/O₂/kg)

Women					
Age	17–26	27–39	40–49	50–59	60–69
High performance zone	46+	40+	38+	35+	32+
Good fitness zone	36–45	33–39	30–37	28–34	24–31
Marginal zone	30–35	28–32	24–29	21–27	18–23
Low zone	<30	<28	<24	<21	<18
Men					
Age	17–26	27–39	40–49	50–59	60–69
High performance zone	50+	46+	42+	39+	35+
Good fitness zone	43–49	35–45	32–41	29–38	26–34
Marginal zone	35–42	30–34	27–31	25–28	22–25
Low zone	<35	<30	<27	<25	<22

Source: Data from P. O. Astrand and K. Rodahl, *Textbook of Work Physiology*, 1986.

Chart 5.6 Walking Ratings for Females

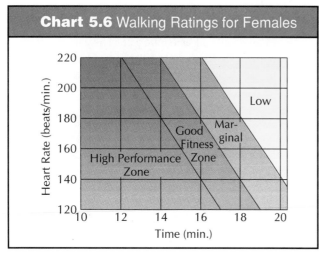

The ratings in chart 6 are for ages 20–29. They provide reasonable ratings for people of all ages.
Adapted from the *One Mile Walk Test,* with permission of the author, James M. Rippe, M.D.

Chart 5.7 Ratings of Perceived Exertion (RPE)

Scale	Verbal Rating
6	
7	Very, very light
8	
9	Very light
10	
11	Fairly light
12	
13	Somewhat hard
14	
15	Hard
16	
17	Very hard
18	
19	Very, very hard
20	

Source: Data from G. Borg, "Psychological Bases of Perceived Exertion" in *Medicine and Science in Sports and Exercise,* 14:377, 1982, the American College of Sports Medicine.

Chart 5.8 Threshold of Training and Target Zone Heart Rates

Resting Heart Rate		Less than 25	25–29	30–34	35–39	40–44	45–49	50–54	55–59	60–64	Over 65
below 50	Threshold	123	122	119	117	114	112	109	107	104	103
	Target Zone	123–173	122–172	119–167	117–163	114–159	112–155	109–150	107–146	104–142	103–139
50–54	Threshold	124	123	120	118	115	113	110	108	105	104
	Target zone	124–174	123–172	120–168	118–163	115–160	113–1551	110–151	108–146	105–143	104–140
55–59	Threshold	126	125	123	120	117	115	112	110	107	106
	Target zone	126–174	125–173	123–168	120–164	117–160	115–156	112–151	110–147	107–143	106–140
60–64	Threshold	129	128	125	123	120	118	115	113	111	109
	Target zone	129–175	128–174	125–169	123–165	120–161	118–156	115–152	113–148	111–144	109–141
65–69	Threshold	131	130	128	125	123	120	118	115	113	111
	Target zone	131–176	130–173	128–170	125–165	123–161	120–157	118–153	115–149	113–144	111–142
70–74	Threshold	134	133	131	128	125	123	120	118	116	114
	Target zone	134–177	133–173	131–171	128–166	125–162	123–158	120–154	118–150	116–145	114–143
75–79	Threshold	136	135	133	130	128	125	123	120	118	116
	Target zone	136–177	135–174	133–171	130–167	128–163	125–159	123–154	120–150	118–146	116–143
80–85	Threshold	139	138	135	133	130	128	126	123	121	119
	Target zone	139–178	138–175	135–172	133–168	130–164	128–159	126–155	123–151	121–147	119–144
86 and over	Threshold	141	140	137	135	132	130	127	125	123	121
	Target zone	141–179	140–176	137–173	135–169	132–164	130–160	127–156	125–152	123–147	121–145

CONCEPT
·6·

Lifestyle, Aerobic, and Anaerobic Physical Activity

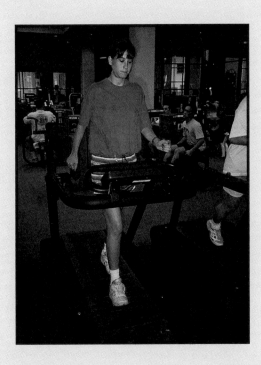

Concept 6

Lifestyle and aerobic activities are effective in promoting health benefits and aerobic and anaerobic activities are effective in developing physical fitness and enhancing performance in sports and other activities.

Introduction

There are many forms of lifestyle physical activities, aerobic physical activities, and anaerobic physical activities from which an individual can choose. Some of the more popular activities are described in this concept.

Health Goal for the Year 2000

■ Increase proportion of people who engage in regular physical activity to improve cardiovascular fitness. (↑)

Note: (↑) indicates progress toward goal, (↓) indicates regression from goal, and (<>) indicates either no change or lack of new data since 1990.

Terms

■ **Aerobic Physical Activity or Exercise**   Aerobic means "in the presence of oxygen." Aerobic activity is activity in which the body is able to supply adequate oxygen to sustain performance for long periods.

■ **Anaerobic Exercise**   Anaerobic means "in the absence of oxygen." Anaerobic exercise is performed at an intensity so great that the body's demand for oxygen exceeds its ability to supply it.

■ **Continuous Aerobic Activity**   Activity that is slow enough to be sustained for relatively long periods without frequent rest periods.

■ **Intermittent Aerobic Activity**   Activity that is alternated with frequent rest periods, often of relatively high intensity.

■ **Lifestyle Physical Activity**   Activities done as part of the normal daily routine such as walking to work, raking leaves, climbing the stairs, and shoveling snow are considered to be lifestyle physical activities.

Some Facts About Lifestyle Activity

The physical activity pyramid includes **lifestyle physical activities** at its base because virtually all people could benefit from performing these activities.

It is now clear that when it comes to physical activity, "something is better than nothing." Even modest physical activity yields many benefits. Nevertheless about one quarter of all adult Americans do no physical activity. They are totally sedentary. One possible solution is to get more Americans to do physical activity as part of their daily activities (Lifestyle Activity). The physical activity pyramid (see figure 6.1) includes lifestyle activities at its base because it is appropriate for all people. By simply walking rather than riding, climbing the stairs rather than taking an

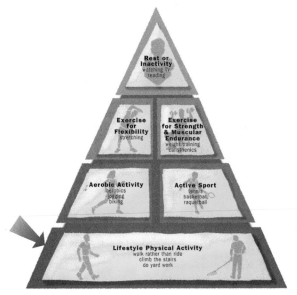

Figure 6.1
Lifestyle activities are appropriate for virtually all people.

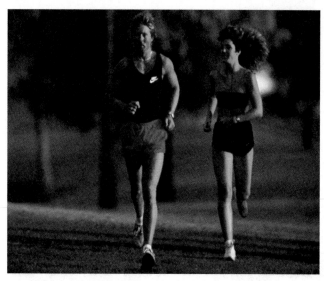

Jogging is a good example of an aerobic exercise.

elevator, mowing the grass, parking the car farther from the office, or riding a bike to the store Americans could expend the calories necessary to get many health benefits and could achieve the minimal cardiovascular fitness necessary for good health and wellness. All Americans are encouraged to do daily lifestyle activities.

Some Facts About Aerobic Activity

> Aerobic physical activities are included in the second level of the activity pyramid because they are recommended for regular participation in addition to lifestyle activities.

Most of the activities classified as lifestyle activities are also aerobic activities because your body can adequately supply the oxygen necessary to perform them for relatively long periods of time. Examples of these activities are walking and biking. These activities are also included in the aerobic physical activity category of the activity pyramid because they are often done during leisure time as well as a part of daily living. When done following the guidelines outlined in concept 5, aerobic physical activities are considered to be the most effective of all activities in developing cardiovascular fitness and the health benefits associated with it. Some of the more popular aerobic activities are described later in this concept.

> **Aerobic physical activities** are exceptionally popular among adults.

Activities that have a strong anaerobic component, such as sprinting, football, baseball, and sprint swimming, are very popular among youth, whereas aerobic activities are more popular among adults. Adults report that they are most often involved in continuous swimming, jogging, cycling, walking, and calisthenics. All but vigorous calisthenics, sprint running, or sprint swimming are aerobic. When done at a slow or moderate pace, calisthenics are aerobic; when done continuously, they can be effective in producing the same benefits as jogging, swimming, and other aerobic activities.

> Aerobic exercise can be done either continuously or intermittently.

We generally think of aerobic exercise as being continuous in nature. Jogging, swimming, and cycling at a steady pace for long periods are classic examples of aerobic exercise. Experts have shown that aerobic exercise can be done intermittently as well as continuously. Both **continuous** and **intermittent aerobic exercise** can build cardiovascular fitness. For example, one recent study showed that three ten-minute exercise sessions in the target zone were as effective as one thirty-minute exercise session. Still, experts recommend bouts of 30 minutes in length with several 10–15 minute bouts an acceptable alternative when 30 minute activity sessions are not possible.

Aerobic interval training and interval dance exercise are examples of intermittent aerobic exercise. Sports such as basketball, tennis, and racquetball that are intermittent are often considered to be aerobic activities when they are performed for long periods without stopping. Though they are considered to be aerobic, they also involve periodic anaerobic exercise.

> There are advantages and disadvantages of continuous and intermittent exercise.

The advantages and disadvantages of continuous and intermittent exercise are presented in table 6.1.

Table 6.1
Continuous versus Intermittent Exercise: Advantages and Disadvantages

Continuous	Intermittent
• Is done slowly and continuously, rather than in short, vigorous bursts; therefore, many people consider continuous exercise to be less demanding and more enjoyable.	• When done in the target zone, it has the same benefits as continuous exercise. If done intensely it can increase risk of soreness and injury for beginners.
• Is less intense and because of lower injury risk may be best for beginners, especially for those who are older and those who are just starting an exercise program after a long layoff.	• Three ten-minute or two fifteen-minute exercise sessions might be easier to schedule for busy people than one longer exercise period.
• Provides health benefits associated with cardiovascular fitness.	• May be more interesting to some people.
• May not provide optimal performance benefits for competitors.	• If done at relatively high intensity with alternating rest periods, it can be beneficial in preparing for competition.

Table 6.2
Risk of Injury in Exercise

Activity	Injury per 1000 Hrs. of Activity
Skating	20
Basketball	18
Avg. competitive sports	16
Running/jogging	16
Racquetball	14
Avg. aerobic activity	10
Tennis	8
Cycling	6
High impact dance aerobics	6
Step aerobics	5
Aerobic exercise machines	3
Walking	2
Low impact dance aerobics	2

Source: Data from the Center for Sports Medicine at St. Francis Hospital, San Francisco, CA.

Not all aerobic exercise is equally safe.

Sports medicine experts indicate that certain types of aerobic exercise are more likely to result in injury than others. As shown in table 6.2, walking and low impact dance aerobics are among the least risky activities. Skating, an aerobic activity, is even more risky than most competitive sports. Among the most popular aerobic activities, running has the greatest risk, with cycling, high impact dance aerobics, and step aerobics having moderate risk of injury.

There Are Many Popular Forms of Aerobic Exercise

Some of the most popular forms of aerobic exercise are discussed briefly here.

Aerobic Exercise Machines

There are many kinds of aerobic exercise machines, including stairclimbers, cross-country ski machines, and stationary bicycles. Advantages of such machines are that they can be used in the home or in most fitness clubs and do not require excessive amounts of skill. There is some evidence that use of these machines is fun and interesting initially, but that interest decreases with repeated use. Ski machines would seem to be most useful for people who ski on a regular basis, and bicycles would seem to be most interesting to those who do cycling. Aerobic exercise machines can be useful in developing cardiovascular fitness for those who use them to exercise in the target zone for fitness. The key to the effectiveness of the machines is persistent use over long periods of time.

Aerobic Interval Training

Interval training is one of the most common forms of intermittent exercise. Short bursts of energy, commonly referred to as *sprints,* are alternated with rest periods. For many years interval training was considered to be exclusively a form of anaerobic training, and as noted later in this concept, it is an excellent form of anaerobic training. However, athletes and coaches now feel that *aerobic interval training* may be quite important for competitors in sports such as swimming, running, and cycling. In aerobic interval training, repeated performances of relatively short exercise bouts are alternated with brief rest periods. The exercise bouts are performed at slower than race (for racers) pace and not so intensely as anaerobics. Proponents of aerobic interval training suggest that this procedure allows a greater volume of training in a shorter period. To date, the evidence supporting the superiority of this form of training for competitors is principally based on the testimony of coaches and athletes. Additional research is necessary.

An example of a schedule of aerobic interval training for a 10-km runner is illustrated in table 6.3. To use the schedule, locate your typical 10-km time in the left-hand

Table 6.3

Aerobic Interval Training Schedules
for a Ten-Kilometer Runner

Best 10–km Time (Min: Sec)	Reps	Distance (Meters)	Rest (Sec)	Pace (Min: Sec)
46:00	20	400	10–15	2:00
43:00	20	400	10–15	1:52
40:00	20	400	10–15	1:45
37:00	20	400	10–15	1:37
34:00	20	400	10–15	1:30

From Jack H. Wilmore and David L. Costill, *Training for Sport and Activity*, 3d ed. Copyright © 1988 Times Mirror Higher Education Group, Inc., Dubuque, Iowa. All Rights Reserved. Reprinted by permission.

column. Perform 400-meter runs at the time specified in the "pace" column. Repeat twenty times with intervals of ten to fifteen seconds between runs. Similar schedules can be developed with other activities such as swimming and cycling. This activity, however, is not recommended for those just beginning exercise.

Bicycling

Bicycling, when done continuously, is a form of aerobic exercise. This activity requires only a bicycle and some safety equipment, such as a helmet and a light and reflectors if done after dark. A tall flag is needed if biking in traffic. To be most effective in building physical fitness, you should pedal continuously, rather than coasting for long periods. Maintaining a steady pace is recommended. Riding a different course periodically can increase enjoyment of the activity.

Circuit Resistance Training (CRT)

Originally, circuit training was a type of physical training involving movement from one exercise station to another. A different type of exercise was performed at each station. In order to complete the circuit, you had to complete all the exercises at the different stations. Your goal was to perform the circuit in progressively shorter periods.

Recently, however, circuit training has been modified by some to include several strength overload stations. These stations may involve resistance exercises with free weights or exercise machines. There is some evidence that when CRT is done with high repetitions and moderate loads, it can make modest contributions to cardiovascular fitness. When aerobic exercise such as rides on stationary bicycles and running on treadmills is incorporated in the continuous exercise circuit, the contribution of this type of exercise to cardiovascular fitness increases. The key is continuous exercise. When repetitions of resistance training exercises are followed by relatively long rest periods (longer than the exercise time) they do little for cardiovascular fitness. One problem with this form of exercise, if cardiovascular fitness is the goal, is that the best of programs are ineffective if they cannot be performed properly. Some exercise clubs promote exercise circuits as a method of building both strength and cardiovascular fitness. Yet exercise stations are often crowded, and it is next to impossible to perform the circuit without long waiting periods. You may want to add aerobic exercise to your circuit during periods of waiting.

Cooper's Aerobics

Based on the needs of military personnel, Dr. Kenneth Cooper developed a physical activity program that he called aerobics. In fact, he popularized the term. His program includes a variety of aerobic activities that have point values for the different types of exercise involved. For example, walking a mile in 14½ to 20 minutes would earn one point while running a mile in less than 6 minutes and 30 seconds would earn five points. Examples of other activities that will earn one aerobic point are cycling two miles at 10–15 mph and swimming 300 yards in 8 to 10 minutes. To develop fitness—especially cardiovascular fitness—using the aerobics point system, it is necessary to earn thirty "aerobic points" per week. Aerobic points are part of Cooper's system for helping people know when they are exercising frequently enough, intensely enough, and long enough. Though earning thirty points per week is a good way of achieving fitness, we now know that earning less than thirty points can be beneficial to health. For more complete details on the Cooper aerobic points program, the reader is encouraged to read one of Cooper's books (see Suggested Readings).

Continuous Calisthenics

Survey results repeatedly indicate that calisthenics are among the top two or three participant activities performed. Calisthenics, exercises such as the crunch and push-ups, are designed to build flexibility, strength, or muscular endurance in specific muscle groups. Even though most calisthenics are aerobic, they are usually done intermittently. That is, calisthenic exercises are done a few at a time followed by a rest period. They will do little for cardiovascular fitness or fat control unless they are done continuously.

Continuous calisthenics, or calisthenics that are done without stopping or with walking, jogging, rope jumping, or some other aerobic activity performed during the rest period, can develop virtually all health-related aspects of physical fitness. Fitness pioneer Dr. Thomas Cureton long advocated the use of continuous calisthenics, or what he referred to as "continuous rhythmical endurance exercise." Almost everyone can plan a continuous calisthenic program by selecting exercises for each fitness part that will elevate the heart rate to the optimal level and sustain this intensity an adequate length of time. As is the case with CRT, it is essential that resting between exercises be kept to a minimum. Continuous calisthenics can be done individually, but are also excellent for group use.

Cross-Country Skiing

In Europe, cross-country skiing is one of the most popular aerobic activities. Of course, this sport requires snow and a certain amount of specialized equipment. For those who can cross-country ski on a regular basis, studies show that it is one of the most effective types of cardiovascular fitness exercise.

Dance and Step Aerobics

This activity was first popularized by Jackie Sorensen in the 1970s as "aerobic dance." Since then, other versions of the activity have been promoted as rhythmic aerobics, jazzercise, and dancercize, to note but a few of the popular names. In most cases, dance aerobics consists of a pre-planned or choreographed series of dance steps and exercises done to music. Most of the early programs were considered to be "high impact" because they included jumping, leaping, and hopping dance steps that resulted in stress on the feet and legs.

In an attempt to reduce the risk of injury or soreness, "low impact" dance aerobics were developed. In low impact dance aerobics, one foot stays on the floor at all times. Low impact dance aerobics are an especially wise choice for beginners and older exercisers. "Step aerobics," also known as "bench stepping," is another adaptation of dance aerobics. In this activity the performer steps up and down on a bench when performing the various dance steps. In most cases step aerobics is still considered to be low impact but higher in intensity than many forms of dance aerobics. Dance and step aerobics, when planned appropriately for individual participants, can be very effective in building cardiovascular fitness for both men and women.

One problem with dance aerobics is that it is a pre-planned exercise program; therefore, it requires all participants to do the same activity regardless of their fitness or activity levels. A vigorous routine can cause unfit people to overextend themselves, whereas an easy routine may not result in fitness gains for those who are already quite fit. Also, some dance aerobic routines have been known to include contraindicated exercises. Good instructors encourage participants to adapt the steps and movements to meet their individual needs.

Hiking and Backpacking

Like walking and jogging, hiking is an excellent form of exercise. Hiking has the advantage of an out-of-doors setting, often in a very scenic environment. It does require some equipment, such as a rucksack and good hiking shoes, but highly specialized skills are not needed.

Backpacking is a form of hiking that usually covers longer distances and involves an overnight stay, often in the mountains. When done continuously, backpacking is excellent for building muscular endurance as well as cardiovascular fitness. Like other aerobic activities, it can be helpful in controlling body fatness. In recent years, it has become a popular activity; nearly eleven million American adults report regular involvement in backpacking.

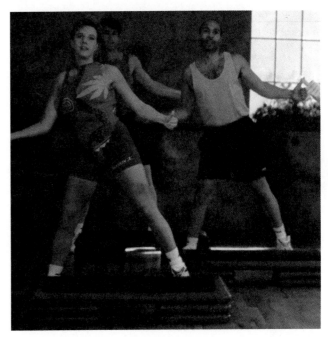

Dance aerobics is a popular form of exercise.

Jogging/Running

An aerobic activity that has rapidly grown in popularity in recent years among both adult men and women is jogging or running. Though there is no official distinction between jogging and running, those who run more than a few miles per day, who participate in races, and who are concerned about improving the time in which they run a certain distance often prefer to be called runners rather than joggers. Fifteen to twenty million American adults report that they jog or run on a regular basis.

The major advantage of jogging/running is that it requires only a good pair of running shoes, some inexpensive exercise clothing, and very little skill. With effort, almost anyone can benefit from the activity and even improve performance if that is the goal.

There are some techniques that every jogger should be familiar with before starting a jogging program.

- *Foot Placement*—The heel of the foot hits the ground first in jogging. Your heel should strike before the rest of your foot (but not hard), then you should rock forward and push off with the ball of your foot. Contrary to some opinions, you should *not* jog on your toes. (A flat foot landing can be all right as long as you push off with the ball of your foot.) Your toes should point straight ahead. Your feet should stay under your knees and *not* swing out to the sides as you jog.

- *Length of Stride*—For efficiency, you should have a relatively long stride. Your stride should be several inches longer than your walking stride. If necessary, you may have to reach to lengthen your stride. Most older people find it more efficient to run with a shorter stride.

- *Arm Movement*—While you jog, you should swing your arms as well as your legs. The arms should be bent at about 90 degrees and should swing freely and alternately from front to back in the direction you are moving, not from side to side. Keep your arms and hands relaxed.
- *Body Position*—While jogging, you should hold your upper body nearly erect and your head and chest up. There should not be a conscious effort to lean forward as is the case in sprinting or fast running.

Rope Jumping

Rope jumping is aerobic if done at a slow or moderate pace, but is anaerobic if done vigorously. One study shows that typical exercisers jump very briskly, and for this reason cannot maintain the jumping continuously. Even those who are highly trained or who jump at a moderate pace find it difficult to continue this exercise long enough to build cardiovascular fitness because of leg fatigue, high heart rate, or loss of interest in the activity. To be most effective, a continuous routine involving several different jump steps should be used in combination with other forms of exercise. For example, rope jumping could be a part of a circuit resistance training program or a dance aerobics program.

Skating

Ice skating tends to be regional in its appeal, roller skating is often limited to roller rinks or amusement areas, and roller blades are most frequently used by young people. However, all three are examples of aerobic exercise that can be useful in promoting cardiovascular fitness when done regularly. In-line (rollerblades) skates, originally developed for training skiers in the off-season, have been improved through recent technology and are now a popular form of aerobic exercise. Because the risk of injury is greater for skating than for many other aerobic activities, special precautions should be taken when doing this activity, including wearing a helmet and knee and elbow pads. Some degree of fitness and skill is necessary to perform skating safely and effectively.

Sports (Continuous)

As noted earlier in this concept, some activities that are at least partially anaerobic are considered aerobic if they are done at a continuous pace. Many sports have extended rest periods and do not allow for continuous involvement. Some sports considered to be good aerobic activities when performed continuously are basketball, handball, racquetball, and soccer.

Swimming and Water Exercises

The most recent exercise polls rank swimming as the first or second most popular form of regular physical activity among adults. Most of those who swim for exercise swim laps or do water exercises. When done at a mild or moderate pace, both of these can be aerobic. When done continuously,

Table 6.4
Walking Time for Expending 1000 Calories per Week

Days per Week	Pace	Minutes per Day		
		*100 lb. (45 kg)	*150 lb. (68 kg)	*200 lb. (90 kg)
5	2 mph (3.2 kph)	96	62	46
	3 mph (4.8 kph)	44	48	38
	4 mph (6.4 kph)	48	36	24
6	2 mph	80	52	40
	3 mph	62	40	32
	4 mph	40	26	20
7	2 mph	68	44	34
	3 mph	54	36	26
	4 mph	34	24	18

*Body weight

these are excellent forms of cardiovascular exercise. Another popular but more structured program for this type of exercise is Aquadynamics, prepared by the President's Council on Physical Fitness and Sports.

Walking

Approximately one-quarter of all adults report that they walk regularly for exercise. This exercise is probably popular because it can be done easily by people of all ages and of all ability levels. In previous years the value of walking has been minimized. Because less than very brisk walking may not produce heart rates in the cardiovascular fitness target zone, it was sometimes considered to be a less than desirable form of exercise. Given the recent evidence that regular calorie expenditure is important in reducing the risk of heart disease, walking is viewed in a different light. Walking is an excellent way to expend calories because it can be done for long periods. The calories expended also help in maintaining optimal body fatness. Since controlling fatness is associated with health benefits, walking has a double benefit.

Table 6.4 illustrates the minutes per day and days per week necessary to accumulate an expenditure of 1000 calories per week at different rates of walking. Walkers could begin at lower levels (expending a minimum of 500 calories per week, for example), and gradually increase to the levels shown in table 6.4—the amounts of walking that would produce a health benefit. Ideally, walkers would then continue to increase until they are regularly expending 2000 calories per week. Of course, walking can be combined with other more vigorous activities to expend greater amounts of calories in a shorter period of time.

Table 6.5
Fitness Benefits Achieved through Aerobic Exercise

Program Type	Cardio-vascular Fitness	Strength and Muscular Endurance	Flexi-bility	Fat Control	Skill-Related Fitness	Enjoyment or Fun[1]
Aerobic exercise machines	***	**	*	***	—	—
Aerobic interval training	***	**	—	***	—	—
Bicycling	***	**	*	***	*	**
Circuit resistance training	*	***	*	**	*	**
Cooper's aerobics	***	*	*	***	*	**
Continuous calisthenics	***	**	***	***	*	**
Cross-country skiing	***	**	*	***	**	**
Dance aerobics	***	**	***	***	*	**
Hiking and backpacking	**	**	*	**	*	**
Jogging/running	***	*	*	***	—	**
Rope jumping	**	*	—	**	*	*
Skating	***	*	—	***	**	**
Swimming and water exercises	**	**	**	**	**	**
Walking	**	*	*	**	*	**

Key: *** = Very good, ** = Good, * = Minimum, — = Low

[1]Enjoyment and fun are relative, and for this reason it is impossible to classify activities accurately. However, for the average person some activities seem to be more enjoyable than others. The above listed classifications reflect the opinions of the typical person. Any of the activities listed above can be fun and enjoyable for a given person in the right circumstances.

If cardiovascular fitness benefits as evidenced by an increase in $\dot{V}O_2$ are desired, walking must be done intensely enough to elevate the heart rate to threshold levels. Walking is often most enjoyable when done with other people and when different walking routes are used to provide variety.

> Different aerobic activities have different health-related benefits.

The health-related benefits of various aerobic activities are summarized in table 6.5.

The Facts About Anaerobic Exercise

> **Anaerobic exercise** is especially useful for building anaerobic fitness.

Anaerobic exercise does contribute to the development of various parts of health-related physical fitness (see table 6.6). Nevertheless, it is not included in the physical activity pyramid because it is not a type of activity that is recommended for the masses. Anaerobic exercise contributes most to the development of anaerobic fitness or anaerobic capacity which allows interested people to perform at high levels in sports requiring it. Some anaerobic exercise programs are described here for those interested in performing them.

Anaerobic Exercise Programs

Fartlek or "Speed Play"

Fartlek is a Swedish word for "speed play." This exercise was developed in Scandinavia where pinewood paths follow curves of lakes and up and down many hills, where the scenery takes your mind off the task at hand. The idea is to get away from the regimen of running on a track and to enjoy the woods, lakes, and mountains. Because of the terrain, the pace is never constant. The uphill path requires a slow pace, while a straight stretch or downhill trail allows for speed. In the "speed play," or fartlek system, you run easily for a time at a steady, hard speed, walk rapidly following that, alternate short sprints with walking, go full speed uphill, and perhaps at

Table 6.6

Fitness Benefits Achieved through Anaerobic Exercise

Program Type	Cardio-vascular Fitness	Strength and Muscular Endurance	Flexi-bility	Fat Control	Skill-Related Fitness	Enjoyment or Fun[1]
Fartlek or "speed play"	**	**	—	***	**	*
Interval dance	**	**	—	***	*	*
Interval training (anaerobic)	**	**	—	***	***	*

Key: *** =Very good, ** = Good, * = Minimum, — = Low

[1]Enjoyment and fun are relative, and for this reason it is impossible to classify activities accurately. However, for the average person some activities seem to be more enjoyable than others. The above listed classifications reflect the opinions of the typical person. Any of the activities listed above can be fun and enjoyable for a given person in the right circumstances.

a fast pace for a while. You can plan your own speed play program using your own course, which may include both up-hill and downhill running with other variations.

Interval Dance

Recently, interval dance exercise has become more popular. This is simply more intense dance exercise alternated with more frequent rest periods. In some cases, other forms of exercise, such as running, are alternated with dance exercise bouts. When properly planned, this form of exercise can be effective in producing cardiovascular fitness. Because it is a type of intermittent exercise, it has some advantages and disadvantages compared to traditional dance exercise (see table 6.1).

Interval Training Program (Anaerobic)

An anaerobic interval training program involves repeated fast anaerobic running or swimming for short periods of time, alternated with intervals of slow recovery jogging or swimming. Developed by Gerschler of Germany, the stress of anaerobic running raises the heart rate to near maximal from which it drops to a moderate level during recovery. This program controls distance, pace, number of repetitions, and recovery interval, allowing for a wide variety of programs of various intensities.

Research suggests that short interval workouts should use maximum speed with rest intervals lasting from ten seconds to two minutes. These should be repeated eight to thirty times. Anaerobic interval training having long intervals uses 90 to 100 percent speed with rest intervals lasting from three to fifteen minutes. These should be repeated four to fifteen times. A sample short anaerobic interval program and a sample long interval running program are presented in table 6.7, which can be used to plan your own anaerobic interval training program.

Table 6.7

Sample Anaerobic Interval Training Program (Moderate Intensity)

Short Intervals	Long Intervals
1. Do a flexibility and cardiovascular warm-up.	1. Do a flexibility and cardiovascular warm-up.
2. Run at 100% speed for 10 seconds (approximately 70 to 100 yards).	2. Run at 90% speed for one minute (approximately 300 to 500 yards).
3. Rest for 10 seconds by walking slowly.	3. Rest for 4 minutes by walking slowly.
4. Alternately repeat steps 2 and 3 until 20 runs have been completed.	4. Alternately repeat steps 2 and 3 until 5 runs have been completed.

Suggested Readings

Allsen, P. E., and P. Witbeck. *Racquetball*. 6th ed. Dubuque, IA: Brown & Benchmark Publishers, 1996.

Brown, R., and J. Henderson. *Fitness Running*. Champaign, IL: Human Kinetics Publishers, 1994.

Carmichael, C., and E. Burke. *Fitness Cycling*. Champaign, IL: Human Kinetics Publishers, 1994.

Cooper, K. H. *The Aerobics Program for Total Well-Being*. New York: M. Evans & Co. 1982.

Johnson, J. D., and P. Xanthos. *Tennis*. 6th ed. Dubuque, IA: Brown and Benchmark Publishers, 1993.

Kluka, D., and P. Dunn. *Volleyball*. 3rd ed. Dubuque, IA: Brown & Benchmark Publishers, 1996.

McIntosh, M. *Lifetime Aerobics*. Dubuque, IA: Wm. C. Brown Publishers, 1990.

Rasch, P. J. *Weight Training*. 5th ed. Dubuque, IA: Wm. C. Brown Publishers, 1990.

Seaborg, E., and E. Dudley. *Hiking and Backpacking*. Champaign, IL: Human Kinetics Publishers, 1994.

Seiger, L. H., and J. Hesson. *Walking for Fitness*. 2nd ed. Dubuque, IA: Wm. C. Brown Communications, 1994.

Vickers, B., and W. Vincent. *Swimming*. 6th ed. Dubuque, IA: Brown & Benchmark Publishers, 1994.

White, M. *Water Exercise*. Champaign, IL: Human Kinetics Publishers, 1995.

LAB RESOURCE MATERIALS

Chart 6.1 Jogging Technique			
Body Segment	**(Check Appropriate Boxes Below)**		**Technique**
	Correct	Incorrect	
Foot placement	☐	☐	Heel hits ground first
	☐	☐	Rock forward, push off ball of foot
	☐	☐	Toes point straight ahead
	☐	☐	Feet under knees, do not swing side to side
Length of stride	☐	☐	Stride is several inches longer than regular step
Arm movement	☐	☐	Arms bent at 90°
	☐	☐	Arms swing front to back, not side to side
	☐	☐	Arms alternate opposite striding leg
	☐	☐	Hands and arms are relaxed
Body position	☐	☐	Upper body nearly erect
	☐	☐	Head and chest are up

CONCEPT
·7·
Flexibility

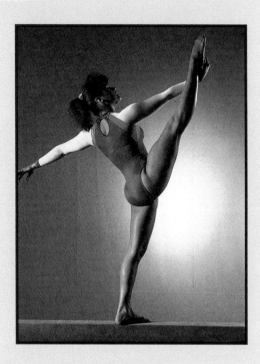

Concept 7

Adequate flexibility permits freedom of movement and may contribute to ease and economy of muscular effort, success in certain activities, and less susceptibility to some types of injuries or musculoskeletal problems.

Introduction

Flexibility is a measure of the range of motion available at a joint or group of joints. It is determined by the shape of the bones and cartilage in the joint, and by the length and extensibility of muscles, tendons, ligaments, and fascia that cross the joint. Traditionally, flexibility has been the most neglected of the five health-related components of physical fitness. However, there has been a recent surge of interest in stretching exercises by athletes, fitness buffs, and researchers.

The range of movement at a joint may vary. It may be restricted so that the joint will not bend or straighten, and is said to be "tight" or "stiff," or to have "contractures." The deformed hand of an arthritic is an example of this extreme. At the other end of the spectrum is a high degree of flexibility referred to as "loose jointedness," "hypermobility," or erroneously, as "double-jointedness." An example of this extreme is the contortionist seen at the circus. Each person, depending upon his or her individual needs, must have a reasonable amount of flexibility to perform efficiently and effectively in daily life.

Health Goal for the Year 2000

- Increase the proportion of people who engage in activity to enhance muscular strength, muscular endurance, and flexibility. (< >)

Note: (↑) indicates progress toward goal, (↓) indicates regression from goal, and (< >) indicates either no change or lack of new data since 1990.

Terms

- **Active Stretch**   Muscles are stretched by the active contraction of the opposing (antagonist) muscle. For example, when doing a calf stretch exercise, the muscles on the front of the shin contract to cause a stretch of the muscles on the back of the leg. (See figure 7.1A.)
- **Agonist Muscles**   In this concept, agonist refers to the muscle group being stretched.
- **Antagonist Muscles**   In this concept, antagonist refers to the muscle group opposing (on the opposite side of the limb from the agonist) the group being stretched.
- **Ballistic Stretch**   Muscles are stretched by the force of momentum of a body part that is bounced, swung, or jerked, as in the calf stretch shown in figures 7.1D, E, and F. The foot is bounced forward either by antagonist muscle force or by an assist from another person, or gravity, or another body part.
- **Flexibility**   Range of motion (ROM) in a joint or group of joints. Because muscle length is a major factor

limiting the range of motion, those having long muscles that allow for good joint mobility are considered to have good flexibility.

- **Hamstrings**   Three long muscles that cross both the back of the hip joint and the back of the knee joint, causing hip extension and knee flexion. They make up the bulk on the back of the thigh.

- **Hypermobility**   Looseness or slackness in a normal plane of the muscles and ligaments (soft tissue) surrounding a joint.

- **Laxity**   Motion in a joint outside the normal plane for that joint, due to loose ligaments (Steiner 1987).

- **Ligaments**   Bands of tissue that connect bones.

- **Lumbar Muscles**   Erector spinae and other muscles of the lower back (lumbar region of the spine); the muscles in the small of the back. These muscles are used to arch (hyperextend) the lower back.

- **Passive Stretch**   Stretch imposed on a muscle by a force other than the opposing muscle, for example by another person (figure 7.1B), another body part (figure 7.1B), gravity (figure 7.1C), weights, or pulleys.

- **PNF Exercise (Proprioceptive Neuromuscular Facilitation)**   Special exercise techniques to increase the contraction or the relaxation of muscles through reflex mechanisms (figure 7.1G, H, and I).

- **Range of Motion (ROM)**   The full motion possible in a joint.

- **Range of Motion Exercise**   Exercises used to maintain existing joint mobility (to prevent loss of ROM).

- **Reciprocal Inhibition**   Reflex relaxation in the muscle being stretched during the contraction of the antagonist.

- **Static Stretch**   A muscle is slowly stretched and then held in that stretched position for several seconds.

- **Stiffness**   Elasticity of the muscle—tendon unit.

- **Stretching (Flexibility) Exercise**   Exercise used to increase the existing ROM at a joint by elongating muscles and other soft tissue.

- **Trigger Point**   An especially irritable spot, usually a tight band or knot in a muscle or fascia. This often refers pain to another area of the body. For example, a trigger point in the shoulder might cause a headache. This condition is referred to as "myofascial pain syndrome" and is often caused by muscle tension, fatigue, or strain.

Some General Facts About Flexibility

There is no ideal standard for **flexibility.**

It is not known how much flexibility any one person should have in a joint. There are test norms available that list how hundreds of subjects of various ages, of both sexes, and in many walks of life have performed. But there is little scientific evidence to indicate that a person who can reach two inches past his or her toes on a sit-and-reach test is less fit than a person who can reach eight inches past the toes. Too much flexibility could be as detrimental as too little. The standards presented in chart 7.1 of the lab Resource Materials are based on the best available evidence.

Lack of use, injury, or disease can decrease joint mobility.

Arthritis and calcium deposits can damage a joint, and inflammation can cause pain that prevents movement. Failure to move a joint regularly through its full range of motion can lead to a shortening of muscles and **ligaments.** Static positions held for longer periods, such as in poor posture, working postures, and when a body part is immobilized by a cast, lead to shortened tissue and loss of mobility. Improper exercise that overdevelops one muscle group while neglecting the opposing group results in an imbalance that restricts flexibility.

Some people are unusually flexible because of a genetic trait that makes their joints "hypermobile."

In some families, the trait for loose joints is passed from generation to generation. This **hypermobility** is sometimes referred to as joint looseness. Studies show that those with this trait may be more prone to dislocated patellas. There is not much research evidence, but some experts believe that people with hypermobility or **laxity** may also be more susceptible to athletic or dance injuries, especially to the knee and ankle, and may be more apt to develop premature osteoarthritis. One recent study found that subjects who were "loose jointed" used more energy in walking and jogging than those who were medium or "tight jointed."

In the fifth century, Hippocrates noted the disadvantage of hyperextension of the elbow in archery. The hyperextended position for elbows and knees is not an efficient position from which to move because of a poor angle of muscle pull. For example, it is difficult to perform push-ups when the elbows lock into hyperextension because extra effort is required to unlock the joint. It may be advantageous for loose-jointed people to take extra care to strengthen muscles around the joints most used.

> To maintain the **range of motion (ROM)** you presently have in your joints, you must regularly perform **"range of motion exercises."**

The adage: "If you don't use it, you'll lose it!" applies particularly to flexibility. Failure to use the joints regularly through their normal range results in loss of flexibility in a fairly short period. To maintain what you have, you should do ROM exercises. Some athletes prefer to do this during the warm-up prior to a workout and save their stretching exercises until the end of the workout.

> To increase the length of a muscle, you must stretch it (overload) more than its normal length.

There is much that is not known about flexibility, but the best evidence suggests that muscles should be stretched to about 10 percent beyond their normal length to bring about an improvement in flexibility. Exercises that do not cause an overload by stretching beyond normal will not increase flexibility.

> Flexibility is specific to each joint of the body.

No one flexibility test will give an indication of your overall flexibility. For example, tight **hamstrings** and lumbar muscles might be revealed by a toe-touch test, but the range of motion in other joints may be quite different. The toe-touch test, done with both legs extended, does not distinguish between flexibility of the hamstrings and the lower back muscles, so it lacks specificity in its measurement.

> Flexibility is influenced by several factors, including age, sex, and race.

As children grow older, their flexibility increases until adolescence when they become progressively less flexible. As a general rule, girls tend to be more flexible than boys. This is probably due to anatomical differences in the joints, as well as to differences in the type and extent of activities the two sexes tend to choose. In adults, there is less difference between the sexes. Some races and ethnic groups have been reported to have specific joints that are hypermobile. For example, the thumb and finger joints of Middle Eastern people and East Indians tend to be more flexible.

> Scores on flexibility tests may be influenced by several factors.

Your range of motion at any one time may be influenced by your motivation to exert maximum effort, your warm-up preparation, the presence of muscular soreness, your tolerance

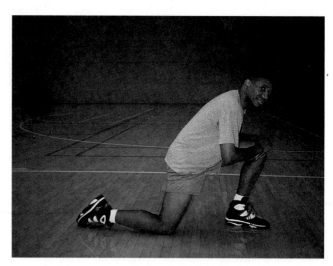

Athletic performance requires good flexibility.

for pain, the room temperature, and your ability to relax. Recent studies have found a relationship between leg or trunk length and the scores made on the sit-and-reach test. For those of average build, this is not a factor, but for a small percentage of people it makes a significant difference unless the test specifically allows for differences in body build.

> Studies of the influence of the temperature of the muscle on the effectiveness of a stretching exercise have produced contradictory results.

Some studies have shown that increasing the temperature of the muscle through warm-up exercises or the application of heat packs has resulted in improved scores on flexibility tests. Other studies have failed to find a difference between the flexibility of subjects who warmed up and those who did not warm up.

Furthermore, some people believe that cooling the muscle with ice packs in the final phase of a stretch aids in lengthening the muscle, but a recent study has failed to confirm this (Lentell et al. 1992). Until scientists reach a consensus, it seems wise to continue the practice of the warm-up and cool-down with careful static stretching.

> It is not necessary to sacrifice flexibility in order to develop strength.

A person with bulging muscles may become muscle-bound or have a restricted range of motion if strength training is done improperly. In any progressive resistance program, both agonists and antagonists should receive equal training, and all movements should be carried through the full range of motion. Properly conducted strength training does not cause a person to be muscle-bound. Furthermore, there is no evidence that a long muscle is any weaker than a short one. A good rule of thumb is: "Stretch what you strengthen and strengthen what you stretch."

Facts About the Benefits of Flexibility Exercises

Adequate flexibility may help prevent muscle strain and such orthopedic problems as backache.

Short, tight muscles are more likely to be injured by over-stretching than are long muscles. One common cause of back-ache is shortened **lumbar muscles** and hip flexor muscles. Short hamstrings are also associated with lower back problems. (See concept 16 for more discussion on back problems.) **Stretching (flexibility) exercises** may help prevent or alleviate some backaches, muscle cramps, and muscle strains.

Trigger points may sometimes be prevented or inactivated by static, or PNF stretching, of the muscles involved.

When body parts are held in static positions for long periods, or when muscles are chronically overloaded, fatigued, or chilled, myofascial **trigger points** may cause stiffness and local or referred pain. Often, the trigger point can be deactivated and the pain relieved by gentle but persistent stretching of the muscle, especially if accompanied or followed by the application of heat or cold.

Good flexibility may bring about improved athletic performance.

A hurdler must have good back and hip joint mobility to clear the hurdle. A swimmer requires shoulder and ankle flexibility for powerful strokes. A diver must be able to reach his or her toes in order to perform a good jackknife. Low back flexibility allows a runner to lengthen the stride. The fencer needs long hamstrings and hip adductors in order to lunge a long distance.

Even weight lifters have been shown to improve their performances by flexibility training. Those who trained were significantly better in the amount of weight they could bench press when it was performed with a "rebound" (no pause between the lowering and lifting phase) to take advantage of the elastic "snap-back" force. It has been hypothesized that the stretching exercises not only increase the length of the muscle, but can also decrease its **stiffness.** Power athletes who use ballistic movements, such as baseball pitchers, high jumpers, and shot putters may benefit from this type of training.

It is widely believed that static muscle stretching is effective in relieving muscle spasms, muscle soreness, and shin splints.

One theory suggests that local muscle soreness may be caused by slight reflex contractions. It is believed that a **static stretch** of the affected muscle may relieve these slight contractions and thus relieve the pain. Even some cases of non-pathological shin splints may be relieved by such exercise.

Research studies to date do not support the conventional wisdom that stretching during a cool-down will *prevent* muscular soreness. In a controlled study, muscle soreness was deliberately induced in a group of subjects. When half of the group stretched immediately afterward and at intervals for 48 hours, they had no less soreness than the group who did not stretch (Buroker and Schwane 1989).

Stretching exercises are useful in preventing and remediating some cases of dysmenorrhea in women.

Painful menstruation (dysmenorrhea) of some types can be prevented or reduced by stretching the pelvic and hip joint fascia. Billig's exercise is an example of an effective exercise for this condition (See concept 8, exercise 6 for this condition).

Flexibility training has been shown to improve spinal mobility and the driving ability of older adults.

When older drivers performed stretching exercises, they improved their range of motion and were better able to look over their shoulders for blind spots, parallel parking, and backing into parking spaces (*Senior World of Orange, County,* 1991).

It is normal for tissue to lose its elasticity with age, but a sedentary lifestyle is probably the greatest contributor to loss of flexibility with aging. Fortunately, the elderly do respond to training. Spinal mobility is important not only for driving, but also for daily activities such as tying one's shoes and reaching and twisting.

Facts About the Types of Flexibility Exercises

To develop flexibility it is necessary to do exercises from the flexibility section of the Physical Activity Pyramid.

The activities in the first two levels of the physical activity pyramid do little to develop flexibility. To build this important part of fitness, flexibility exercises from the third level of the pyramid are essential.

Three commonly used types of flexibility exercises are static stretch, **ballistic stretch,** and **PNF exercise (proprioceptive neuromuscular facilitation).** Each of these can be performed as an **active stretch** or as a **passive stretch.** All are effective in developing flexibility.

Because static stretching is done slowly and held for a period, there is less probability of tearing the soft tissue, particularly if the force comes from your own muscles. Many believe static stretching is also less likely to cause delayed-onset muscle soreness, but one study found it caused greater soreness than ballistic stretching (Smith, et al., 1993).

When active stretch is used (see figure 7.1A), the opposing muscles contract. This produces a reflex (**reciprocal inhibition**) relaxation in the muscles that you are trying to stretch. On the other hand, when a muscle is stretched passively by an outside force, there is no reflex relaxation. A muscle that is not relaxed cannot be stretched as far, and there is potential for injury.

There is one problem, however, with an active stretch. It is almost impossible to produce an overload by simply contracting the opposing muscles. Therefore, it is best to combine the active stretch with a passive assist (see figures 7.1B and C). This gives the advantage of a relaxed muscle and a sufficient force to provide an overload to stretch it.

A ballistic stretch uses momentum to produce the stretch. Momentum is produced by vigorous motion, such as flinging a body part or rocking it back and forth to create a bouncing movement. Because this may stretch the muscle farther than some other methods, there is the potential for injury. Some opponents argue that the sudden stretch of the ballistic motion elicits a myotatic reflex (stretch reflex), which then causes the muscle to contract and thus get shorter and stronger instead of longer. It is true that a myotatic reflex occurs (it also occurs in a static stretch), but the momentum is already spent so there is no overload on the muscle; therefore, *no* strength is developed. It should also be recognized that the active contraction of the **antagonist muscles** (opposite the muscle being stretched) causes a desirable reciprocal inhibition in the muscle being stretched.

Although not everyone agrees that the advantages of ballistic stretch outweigh the disadvantages, most experts do believe that static stretch is the preferred method for beginners, those with a history of muscle injury, and those who do not need exceptional levels of flexibility for athletic performances.

Since many athletic activities are ballistic in nature, sport-specific ballistic stretch is deemed appropriate for some athletes. The *principle of specificity* implies that one should train with the type of movements that are most likely to occur in the activity for which one is training. Since ballistic movement is very much a part of most athletic events (those requiring speed and power), it is appropriate to train using this type of movement. Even among athletes, however, static stretching is recommended prior to the use of ballistic stretching during a workout. Ballistic exercises are illustrated in figures 7.1D, E, and F. Examples of sport-specific ballistic stretches are shown in concept 8). Passive ballistic stretching is particularly risky and is *not* recommended for use outside of a clinic.

PNF has been popular for rehabilitation since the 1960s. It consists of dozens of techniques to stimulate muscles to contract more strongly or to relax more fully so that they can be stretched. Three of the techniques that have become popular in fitness programs to improve the flexibility of healthy people are: contract-relax-antagonist-contract (CRAC), slow-reversal-hold-relax (SRHR), and contract-relax (CR).

The contract-relax-antagonist-contract technique involves three steps: (1) move the limb so the muscle to be stretched is elongated initially, then contract the **agonist muscles** isometrically against an immovable object or the resistance of a partner for three seconds; (2) relax the muscle two seconds; and (3) stretch the muscle immediately by contracting the antagonist for 10 to 15 seconds with an assist from a partner, gravity, or other body part (see figure 7.1G, H, I). Research shows that this and other types of PNF stretch are more effective than a simple static stretch. The SRHR procedure is the same as CRAC except that the agonist is passively stretched prior to step 1 (figure 7.1G) and again after step 3 (figure 7.1I).

A variation of this PNF procedure is contract-relax. This is the same procedure as the CRAC technique except that the static stretch is done passively. Following the isometric contraction, another body part, person, or gravity applies force to stretch the muscles. There is no contraction of the opposing muscles during the stretch. CRAC and SRHR are believed to be superior to CR in their effectiveness.

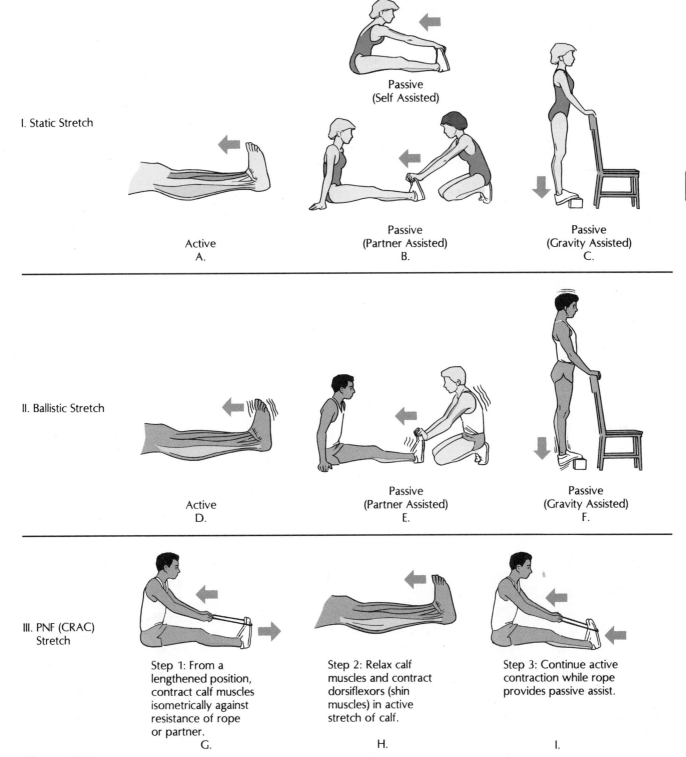

I. Static Stretch

Active
A.

Passive
(Self Assisted)

Passive
(Partner Assisted)
B.

Passive
(Gravity Assisted)
C.

II. Ballistic Stretch

Active
D.

Passive
(Partner Assisted)
E.

Passive
(Gravity Assisted)
F.

III. PNF (CRAC) Stretch

Step 1: From a lengthened position, contract calf muscles isometrically against resistance of rope or partner.
G.

Step 2: Relax calf muscles and contract dorsiflexors (shin muscles) in active stretch of calf.
H.

Step 3: Continue active contraction while rope provides passive assist.
I.

Figure 7.1
Examples of static, ballistic, PNF, active, and passive stretches of the calf muscles (gastrocnemius and soleus). Muscles shown in dark pink are the muscles being contracted. Muscles shown in pink are those being stretched.

Each form of flexibility exercise has its advantages and disadvantages.

The advantages and disadvantages of unassisted ballistic, static, and PNF exercises using active stretch with passive assist are summarized in table 7.1. The best method or methods for you may depend upon your physical condition, whether you wish to increase your range of motion or just maintain it, whether you have a partner to assist, and whether you are training for speed or power athletic events.

Facts About How to Increase Flexibility

For maximal effectiveness and minimal harm, there are guidelines that should be followed in performing flexibility exercises.

There is a correct and an incorrect way to exercise, and some exercises can even be harmful. Concept 8 presents guidelines for flexibility exercises and some samples of the exercises defined in this concept.

There is a minimum amount of exercise (threshold of training) and an optimal amount of exercise (target zone) necessary for developing flexibility.

The threshold of training and target zones for static, ballistic, and PNF stretching are presented in table 7.2. The time required to stretch tissue varies inversely with the force used. Low force requires more time whereas high force requires less time.

Table 7.1
Comparison of Advantages and Disadvantages of Three Types of Flexibility Exercises

Advantages	Static-Active, Assisted	Ballistic-Active	PNF (CRAC), Assisted
		Rating	
Less danger of overstretch	Good–Excellent	Poor–Fair	Good–Excellent
Useful to relieve muscle cramps or soreness	Excellent	Poor	Good
Strength may be developed	Poor	Poor	Good
Utilizes reflexes to relax the stretched muscle	Good	Fair	Excellent
Specific to most athletics and daily activities such as speed and power skills	Poor	Excellent	Poor
Convenient; less apt to need another person to assist	Fair	Excellent	Poor–Fair
Efficient; requires less time	Fair	Fair	Poor
Effective in lengthening muscles	Good	Good	Excellent

Table 7.2
Flexibility Threshold of Training and Fitness Target Zones

	Threshold of Training			Target Zones		
	Static	Ballistic	PNF (CRAC)	Static	Ballistic	PNF (CRAC)
Frequency	• 3 days per week for all methods.			• 3 to 7 days per week for all methods.		
Intensity	• Stretch as far as you can go without pain; with slow movement, hold at the end of the range of motion.	• Stretch muscle beyond normal length with gentle bounce or swing, but do not exceed 10 percent of active-static range of motion.	• Same as static except use a maximum isometric contraction of the muscle prior to stretch.	• Add assist. • Avoid overstretch and pain for all methods.	• Same as threshold.	• Same as static. • Add assist.
Time	• Hold stretch 15 sec.; • 3 reps; rest 30 sec. between.	• Continuous reps for 30 sec. (this is 1 set).	• Hold isometric contraction 3 sec; • Hold stretch 10–15 sec.; • 3 reps; • 30 sec. rest between reps.	• Hold 10–15 sec.; • 3 reps; 3 sets; • 30 sec. rest between reps; • 1 min. rest between sets.	• 1–3 sets; • Rest 1 min. between sets.	• 1–3 reps of 3 sec. contraction and 10–15 sec. hold; • 30 sec. rest between reps; • 1 min. rest between sets.

Facts About Exercise Precautions

Overstretching may make a person more susceptible to injury or hamper performance.

Muscles and tendons have both extensibility and elasticity. Ligaments and the joint capsule are extensible but lack elasticity. When stretched, they remain in the lengthened state. If this occurs, the joint may lack stability and is susceptible to chronic dislocation or movement in an undesirable plane. This is particularly true of weight-bearing joints, such as the hip, knee, and ankle. Loose ligaments may allow the joint to twist abnormally, tearing the cartilage and other soft tissue. Remember these precautions:

- Don't force it to the point of pain.
- Elderly people or those with osteoporosis or arthritis should use special care.
- Avoid vigorous stretching after a body part has been immobilized (such as in a sling or cast) for a long period.
- Avoid stretching swollen joints.
- Avoid overstretching weak muscles.
- Use great care in applying passive stretch to a partner; go slowly and ask for feedback.

- Some (but not all) people with high blood pressure should avoid the PNF techniques because the isometric contractions may increase arterial blood pressure excessively.
- Beginners should use static or PNF stretching rather than ballistic stretching.
- Athletes who use sport-specific ballistic stretching should precede this type of stretching with static stretching.

Suggested Readings

Alter, M. J. *Science of Stretch*. Champaign, IL: Human Kinetics Publishers, 1996.

Buroker, K. C., and J. A. Schwane. "Does Post-Exercise Static Stretching Alleviate Delayed Muscle Soreness." *Physician and Sportsmedicine* 17(1989):65.

"Fitness Improves Driving." *Senior World of Orange County* 17(Jan. 1991).

Hardy, L., and D. Jones. "Dynamic Flexibility and Proprioceptive Neuromuscular Facilitation." *Research Quarterly for Exercise and Sport* 57(1986):150.

Hoeger, W., & Hopkins, D. "Assessing Muscular Flexibility." *Fitness Management* 6(20:34–36, 42, 1990).

Lentell, G. et al. "The Use of Thermal Agents to Influence the Effectiveness of a Low Load Prolonged Stretch." (Platform presentation 1992 APTA Combined Sections Meeting, San Francisco). Abstract. *Journal of Orthopaedic and Sports Physical Therapy* 15(Jan. 1992):48.

McAtee, R. *Facilitated Stretching*. Champaign, IL: Human Kinetics Publishers, 1993.

Smith, L. L., et al. "The Effects of Static and Ballistic Stretching on Delayed Onset Muscle Soreness and Creatine Kinase." *Research Quarterly for Exercise and Sport* 64(1993):103.

LAB RESOURCE MATERIALS

Flexibility Tests

Because it is impractical to test the flexibility of all joints, perform these tests for joints used frequently. Follow instructions carefully.

Test

1. *Modified Sit-and-Reach* (Flexibility Test of Hamstrings)
   a. Remove shoes and assume the position for the "back-saver toe touch," (fig. 4.2, p. 93) except place the sole of the foot of the extended leg flat against the box or bench, and place the head, back, and hips against a wall; 90-degree angle at the hips.
   b. Place one hand over the other and slowly reach forward as far as you can with arms fully extended; head and back remain in contact with the wall. A partner will slide the measuring stick on the bench until it touches the fingertips.
   c. With the measuring stick fixed in the new position, reach forward as far as possible, three times, holding the position on the third reach for at least two seconds while the partner reads the distance on the ruler. Keep the knee of the extended leg straight (see illustration).
   d. Repeat the test a second time and average the scores of the two trials.

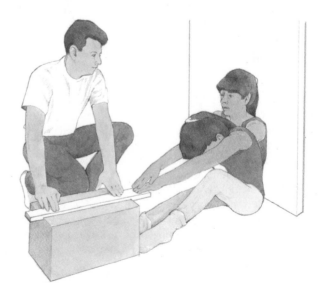

Test

2. *Shoulder Flexibility* ("Zipper" Test")
   a. Raise your right arm, bend your elbow, and reach down across your back as far as possible.
   b. At the same time, extend your left arm down and behind your back, bend your elbow up across your back, and try to cross your fingers over those of your right hand as shown in the accompanying illustration.
   c. Measure the distance to the nearest half-inch. If your fingers overlap, score as a plus; if they fail to meet, score as a minus; use a zero if your fingertips just touch.
   d. Repeat with your arms crossed in the opposite direction (left arm up). Most people will find that they are more flexible on one side than the other.

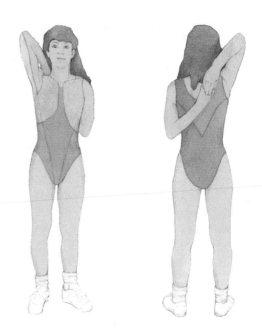

Test

3. *Hamstring and Hip Flexor Flexibility*
   a. Lie on your back on the floor beside a wall.
   b. Slowly lift one leg off the floor. Keep the other leg flat on the floor.
   c. Keep both legs straight.
   d. Continue to lift the leg until either leg begins to bend or the lower leg begins to lift off the floor.
   e. Place a yardstick against the wall and underneath the lifted leg.
   f. Hold the yardstick against the wall after the leg is lowered.
   g. Measure the angle created by the floor and the yardstick using a protractor. The greater the angle, the better your score.
   h. Repeat with the other leg.

Note: For ease of testing, you may want to draw angles on a piece of posterboard as illustrated. If you have goniometers, you may be taught to use them instead.

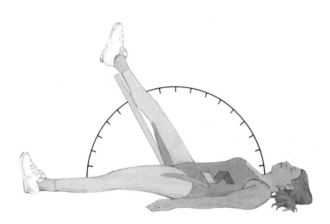

Test

4. *Trunk Rotation*
   a. Stand with your right shoulder an arm's length (fist closed) from the wall. Toes should be on the line (which is perpendicular to the wall and even with the 15-inch mark on the ruler).
   b. Drop the right arm and raise the left arm to the side, palm down, fists closed.
   c. Without moving your feet, rotate the trunk to the left as far as possible, reaching along the ruler, and hold it two seconds. Do not move the feet nor bend the trunk. Your knees may bend slightly.
   d. A partner will read the distance reached to the nearest ½ inch. Record your score.
   e. Repeat the test, facing the opposite direction and rotating to the right.
   f. Record your score.
   g. Average the two scores.

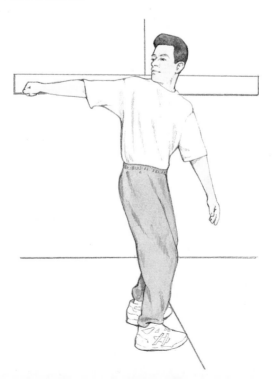

Chart 7.1 Flexibility Rating Scale for Tests 1,2,3,4

Classification	Men					Women				
	Test 1	Test 2 Right Up	Test 2 Left Up	Test 3	Test 4	Test 1	Test 2 Right Up	Test 2 Left Up	Test 3	Test 4
High performance zone	16+	5+	4+	111+	20+	17+	6+	5+	111+	20.5 or >
Good fitness zone	13–15	1–4	1–3	80–110	16–19.5	14–16	2–5	2–4	80–110	17–20
Marginal zone	10–12	0	0	60–79	13.5–15.5	11–13	1	1	60–79	14.5–16.5
Low zone	<9	<0	<0	<60	13 or less	<10	<1	<1	<60	14 or <

CONCEPT
·8·

Flexibility Exercises

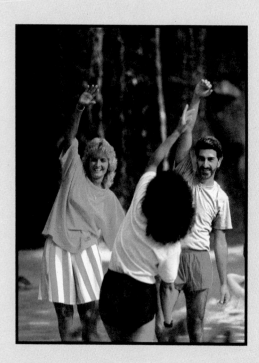

Flexibility exercises are designed to maintain or increase flexibility by stretching the muscles and other soft tissue around the joints. This stretch may, in turn, prevent or alleviate some musculoskeletal problems.

Introduction

There are many ways to stretch muscles and improve flexibility through exercise (see concept 7). The major types of muscle stretching exercises are static stretching, ballistic stretching, and PNF. These exercises can be done by yourself, using only your own muscles to stretch, gravity (body weight), or the assistance of other body parts or a partner. To increase flexibility, the muscles must be stretched beyond their normal range.

Health Goal for the Year 2000

- Increase the proportion of people who engage in activity to enhance muscular strength, muscular endurance, and flexibility. (<>)

Note: (↑) indicates progress toward goal, (↓) indicates regression from goal, and (<>) indicates either no change or lack of new data since 1990.

Terms

- **Ballistic Stretch** Muscles are stretched by the force of momentum of a body part that is bounced, swung, or jerked, either by antagonist muscle force or by an assist from another person, gravity, or another body part.
- **Passive Stretch** Stretch imposed on a muscle by a force other than the opposing muscle; for example, by another person, another body part, gravity, weights, or pulleys.
- **PNF Exercise (Proprioceptive Neuromuscular Facilitation)** Special exercise techniques to increase the contraction or the relaxation of muscles through reflex mechanisms.
- **Static Stretch** A muscle is slowly stretched and then held in that stretched position for several seconds.

The Facts

There is a correct way to perform flexibility exercises.

Remember that stretching can *cause* muscle soreness, so "easy does it." Start below your threshold if you are unaccustomed to stretching a given muscle group, then work up to your target zone. The guidelines that follow will help you to gain the most benefit from your exercises:
- Warm the muscles *before you attempt to stretch them.*
- Exercises that do not cause a muscle to lengthen beyond normal may maintain, but will not increase, flexibility.
- To increase flexibility, the muscle must be overloaded (stretched beyond its normal length), but not to the point of pain. Remember, you want to stretch muscles, not joints!

- Exercises must be performed for each muscle group and at each joint where flexibility is desired.
- To protect adjacent joints, make certain the adjacent body parts are stabilized to prevent undesirable movement and are in good alignment to avoid strain.
- Stretch muscles of small joints in the extremities first, then progress toward the trunk with muscles of larger joints.
- Stretch muscles over joints one at a time before stretching at multiple joints simultaneously; for example, stretch muscles at the ankle, then the knee, then the ankle and knee simultaneously.
- If sport-specific ballistic stretching is used, precede it with static or **PNF exercise.**
- Avoid **ballistic stretches** of previously injured muscles or joints, especially the lower back muscles.
- Avoid **passive** ballistic **stretches** unless you are under the supervision of a registered or certified therapist or a trainer.
- If ballistic stretches are used, the bounces should be gentle and probably not exceed 10 percent of the normal **static stretch** range of motion. Avoid high-risk stretching exercises (see concept 12).
- For static stretches, use "what is called developmental stretch": stretch until you begin to feel pain, back off slightly and hold the position several seconds, then gradually try to stretch a little farther, back off, hold, etc. The stretch should feel slightly uncomfortable but should *not* be painful.
- For static stretches, increase the intensity of the stretch slowly, and also decrease it slowly after the hold.

There are certain areas of the body that especially need to be stretched for good health and fitness.

Areas of the body that are most likely to need stretching include:
- the muscles on the back of the legs (hamstrings) in order to prevent soreness, injury in sports, and referred back pain.
- the muscles on the inside of the thigh in order to prevent back, leg, and foot strain.
- the calf muscles in order to prevent soreness and Achilles tendon injuries in jogging/running.
- the muscles on the front of the hip joint in order to prevent lordosis and backache.
- the low back muscles in order to help prevent soreness and pain, as well as back injuries.
- the muscles on the front of the chest and shoulders in order to prevent rounded shoulders and limited range of movement in the shoulder joint.

The exercises pictured in this concept focus on these body areas.

Certain flexibility exercises are good for therapeutic purposes, as well as for fitness.

Stretching exercises can be prescribed specifically to alleviate pain. Usually, the same exercise, if done regularly, can prevent the condition that originally caused the pain. Examples of "therapeutic exercises" include exercise 1 (or some variation of it) to stretch the calf muscle. This will relieve muscle cramps in the lower leg. Exercise 6, Billig's exercise, can be used to relieve menstrual cramps (dysmenorrhea). The shin stretcher (exercise 10) may relieve shin splints.

Sample Flexibility Exercises

The following stretching exercises are intended primarily to develop flexibility. Exercises for different body parts are presented here. They include static and PNF type exercises. These exercises should be held for ten to sixty seconds. Muscles depicted in pink color are those primarily being stretched by the exercises.

1. Lower Leg Stretcher

Purpose

To stretch the calf muscles and Achilles tendon.

Position

Stand with the toes on a thick book or lower rung of a stall bar. Keep toes pointed straight ahead or slightly inward. Hold on to a support with the hands.

Movement

Rise up on toes (**contract**) as far as possible and hold for three seconds. **Relax** and lower heels to floor as far as possible; **hold.**

Note

Static stretch may alleviate spasms or cramps in calf muscles.

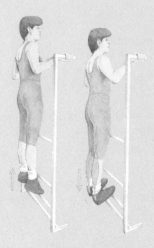

2. Sitting Stretcher

Purpose

To stretch muscles on inside of thighs.

Position

Sit with soles of feet together; place hands on knees or ankles and lean forearms against knees; resist (**contract**) by attempting to raise knees.

Movement

Hold three seconds; then **relax** and press the knees toward the floor as far as possible; **hold.**

Note

Useful for pregnant women and anyone whose thighs tend to rotate inward causing backache, knock-knees, and flat feet.

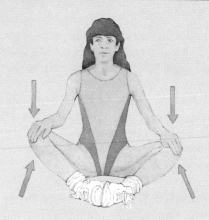

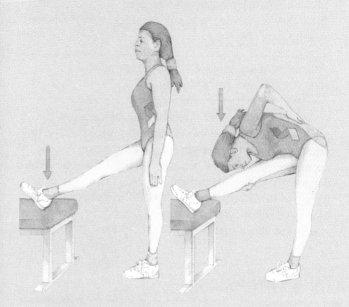

3. One-Leg Stretcher

Purpose

To stretch lower back and hamstring muscles.

Position

Stand with one foot on a bench, keeping both legs straight.

Movement

Contract hamstrings and gluteals by pressing down on bench with the heel for three seconds, then **relax** and bend the trunk forward, trying to touch the head to the knee. **Hold** for 10–15 seconds. Return to starting position and repeat with opposite leg. As flexibility improves, the arms can be used to pull the chest toward the legs. Do not allow either knee to lock.

Note

This is useful in relief of backache and correction of lordosis (swayback).

4. Leg Hug

Purpose

To stretch lower back and gluteals.

Position

Hook-lying position.

Movement

Contract gluteals and lumbar muscles. Lift hips. Hold for three seconds. **Relax** and pull knees to chest with arms as hard as possible; **hold.**

Note

Useful for backache and lordosis (also see concept 12). Do not place the hands over the knees to apply stretch.

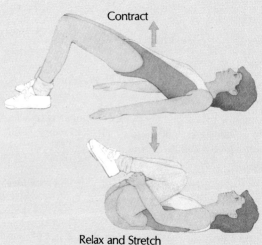

Contract

Relax and Stretch

5. Pectoral stretch

Purpose

To stretch pectorals.

Position

Stand erect in doorway with arms raised 45°, elbows bent, and hands grasping doorjambs; feet in front stride position.

Movement

Press forward on door frame, **contracting** the arms maximally for three seconds. **Relax** and shift weight forward on legs; lean into doorway so muscles on front of shoulder joint and chest are stretched; **hold.** Repeat with arms raised 90°. Repeat with arms raised 135°.

Note

Useful to prevent or correct round shoulders and sunken chest.

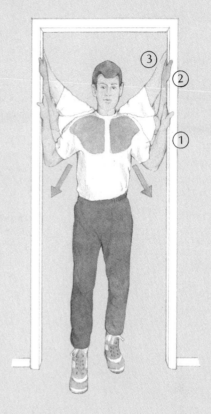

7. Lateral Trunk Stretcher

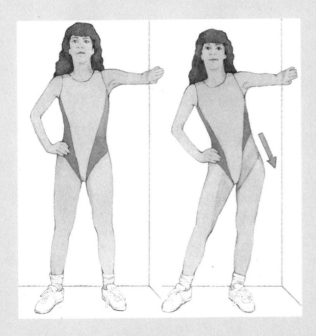

Purpose

To stretch trunk muscles.

Position

Sit on the floor.

Movement

Stretch left arm over head to right. Bend to right at waist, reaching as far to right as possible with left arm and as far as possible to the left with right arm; **hold.** Do not let trunk rotate. Repeat on opposite side. For less stretch, overhead arm may be bent at elbow.

Note

This exercise can be done in the standing position but is less effective.

6. Billig s Exercise

Purpose

To stretch pelvic fascia, hip flexors, and inside of thigh.

Position

Stand with side to a wall and place the elbow and forearm against the wall at shoulder height. Tilt the pelvis backward, tightening the gluteal and abdominal muscles.

Movement

Place opposite hand on hip and push the hips toward the wall. Push forward and sideward (45°) with the hips. Do not twist the hips. **Hold.** Repeat on opposite side.

Note

Useful for preventing some cases of dysmenorrhea.

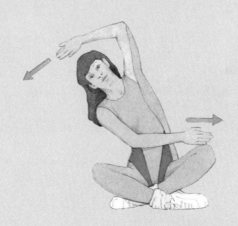

8. Hip and Thigh Stretcher

Purpose

To stretch iliopsoas and quadriceps.

Position

Place right knee directly above right ankle and **stretch** left leg backward so knee touches floor. If necessary, place hands on floor for balance.

Movement

Press pelvis forward and downward; **hold.** Repeat on opposite side. *Caution:* Do not bend front knee more than 90°.

Note

Useful for those who have lordosis or lower back problems.

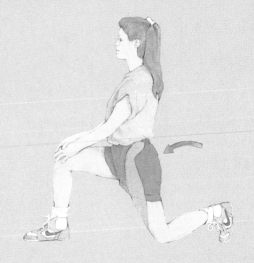

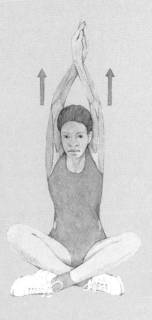

9. Arm Stretcher

Purpose

To stretch arm and chest muscles.

Position

Cross arms and turn palms of hands together. Raise arms overhead behind ears. Extend elbows.

Movement

Stretch as high as possible. **Hold.**

10. Shin Stretcher

Purpose

To relieve shin muscle soreness by stretching muscles on front of shin.

Position

Kneel on both knees, turn to right, and press down and **stretch** right ankle with right hand.

Movement

Move pelvis forward. **Hold.** Repeat on opposite side.

Note

Except when they are sore, most people need to strengthen rather than stretch these muscles.

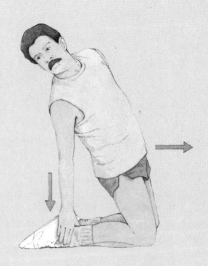

11. Hamstring Stretcher

Purpose

To stretch the muscles on the back of the hip, thigh, knee, and ankle.

Position

Start in a hook-lying position. Bring right knee to chest and grasp toes with right hand. Place left hand on back of right thigh.

Movement

(1) Pull knee toward chest; (2) push heel toward ceiling and pull toes toward shin; (3) attempt to straighten knee. **Stretch** and **hold.** Repeat on left side.

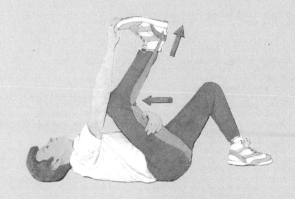

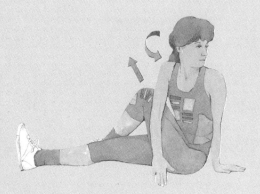

12. Trunk Twister

Purpose

To stretch the trunk muscles and muscles on the outside of hip.

Position

Sit with right leg extended, left leg bent and crossed over the right knee.

Movement

Place right arm on the left side of the left leg and push against that leg while turning the trunk as far as possible to the left; place left hand on floor behind buttocks. **Stretch** and **hold.** Reverse position and repeat on opposite side.

13. Rectus Femoris (Quadriceps) Stretcher

Purpose

To stretch the rectus femoris (two-joint muscle on front of thigh).

Position

Sit in widest possible side-stride position. Lean to left on elbow and bend right knee 90°.

Movement

Place right hand on floor behind right calf and roll trunk backwards. Adjust until a pull is felt on the front of the right thigh, **not** on the inside of the right knee. **Stretch** and **hold.** Repeat on left leg.

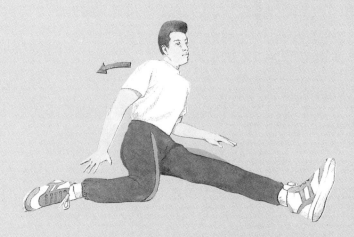

14. Lateral Thigh and Hip Stretch

Purpose

To stretch the iliotibial band and tensor fascia lata.

Position

Stand with left side to wall, left arm extended and palm of hand flat on wall for support. Cross left leg behind right and turn toes of both feet out slightly.

Movement

Bend left knee slightly and shift pelvis toward wall (left) as trunk bends toward right. Adjust until pull is felt down outside of left hip and thigh. **Stretch** and **hold.** Repeat on other side.

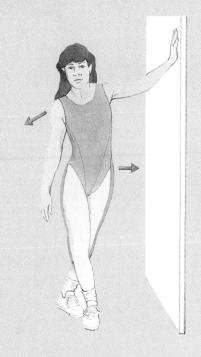

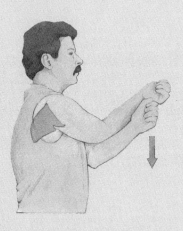

15. Arm Pretzel

Purpose

To stretch lateral rotators of the shoulder.

Position

Stand or sit with elbows flexed at right angles, palms up.

Movement

Cross right arm over left; grasp right thumb with left hand and pull gently downward, causing right arm to rotate laterally. **Stretch** and **hold.** Reverse arm position and repeat on left arm.

16. Spine Twist

Purpose

To stretch trunk rotators and lateral rotators of the thighs.

Position

Start in hook-lying position, arms extended at shoulder level.

Movement

Cross left knee over right; keep arms and shoulders on floor while touching knees to floor on left. **Stretch** and **hold.** Reverse leg position and lower knees to right.

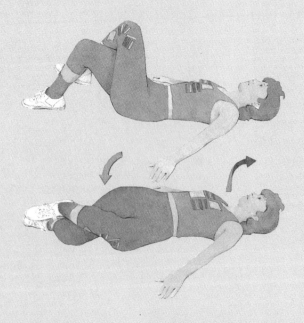

17. Neck Rotation

Purpose

To stretch neck rotators.

Position

Place palm of left hand against left cheek; point fingers toward ear and point elbow forward.

Movement

Try to turn head and neck left while resisting with left hand. Hold six seconds. Relax and turn head to right as far as possible; hold ten seconds. Repeat four times; then repeat on opposite side.

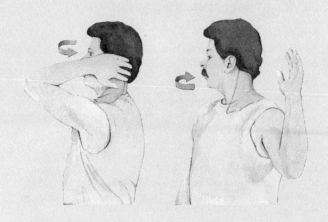

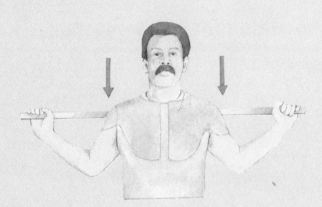

18. Wand Exercise

Purpose

To stretch front of shoulder and chest.

Position

Sit with wand grasped at ends. Raise wand overhead. Be certain that the head does not slide forward into a "poke neck" position. Keep the chin tucked and neck straight.

Movement

Bring wand down behind shoulder blades. Keep spine erect. Hold. Hands may be moved closer together to increase stretch on chest muscles.

Note

If this is an easy exercise for you, try straightening the elbows and bringing the wand to waist level in back of you.

19. Calf Stretcher

Purpose

To stretch the calf muscles and Achilles tendon.

Position

Face a wall with your feet two or three feet away. Step forward on left foot to allow both hands to touch the wall.

Movement

(1) Keep the heel of your right foot on the ground, toe turned in slightly, knee straight, and buttocks tucked in. Lean forward by bending your front knee and arms and allowing your head to move nearer the wall. Hold. (2) Bend right knee, keeping heel on floor. **Stretch** and **hold.** Repeat with other leg.

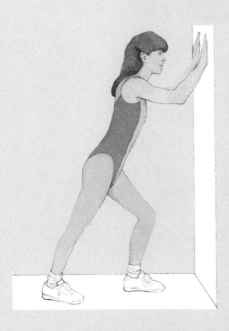

Sample Flexibility Exercises *cont.*

20. Back-Saver Hamstring Stretch

Purpose

To stretch hamstrings and calf muscles, and help prevent or correct backache caused in part by short hamstrings.

Position

Sit on the floor with the feet against the wall or an immovable object. Bend left knee and bring foot close to buttocks. Clasp hands behind back.

Movement

Bend forward from hips, keeping lower back as straight as possible. Let bent knee rotate outward so trunk can move forward. Lean forward keeping back flat; hold and repeat on each leg.

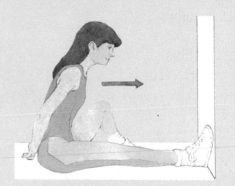

Flexibility Stunts and Sports-Specific Ballistic Stretches

1. Two-Hand Ankle Wrap

Position

Stand with heels together.

Movement

Bend forward and place arms between knees; bend knees and wrap arms around legs, attempting to touch fingers in front of ankles. Hold ten seconds.

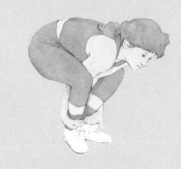

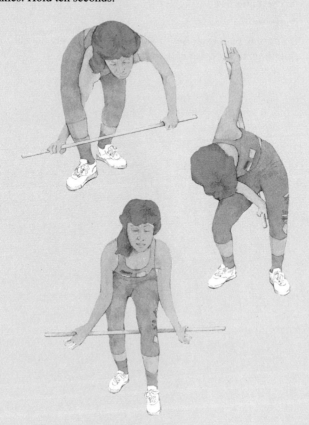

2. Wand Step-Through

Position

Stand; grasp wand with palms down, hands shoulder width apart.

Movement

(A) Bend forward and swing right leg around the outside of the right arm and over the wand (from front to back) into the "hole" made by the arms and wand. (B) Slide the wand around the back of the body by bringing the left arm over the head; then slide the wand under the hips and (C) step over the wand (from front to back) with the left foot, stepping out of the "hole."

Note

Arms finish in a palms-up position. Do not release the wand at any time.

3. Wring the Dishrag (with a partner)

Position

Partners stand facing each other, holding opposite hands.

Movement

Number one starts with the left leg and number two starts with the right leg. Each lifts the leg over the near arm and steps into the middle of the "hole" (formed by the arms); turn back to back while swinging the opposite arms overhead; step out of the hole with the opposite legs and end facing each other, hands still grasped.

Purpose

To aid one-handed throwing and striking skills (for example, racket sports forehand, backhand, and serve; baseball throw, or discus and shot put); and/or two-handed throwing or striking skills (for example, batting a softball or executing a golf drive or hammer throw).

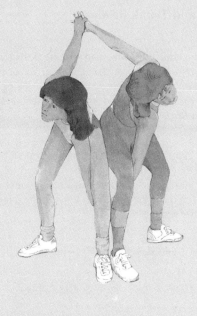

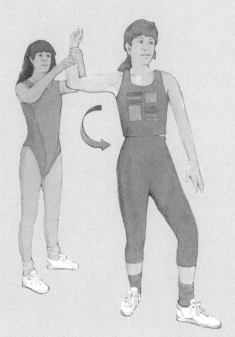

4. Trunk Motions (with a partner)

Purpose

To aid one-handed throwing and striking skills (for example, racket sports forehand, backhand, and serve; baseball throw, or discus and shot put); and/or two-handed throwing or striking skills (for example, batting a softball or executing a golf drive or hammer throw).

Movement

Assume a position at the end of the backswing for any skill listed above. Partner grasps hand(s) and resists movement while the performer turns the trunk away from the partner, making a series of gentle bouncing movements, attempting to rotate the trunk as if performing the skill. Alternate roles with the partner.

Note

Avoid overstretching by too vigorous bouncing. If no partner is available, use a door frame for resistance or these sports actions can be practiced using elastic bands or inner tubes (attached to fixed objects) as resistance.

5. Arm and Trunk Motions

Purpose

To aid one-handed throwing and striking skills (for example, racket sports forehand, backhand, and serve; baseball throw, or discus and shot put); and/or two-handed throwing or striking skills (for example, batting a softball or executing a golf drive or hammer throw).

Movement

Stand and swing the racket, club, bat, or arm with or without a weight on the implement or on the wrist. Start by swinging backward and forward rhythmically and continuously. Gradually increase the speed and vigor of the swing to finally resemble the actual skill.

Note

If a weight is added, swing easily to avoid torn muscles.

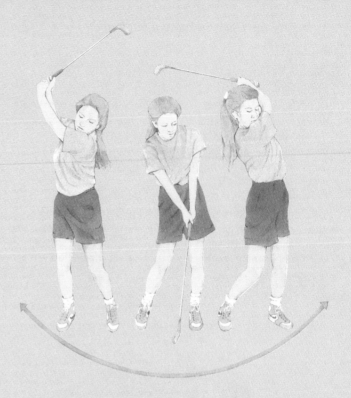

Suggested Readings

Alter, M. J. *The Science of Stretching*. Champaign, IL: Human Kinetics Publishers, 1996.

Alter, M. J. *Sports Stretch*. Champaign, IL: Human Kinetics Publishers, 1990.

McAtee, R. *Facilitated Stretching*. Champaign, IL: Human Kinetics Publishers, 1993.

CONCEPT
·9·

Muscular Strength and Power

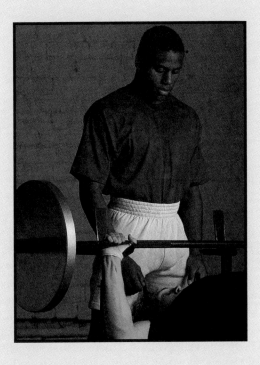

Concept 9

Strength is an important health-related component of physical fitness, whereas power is an important combination of skill-related and health-related components.

Introduction

Strength is measured by the amount of force you can produce with a single maximal effort. You need strength to increase work capacity; to decrease the chance of injury; to prevent low back pain, poor posture, and other hypokinetic diseases; to improve athletic performance; and perhaps to save life or property in an emergency. Strength training increases strength of bones, tendons, and ligaments, as well as muscles. It has been found to be therapeutic for patients with chronic pain.

Power training increases strength and endurance up to a point but is primarily useful in preparing you to perform activities that require power. Examples of activities requiring power are throwing, striking, and jumping skills in sports and dance or throwing heavy loads in farming and industry.

Health Goals for the Year 2000

- Increase the proportion of people who engage in activity to enhance muscular strength, muscular endurance, and flexibility. (<>)
- Reduce the proportion of male high school seniors who use anabolic steroids. (<>)

Note: (↑) indicates progress toward goal, (↓) indicates regression from goal, and (<>) indicates either no change or lack of new data since 1990.

Terms

- **Absolute Strength**   The maximum amount of force one can exert, e.g., maximum number of pounds or kilograms one can lift on one attempt. (See Relative Strength.)
- **Anabolic Steroid**   A synthetic hormone similar to the male sex hormone testosterone. It functions androgenically to stimulate male characteristics and anabolically to increase muscle mass, weight, bone maturation, and virility.
- **Antagonistic Muscles**   The muscles that have the opposite action from those that are contracting (agonists); normally, antagonists reflexly relax when agonists contract.
- **Concentric Contraction**   An isotonic muscle contraction in which the muscle gets shorter as it contracts, such as when a joint is bent and two body parts move closer together. An example is the biceps muscle contraction that occurs when pulling up on a chinning bar.
- **Definition of Muscle**   The detailed external appearance of a muscle.
- **Dynamic Contraction**   A popular name for isotonic exercise.

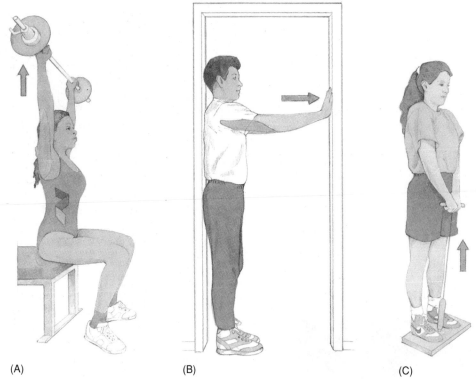

(A)   (B)   (C)

Figure 9.1
Examples of three types of strength exercises (A) isotonic, (B) isometric, and (C) isokinetic

Source: Big Four Exer-Genie from Exergenie, Inc. Glendale, CA.

- **Eccentric Contraction** "Negative exercise." An isotonic muscle contraction in which the muscle gets longer as it contracts; that is, when a weight is gradually lowered and the contracting muscle gets longer as it gives up tension. Lowering the body from a pull-up on a chinning bar is an example of eccentric contraction of the biceps muscle.

- **Hypertrophy** Increase in the size of muscles as the result of strength training; increase in bulk.

- **Isokinetic** Isotonic concentric exercises done with a machine that regulates movement, velocity, and resistance (figure 9.1).

- **Isometric** A type of muscle contraction in which the muscle remains the same length. Isometric exercises are those in which no movement takes place while a force is exerted against an immovable object (also known as "static contraction") (figure 9.1).

- **Isotonic** Type of muscle contraction in which the muscle changes length, either shortening (concentrically) or lengthening (eccentrically). Isotonic exercises are those in which a resistance is raised and then lowered, as in weight training and calisthenics (also called **dynamic** or "phasic") (figure 9.1).

- **Plyometrics** A training technique used to develop explosive power. Referred to as "speed-strength

training" in Eastern Europe and the former Soviet Union, where it originated. It consists of concentric isotonic muscle contractions performed after a prestretch or eccentric contraction of a muscle.

- **PRE** **P**rogressive **R**esistance **E**xercise, such as those done with free weights or weight machines.

- **Relative Strength** Amount of force one can exert in relation to one's body weight or per unit of muscle cross-section; that is, if a 100-pound person lifts 250 pounds, he or she has lifted 2.5 pounds per pound of body weight, and thus has more relative strength than a 250-pound person who lifts 500 pounds, or 2 pounds per pound of body weight. The latter has more absolute strength.

- **RM (Repetitions Maximum)** The maximum amount of resistance one can move a given number of times; for example
1 RM = maximum weight lifted one time;
6 RM = maximum weight one can lift six times.

- **Sticking Point** The point in the range of motion where the weight cannot be lifted any farther without extreme effort or assistance; the weakest point in the movement.

The Basic Facts About Strength

> There are three types of muscle tissue.

The three types of muscle tissue—smooth, cardiac, and skeletal—have different structures and functions. Smooth muscle tissue consists of long, spindle-shaped fibers; each fiber usually contains only one nucleus. The fibers are involuntary and are located in the walls of the esophagus, stomach, and intestines, where they function to move food and waste products through the digestive tract. Cardiac muscle tissue is also involuntary and, as its name implies, it is found only in the heart. Skeletal muscle tissues consist of long, cylindrical, multinucleated fibers. They provide the force needed to move the skeletal system and may be controlled voluntarily. Skeletal muscles are made up of slow- (red), intermediate-, and fast-(white) twitch fibers.

> Some experts suggest that strength training using high resistance exercises tends to selectively develop fast-twitch muscle fibers.

Fast-twitch fibers generate greater tension than slow-twitch fibers, but they fatigue more quickly. They primarily use anaerobic metabolism. These fibers are particularly suited to fast, high-force activities such as explosive weight lifting movements, sprinting, and jumping. Strength training primarily increases the size of fast-twitch fibers though intermediate fibers also increase in size and take on fast-twitch fiber characteristics with training.

An example of fast-twitch muscle fiber in animals is the white meat in the flying muscles of a chicken. The chicken is heavy and must exert a powerful force to fly a few feet up to a perch. A wild duck that flies for hundreds of miles has dark meat (slow-twitch fibers) in the flying muscles for better endurance.

> The amount of force you can exert during a strength test depends upon the speed of contraction, muscle length, warm-up, and other muscle-related factors.

If you want to score high on a strength test, consider some of the secrets of success used by experienced lifters and proven by research. Generally, a muscle exerts the least force as it becomes shorter (toward the end of a movement), and can exert more force during an isometric contraction than when it is shortening. The muscle exerts the most force when it is lengthening (lowering a weight). If a muscle is placed on a slight stretch immediately before it contracts, it can exert more force than it could if it started from a resting length.

Speed of contraction affects the amount of force that can be exerted. A slow contraction can lift a heavier weight than a fast contraction and it is safer. If muscles are warmed up before lifting, more force can be exerted and heavier loads can be lifted.

> Strength capacity differs with gender and age.

Women have less muscle mass than men and typically average 60 percent to 85 percent of the **absolute strength** of men. Women are as strong as men, however, in **relative strength.** Maximum strength is usually reached in the twenties and declines with age. Regardless of age or gender, strength can be improved.

The Facts: Principles of Training

> Strength is best developed by applying the "overload principle" so that exercise is done with a near maximum resistance with only a few repetitions.

In order to increase strength, the muscle must be contracted to at least 60 percent of its maximum. Strength training requires an overload in the amount of the resistance, while muscular endurance training (see concept 10) requires an overload in the number of repetitions. Therefore, according to the law of specificity, when designing a program for strength development, high resistance and low repetitions at a moderately slow speed should be used for maximum effectiveness.

When you begin strength training, there will be marked improvements during the first couple of weeks. This is primarily due to motor learning factors rather than to muscle growth. Thereafter, improvements will be slow and the changes will be the result of hypertrophy of the muscle.

> To develop strength it is often necessary to do exercises from the strength and muscular endurance exercise section of the Physical Activity Pyramid.

The activities in the first two levels of the physical activity pyramid do little to develop strength and very few people do exercise with enough overload to build strength in their normal daily activities. For most people it is necessary to select exercises from the third level of the pyramid if strength development is to occur (see figure 9.2).

> There is a threshold of training and a target zone for muscular strength development.

Experts generally agree that in **progressive resistance exercise (PRE)** using a maximum load (resistance) for three to eight repetitions in one to three sets three or four times per week will develop strength. Experts do *not* agree, however, on the ideal combination of repetitions, sets, and speed. At least one recent study suggests that doing just

there are "peaks" and "valleys" (tapering-off) that are associated with the sports schedule. Training normally begins with high repetitions and low resistance. The resistance is gradually increased and the repetitions are decreased as each climax approaches.

> A strength training program should apply the "principle of specificity" by closely resembling the activity for which the strength is needed.

Specificity of training will enhance performance. If you want your arms to be stronger so you can *carry* heavy loads, or if you want finger strength to *grip* a heavy bowling ball, much of your strength exercise should be done isometrically, using the arm muscles the way you use them to carry loads or using the fingers the same way you hold a bowling ball. On the other hand, if the task for which you are training is performed *isotonically,* your strength program should be primarily isotonic use of the muscles involved in that skill.

If you are training for a particular skill that requires *explosive power,* such as in throwing, striking, kicking, or jumping, your strength exercises should be done with less resistance and greater speed. If you are training for a skill that uses both **concentric** and **eccentric contractions** or is **plyometric,** you should perform strength exercises using these characteristics.

If you are not training for a specific skill, but merely wish to develop pure strength, then consider the advantages and disadvantages of isometrics, isotonics, and isokinetics listed in table 9.2. You may wish to use a variety of methods to avoid boredom.

> Training for cardiovascular endurance at the same time as strength training may prevent maximum results in both.

Studies have shown that simultaneously training for strength and cardiovascular endurance may not produce the same result as one could obtain while training for either one separately. Some people have interpreted this to mean that they interfere with each other. The cause of this is not clear. It may be that the time spent on each one is less or that overtraining occurs rather than the fact that one inhibits the other. Whatever the cause, the differences are relatively minor and it should not prevent an individual from doing both concurrently.

> Strength developed in one limb can be transferred to another unexercised limb.

When the right arm is trained until its strength increases, the unexercised left arm will also increase in strength, though not as much as the exercised arm. This phenomenon is called "transfer of training," "bilateral transfer," or "cross-education." The reason for this is not fully understood, but the phenomenon is sometimes applied in rehabilitation to prevent injured muscles from atrophying.

> Progressive resistance exercise (PRE) is the most effective type of strength training program.

Muscles adapt only to the load placed upon them; therefore, in order to continue increasing strength, you must

Table 9.2
Advantages and Disadvantages of Isometric, Isotonic, and Isokinetic Resistance Exercises[*]

	Isometrics (Statics)	Isotonics (Dynamics)	Isokinetics
In small space	E	F–G	F–G
No equipment or low-cost equipment	E	F–G	F–G
Provides feedback for motivation	P	E	F
Can rehabilitate immobilized joint	E	P	P
Builds strength through full range of motion	P	F–G	E
Less likely to cause soreness	E	F–G	E
Aids dynamic coordination	P	E	G
Safe for hypertensives	P	E	G–E
Amount of strength developed	F	E	E
Dynamic exercises and controlled testing	P	F–G	E
Hypertrophy	P	E	E
Power development	P	G	E
Rapid improvement in strength	E	F–G	F–G
Can accelerate to resemble sport skill	P	E	P

[*]Key: E = Excellent; G = Good; F = Fair; P = Poor

progressively increase the stress on the muscle as it adapts to each new load. Muscle groups differ in their strength potential, so each muscle group must have an individualized program (target zone). For example, the legs and trunk can usually lift greater loads than the arms.

> The "double progressive system" is an effective variation of the PRE system.

The double progressive system of progression periodically adjusts both the resistance and the number of repetitions. For example, you may begin with three repetitions for the arms. Once a week, you add one repetition. When you have progressed to eight repetitions, increase the weight by five pounds. Decrease the repetitions to three and begin the progression again.

Facts About Types of Resistance Training

> There are several good PRE programs for strength development, each having advantages and disadvantages.

Progressive resistance exercise can be performed in properly designed programs using free weights, constant resistance machines, variable (accommodating) resistance machines, isometrics, pulleys, calisthenics, springs, latex tubing, or isokinetic dynamometers. Machines may offer resistance by weight stacks, hydraulic or pneumatic pressure, or electrical resistance. (In concept 11 some sample exercises are described and some of these programs are compared). Weight training is considered the fastest and best method of improving strength. However, properly designed calisthenics are adequate for developing strength in most people.

> The most popular form of strength exercise utilizes isotonic contractions of the muscles.

Isotonic (also called **dynamic**) exercise refers to such activities as weight training, calisthenics, and pulley weights, in which the muscles alternately shorten concentrically and lengthen eccentrically. Typically, the stress on the muscle in these types of exercises varies with speed, joint position, and muscle length. Thus, the muscle may work harder at the beginning of a lift than it does near the end of the range of motion or as the weight is lowered.

Isokinetics, plyometrics, and "negative" exercises are special forms of isotonic exercise. These are discussed later in this concept.

> "Negative" exercise has no advantage over other types of exercise for strength development.

Contrary to the claims of some enthusiasts, there does not seem to be any difference between eccentric (negative) exercise and concentric (positive) exercise (see definitions) in terms of their effectiveness in developing strength. Eccentric exercise is performed more comfortably even though more weight can be handled. It is particularly useful in rehabilitation settings, but has a tendency to cause more muscle soreness. This type of exercise also requires the assistance of another person or the use of a special machine such as the Kin Com Biodex or Keiser dynamometers.

Eccentric contractions are combined with concentric contractions in most everyday activities and sports skills utilizing strength. For example, if you lift something you also lower it. Thus, to apply the law of specificity, some of the strength training for those activities should include both types of contractions. As noted in concept 3, eccentric contractions are more likely to cause muscle soreness than concentric contractions.

> Isometric strength exercises have advantages and disadvantages.

You can exert 15 percent to 20 percent more force with an isometric contraction than with a concentric one. Isometric exercises are effective for developing strength, require no equipment and only minimal space. They have been found to be quite useful for some athletes, such as wrestlers and gymnasts, and work especially well for people in the early stages of some rehabilitation programs. Research has shown that isotonic training can be enhanced significantly by using isometrics at the **sticking points** during isotonic lifts.

However, isometric exercises do not develop as much strength as isotonic and isokinetic exercises, nor do muscles hypertrophy as much. They work the muscle only at the angle of the joint used in the exercise. Isometrics may be dangerous for those with high blood pressure or cardiovascular disease. (See table 9.2 for a comparison with other types of exercise.)

> Isokinetic exercises are effective for developing strength.

Isokinetic exercises are isotonic-concentric muscle contractions performed on devices such as the Apollo, Exer-Genie, Mini-Gym, Hydra-Fitness (hydraulic machine) or on electromechanical dynamometers, such as the Cybex II. These machines keep the velocity of the movement constant and match their resistance to the effort of the performer, permitting maximal tension to be exerted throughout the range of motion. For example, on the Cybex II,

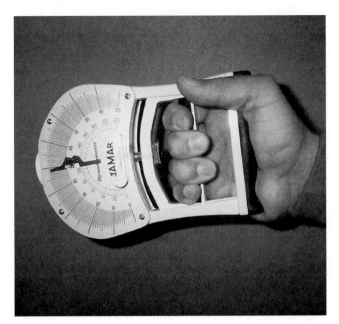
Isometric strength can be measured using a dynamometer.

speeds are possible from 0 to 300 degrees per second. This rate-limiting mechanism prevents the performer from moving faster no matter how much force is exerted.

Thus, isokinetic devices attempt to overcome the basic weakness of isotonics. On the other hand, these devices do not permit acceleration, so it is not possible to train specifically for sports skills, such as throwing or kicking, in which the limb is accelerated while applying maximum force, and some of these devices permit only concentric contractions.

Isokinetic exercise has the advantage of being safer than most other forms of exercise and may be better for developing power (see concept 11). It is not better for developing pure strength, however. More research is needed to determine the best training regimen for isokinetic exercise.

> Variable resistance machines have some advantages over constant resistance machines and free weights.

Some machines, such as Nautilus and Universal, offer what is called "variable" or "accommodating resistance." The Nautilus, for example, uses a cam to adapt the resistance as the performer moves through the range of motion. The Universal Trainer uses a rolling pivot to do the same thing. These adaptations attempt to compensate for the weakness in isotonic constant resistance exercises, but they are only partially successful in adapting to the shapes, sizes, and torques of individual human bodies. There is no evidence that variable resistance machines develop more strength than other devices, although they may strengthen a muscle through more of its range.

Table 9.3
Advantages and Disadvantages of Free Weights and Weight Machines

Free Weights	Weight Machines
• Requires balance and coordination; uses more muscles for stabilization.	• Other body parts are stabilized; easier to isolate particular muscle group.
• Truer to real-life situation, so skills transfer to daily life.	• Controlled path of weight not true to life.
• Creates more possibility of injury.	• Safer because weight cannot fall on participant.
• Requires spotters for safety.	• No spotters required.
• Takes more time to change weights.	• Easy and quick to change weights.
• Unlimited number of exercises possible.	• Restricted to range and angle of movement permitted by the machine.
• Less expensive.	• Expensive; need to go to club if cannot afford equipment; need more than one machine for variety.
• Loose equipment clutters area and may get lost or stolen.	• Machines are stationary but occupy large space.

> Free weights have some advantages and some disadvantages when compared to other methods of strength development.

Free weights include barbells and dumbbells, as well as homemade weights, such as sandbags or bottles filled with water. These are compared with weight machines (for example, Nautilus, Universal, Marcy, Hydra-Gym, Dynacam, and Paramount) in table 9.3. Both free weights and weight-stack machines are compared with other resistance machines in table 9.4.

Facts About Advanced Strength Training

> Resistance training may be used as a competitive sport or as a recreational sport and as a means to improve fitness, especially muscular strength, endurance, and power.

There are three competitive sports associated with resistance training. Olympic weight lifting competitors use free weights and compete in two exercises: the snatch, and the

Table 9.4
Comparison of Selected Resistance Training Devices

	Free Weights	Weight-stack Machine	Compressed Air Machine	Hydraulic Machine	Isokinetic Machine
Concentric resistance	+	+	+	+	+
Eccentric resistance	+	+	+	−	+−
Isometric resistance	+	+	+	+	−
Match resistance to effort through range of motion	−	+−	+	+	+
Isolation of all major muscle groups	−	+−	+	+	+
Safety features	−	+	+	+	+
Durability	+	+	+	+	+

From Wayne L. Wescott, "Strength Training" in *Sportcare & Fitness Magazine*, July/August 1988, page 62. Reprinted by permission of Wayne L. Westcott.

clean and jerk. Power lifting competitors use free weights and compete in three lifts: the bench press, squat, and dead lift. Body building competitors use several forms of resistance training, and are judged on muscular hypertrophy and **definition of muscle.**

Advanced "lifters" use heavier resistance than most people during strength training; therefore, they use some techniques not recommended for the beginner.

The compressive force on the lumbar disks during a half-squat can be six to ten times the body weight. To reduce the spinal compression, prevent abdominal hernias, and aid in lifting more weight, advanced lifters are encouraged to use a belt with a rigid abdominal pad and a wide band across the lumbar spine. At the same time, they hold their breath until they get past the "sticking point" of a lift. The belt must be loosened between reps to breathe and to allow the blood to return to the heart (Lander, et al. 1990). Holding the breath permits "trunk cavity pressurization" to relieve the load on the spine while the belt helps hold the abdominal contents in. Advanced lifting requires advanced training in proper techniques to avoid injury. Beginners should not attempt these lifts nor hold the breath, but they may wish to use the belts if they have a history of back problems.

Training for bulk and "definition" may differ from strength training.

Most body builders use three to seven sets of ten to fifteen repetitions, rather than the three sets of three to eight repetitions recommended for most weight trainers. Body builders are more interested in **hypertrophy** (large muscles) than in strength. Sometimes "definition" is difficult to obtain because it is obscured by fat. It should be noted that those with the largest looking muscles are not always the strongest.

Is There Strength in a Bottle? The Facts

Taking anabolic steroids is not a safe and effective way for normal, healthy people to develop fitness.

Anabolic steroids are prescription drugs—a synthetic reproduction of the male hormone testosterone. Physicians use them to treat such conditions as muscle diseases, breast cancer, severe burns, rare types of anemia, and kidney disease. Because of their dangerous side effects, doctors use them in minimal doses. They are obtained on the black market or from unethical physicians, coaches, or trainers by some body builders, athletes, and an increasing number of nonathletes to enhance their strength or improve their physique or appearance. Two million people are estimated to be using "roids." Steroids may be taken orally or injected. Usually they are taken in massive doses 20–100 times the normal therapeutic dose used for medical conditions. When combined with a resistance training program, they have been found to increase strength and muscle mass, but their *adverse side effects far outweigh any benefits. In women, unlike men, some of these effects are irreversible (see table 9.5).* As can be seen in the table, steroids (like all drugs) are dangerous. They can be addictive and produce more than seventy serious side effects, some of which may be fatal. Unfortunately, some studies show that many athletes who use anabolic steroids are familiar with the adverse effects, but say, "I don't care, I will use them anyway."

Injuries happen more easily and last longer in people who use steroids.

Even though steroids make muscles stronger, tendons and ligaments do not increase in strength proportionately. Therefore a strong muscle contraction can tear a tendon and/or a

Table 9.5
Adverse Effects of Anabolic Steroids

Gender	Physical	Psychological
M/F	• Cancer of liver	• Total personality changes
M/F	• Cardiac disease/early heart attacks	• Hostile and aggressive; violent behavior; sexual crimes
M/F	• Hypertension and increased risk of strokes	
M/F	• Edema (puffy face)	• Addiction (both psychological and physiological)
M/F	• Scalp hair loss** (baldness in men)	
M/F	• Nosebleeds	• Inability to accept failure
M/F	• Premature closure of growth plates of long bones	• Sleep disturbance (when cycled off drug)
M/F	• Immune system may be suppressed	• Depression
M/F	• Decreased HDL	• Apathy
M/F	• Decreased aerobic capacity	• Wide mood swings
M/F	• Altered glucose tolerance	• "Reverse anorexia" (eating compulsion)
M/F	• Severe acne (face, chest, upper back and thighs)*	
M/F	• Oily skin*	
M/F	• Muscle or bone injuries	
M/F	• Injuries take longer to heal	
M/F	• Fever	
M/F	• Frequent headaches	
M/F	• Sterility	
M/F	• Death	
M	• Testicular atrophy	
M	• Prostate enlargement	
M	• Decreased sperm count	
M	• Impotence	
M	• Feminine breast characteristics	
F	• Uterine atrophy	
F	• Decreased breast size	
F	• Menstrual irregularities	
F	• Clitoral enlargement	
F	• Deepening voice**	
F	• Dark facial hair**	

Key: M = Males; F = Females
*In women, only partially reversible when drug is stopped
**In women, irreversible when drug is stopped

ligament. This is made more serious because steroids make the injury heal more slowly. When steroids increase muscle size, the extra muscle can grow around the bones and joints, causing them to break more easily (Peterson, 1990).

> The use of anabolic steroids can cause people to die.

The violent behavior sometimes seen in users often referred to as "roid rage" has led to the serious injury and death of other people. Many users have died from hepatitis or HIV/AIDS infections from shared needles. Others have died from the cancers and heart disease attributable to the use of steroids. Twenty-five Soviet athletes who competed in the 1980 Olympics died because of conditions attributed to steroid use, and the deaths of several American professional athletes have also been attributed to anabolic steroid use. The death of Lyle Alzado, a former professional football star, was one of those attributed to steroid use.

> Human growth hormone (HGH) taken to increase strength may be even more dangerous than taking anabolic steroids.

HGH is produced by the pituitary gland but is made synthetically. Some athletes are taking it in addition to anabolic steroids or in place of anabolic steroids because it is difficult to detect in urine tests of competitors. It is believed to increase muscle mass and bone growth and hasten healing of tendons and cartilage; however, *its adverse effects can be deforming and life threatening*. They include the danger of irreversible acromegaly (giantism) and gross deformities, cardiovascular disease, goiter, menstrual disorder, excessive sweating, lax muscles and ligaments, premature bone closure, decreased sexual desire, and impotence. In addition, the life span can be shortened by as much as twenty years.

Another hormone being used by some male athletes is human chorionic gonadotropin (HCG), a substance found in the urine of pregnant women. It is being used to stimulate testosterone production before competition. The International Olympic (IOC) has banned its use, but no test has been developed to detect it.

> Some athletes have turned to dietary supplements and glandulars, which have been promoted as "safe substitutes" for anabolic steroids.

In an effort to avoid the undesirable side effects of anabolic steroids or the detection of its use by sports governing bodies who have banned it, some athletes or body builders are taking chemicals and supplements such as boron, chromium picolinate, gamma oryzanol and L-carnitine (see concept 22). There is also a considerable market for "glandulars" such as ground-up bull testes, hypothalamus and pituitary glands, hearts, livers, spleens, and brains. These products have been advertised as "steroid alternatives." Dietitians, the F.D.A., and the National Council Against

Health Fraud are alarmed at this practice and consider it potentially dangerous because these products have not been tested on humans or animals for safety and effectiveness. Very little is known about some of them. There is no published scientific evidence to substantiate claims for improved human performance. An article in The *Journal of the American Medical Association* has cautioned people concerning the use of "body building" supplements (Philen, et al. 1992).

The Facts About Proper Resistance Training Technique

There is a proper way to perform resistance training.

The following are some guidelines for safe and effective strength training for beginners:
- Make sure you are prepared from a medical standpoint to begin an exercise program (see concept 3).
- When beginning a weight program, start with weights that are too light so you can learn proper technique and avoid soreness and injury. Novices might, for example, start with one-fourth of their body weight for the military press; ten pounds less than the press for the curl; ten pounds more than the press for the bench press; and half of the body weight for back and leg exercises.
- Progress gradually. For example, use one set of three repetitions with a light weight to begin; add one or two repetitions when it gets easy, then another, until you reach eight repetitions; then drop back to three repetitions and add a second set. Repeat until you can do three sets. After this, the double progressive system (previously described) can be used, increasing the weight and the repetitions.
- Beginning weight trainers should probably train for endurance initially (see concept 10). For example, a reasonable goal might be ten to fifteen repetitions at 50 percent to 70 percent of the maximum amount of weight they can lift for one repetition.
- For health purposes, one set may be adequate for most people. Using up to 15 reps in one set can build modest amounts of both strength and endurance.
- Beginners should not attempt to use advanced techniques. After training for several months, you may wish to experiment with such things as supersets, split routines, and plateau systems used by advanced trainers.
- To ensure overall development, include all body parts and balance the strength of **antagonistic muscles.** For example, the ratio of quadriceps strength to hamstring strength should be 60:40. Exercise large muscles before small muscles.

- Athletes should train muscles the way they will be used in their skill, employing similar patterns, range of motion, and speed (the principle of specificity). This applies to anyone who knows the precise skill for which he or she is training.
- If you wish to develop a particular group of muscles, it is important to remember that it can be worked harder when it is *isolated* than when it is worked in combination with other muscle groups.
- Sports participants should include some eccentric training, such as plyometrics, to prevent injury to decelerating muscles during sports events and to develop power in accelerating muscles. Choose an exercise sequence that alternates muscle groups so muscles have a rest period before being used in another exercise.
- Make all movements through the full range of motion.
- Isometric training should be done at several joint angles.
- To avoid boredom, especially when you reach a plateau or sticking point, use such motivating techniques as music, record keeping, partners, competition, and variation in routine.
- To avoid overtraining, take a break by resting or choosing some other activity after eight to ten weeks. Also, try varying your training days so one is light (75 percent to 80 percent), one is medium (85 percent to 90 percent), and one is heavy (100 percent). It has been estimated that motivation can account for 10 percent to 15 percent of the score on a strength test. Varying the routine helps motivation.
- Lifters may reduce spinal and abdominal injury by using a belt which supports the back and abdomen.
- Unilateral training allows a muscle to exert more force than is possible when both sides of the body work simultaneously (bilaterally).

Most injuries can be prevented by using correct technique and proper care.

Refer to table 9.6 for some tips on injury prevention for the beginner.

The Facts: Common Misconceptions

There are many fallacies, myths, and superstitions associated with strength training.

Some common misconceptions about strength training have been refuted:
- It is *not* true that you will become muscle-bound and lose flexibility just because you do strength training. This could happen only if you train improperly. It has been found, however, that power lifters are less flexible than other weight lifters.

Table 9.6
How to Prevent Injury (for the Beginner)

- Warm up ten minutes before the workout and stay warm during the workout.
- Do not hold your breath while lifting. This may cause blackout or hernia.
- Avoid hyperventilation before lifting a weight.
- Avoid dangerous or high-risk exercises.
- Progress slowly.
- Use good shoes with good traction.
- Avoid arching your back. Keep the pelvis in normal alignment.
- Keep the weight close to the body.
- Do not lift from a stoop (bent-over with back rounded).
- Do not let the hips come up before your upper body when lifting from the floor.
- For bent-over rowing, put the head on a table and bend the knees or use one-arm rowing and support trunk with free hand.
- Stay in a squat as short a time as possible and do not do a full squat.
- Be sure collars are tight on free weights.
- Use a moderately slow, continuous, controlled movement and hold the final position a few seconds.
- Overload but don't overwhelm! A program that is too intense can cause injuries.
- Do not pause between repetitions.
- Try to keep a definite rhythm.
- Do not allow the weights to drop or bang.
- Do not train without medical supervision if you have a hernia, high blood pressure, fever, infection, recent surgery, heart disease or back problems.
- Use chalk or a towel to keep hands dry when handling weights.

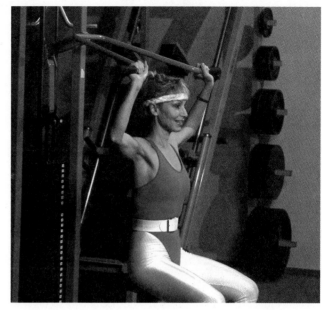

"No pain, no gain" is an exercise myth.

- It is *not* true that women will become masculine looking if they develop strength. Contrary to popular belief, most women will not be able to develop as large and bulky muscles as men, nor will their muscles be as well defined. On a heavy resistance training program, women and men make about the same percentage change in strength and hypertrophy. The greater percentage of fat in most women prevents the muscle definition possible in men and camouflages the increase in bulk. (Until CAT scans were used in research studies, it was not evident that women achieved hypertrophy at the same rate as men.)
- Strength training does *not* make you move more slowly or make you more uncoordinated. Up to a point, increased strength may help to increase speed.
- The expression *"no pain, no gain"* is a fallacy. It may be helpful to strive for a burning sensation in the muscle, but this is not painful. If it hurts, you are probably harming yourself.

- Food supplements are not ergogenic aids and do *not* benefit muscle mass or strength building. You do need a balanced diet, however.
- Drugs do *not* make you fit. Anabolic steroids, growth hormones, diuretics, narcotics, and other drugs taken to enhance performance are extremely dangerous and ultimately produce an unhealthy person rather than a fit one.
- Strength training is *not* effective for cardiovascular fitness, flexibility, or weight loss. Muscles will get firmer, and desirable changes may occur in girth, but other aspects of fitness are specific and require specific training.
- It does *not* require two hours to complete a workout in weight training—unless you are a competitive lifter or body builder. If you are training for athletics, you will need forty-five to ninety minutes; the beginner or the person training for fitness or recreation can complete a circuit in thirty to forty-five minutes.

Facts About Power

> Power is a combination of strength and speed, and is both health-related and skill-related.

Most experts classify power as a skill-related component of fitness (see concept 1) because it is partially dependent on speed. On the other hand, power is also dependent on strength and can be classified as a health-related component to the extent that strength is involved. Thus, power falls somewhere in between the two distinct groups of fitness attributes. Certainly its use is not limited to sports and dance. We use power extensively in our daily activities every time we apply a force to move something quickly. Power is important in protective movements, such as a pedestrian jumping to dodge a car or a driver jerking the steering wheel to avoid a collision or jamming on the brakes to stop in an emergency. A worker heaves a heavy load from a truck to a dock, and a carpenter uses force to hammer a nail.

Power is usually neglected in fitness literature and often in fitness programs as well. Garnica (1986) called it the "most functional mode in which all human motion occurs." If this is true, all fitness programs should consider appropriate exercises that develop power.

> The stronger person is not necessarily the more powerful.

Power is the amount of work per unit of time. To increase power, you must do more work in the same time or the same work in less time. If you extend your knee and move a 100-pound weight through a 90-degree arc in one second, you have twice as much power as a person who needs two seconds to complete the same movement. Power requires both strength and speed. Increasing one without the other limits power. Some "power athletes" (for example, football players) might benefit more by trying for less strength and more speed.

> There is probably no one best training program for developing power, but the law of specificity applies.

If you need power for an activity in which you are required to move heavy weights, then you need to develop *strength-related power* by working against heavy resistance at slower speeds. (See figure 9.2.) If you need to move light objects at great speed, such as in throwing a ball, you need to develop *speed-related power* by training at high speeds with relatively low resistance. There must be trade-offs between speed and power because the heavier the resistance, the slower the movement.

> There is a target zone for optimum power.

Studies show that power is best developed when the force is between 30 and 60 percent of maximum. But the optimum is probably when the load and the speed are about one-third of maximum (see figure 9.3). Stamford (1985) uses the following illustration of the relationship between speed, strength, and power. If your maximum strength is represented by 2 and maximum speed by 2, then your power is $2 \times 2 = 4$. If you double your strength ($4 \times 2 = 8$), your power would be doubled. However, if your strength and speed were increased by only 50 percent, then even more power results ($3 \times 3 = 9$).

> There are several effective techniques for developing power.

For specificity of training, as mentioned previously, much of an athlete's program should closely resemble the activity

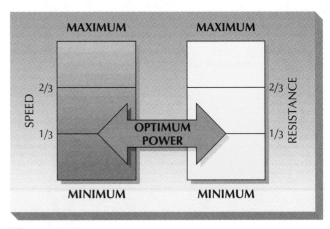

Figure 9.3
Optimum power is produced when the load and speed are each about one-third of maximum.

for which he or she is training, using similar speed, force, angle, range of motion, and so forth. However, if one is striving for all-around fitness or if an athlete is unable to perform the specific skill because of weather or injury or is seeking variety, then plyometrics, isokinetics, and weight training (especially with free weights or pulleys if simulating a sport skill) are effective means of developing power.

> Plyometrics may be useful in athletic training for certain sports events requiring power.

A quick prestretch, or eccentric contraction of a muscle, immediately followed by an isometric or concentric contraction can produce more power. This has been called "preexertion countermovement," "wind up," or "plyometrics." Soviet Olympic coaches pioneered this area, developing drills for their athletes. Track and field athletes may, for example, perform a hopping drill for thirty to one hundred meters. This is called "depth jumping," "drop jumping," or "bounce loading." As the body lands, some of the major leg muscles lengthen in an eccentric contraction, then follow immediately with a strong concentric contraction as the legs push off for the next jump or stride. The prestretch of the muscle during landing adds an elastic recoil that provides extra force to the push-off.

Plyometrics are used to apply the specificity principle to training for certain skills. Because eccentric exercise tends to result in more muscular soreness, it would be wise to proceed slowly with this type of training. It would also be important to have good flexibility before beginning a plyometrics program. Some guidelines are listed in table 9.7.

> Power exercises can increase muscular endurance or strength.

Power exercises done at high speeds have been shown to increase muscular endurance. Likewise, power exercises that use heavy resistance at lower speeds will increase strength.

Table 9.7
Safety Guidelines for Plyometrics

- Adolescents whose bones are still growing should avoid plyometric exercise (to avoid permanent growth-stunting damage to the growth plates).
- Progression should be gradual to avoid extreme muscle soreness.
- Adequate strength should be developed prior to plyometric training. (As a general rule, you should be able to do a "squat" with one and a half times your body weight.)
- Get a physician's approval prior to doing plyometrics if you have a history of injuries or if you are recovering from injury to the body part being trained.
- The landing surface should be semi-resilient, dry, and unobstructed.
- Shoes should have good lateral stability, be cushioned with an arch support, and have a nonslip sole.
- Obstacles used for jumping-over should be padded.
- The training should be preceded by a general and specific warm-up.
- The training sequence should:
  a. precede all other workouts (while you are fresh);
  b. include at least one spotter;
  c. be done no more than twice per week, with 48 hours rest between bouts;
  d. last no more than 30 minutes;
  e. (for beginners) include 3 or 4 drills, with 2 or 3 sets per drill, 10–15 reps per set and 1–2 minutes rest between sets.

Source: Data from G. Brittenham, "Plyometric Exercise: A Word of Caution" in *Journal of Physical Education, Recreation, and Dance,* January 1992: 20–23. American Alliance for Health, Physical Education, Recreation, and Dance, Reston, VA.

> The principle of specificity should be applied to training programs for power events.

Athletes who need explosive power to perform their events should use training that closely resembles the event. Jumpers, for example, should jump as a part of their training programs in order to learn correct timing at the same time they are developing power. This also applies to Olympic weight lifters, shot-putters, jumpers, ballet dancers, and others. These athletes need both strength and endurance; however, studies show that too much of either can have a negative effect on performance. If they use machines, it is better to use the leg press than a knee extension machine because the press more nearly resembles the leg action of the jump.

Suggested Readings

Garnica, R. A. "Muscular Power in Young Women after Slow and Fast Isokinetic Training." *Journal of Orthopaedic and Sports Physical Therapy* 8(1986):1.

Lander, J. E., et al. "The Effectiveness of Weight-Belts During the Squat Exercise." *Medicine and Science in Sports and Exercise* 22(1990):117–26.

Peterson, P. G. *About Steroids.* Santa Cruz, CA: ETR Associates, Network Publications, 1990.

Philen, R., et al. "Survey of Advertising for Nutritional Supplements in Health and Body Building Magazines." *Journal of the American Medical Association* 268(1992):1008.

Stamford, B. "The Differences between Strength and Power." *Physician and Sportsmedicine* 13(1985):155.

Stone, M. H., et al. "Muscle Conditioning and Muscle Injuries." *Medicine and Science in Sports and Exercise* 22(1990):210-31.

Westcott, W., *Strength Fitness.* 4th ed. Dubuque, IA: Brown & Benchmark. 1995.

Yesalis, C. *Anabolic Steroids in Sport and Exercise.* Champaign, IL: Human Kinetics Publishers, 1993.

LAB RESOURCE MATERIALS

Evaluating Isotonic Strength:
One Repetition Max (1 RM)

1. Use a weight machine for the leg press and bench press for the evaluation.
2. Estimate how much weight you can lift two or three times. Be conservative; it is better to start with too little weight than too much. This procedure will *not* work if you select a weight heavier than you can lift ten times. If you lift more than ten times, the procedure should be done again on another day when you are rested.
3. Using correct form (see page 137 concept 11), perform a leg press with the weight you have chosen. Perform as many times as you can up to 10.
4. Use chart 9.1 to determine your 1RM for the leg press. Find the weight used in the left-hand column and then find the number of repetitions you performed across the top of the chart.
5. Your 1RM score is the value where the weight row and the repetitions column intersect.
6. Repeat this procedure for the bench press using the technique described on page 139.
7. Record your 1RM scores for the leg press and bench press in the results section.
8. Next divide your 1RM scores by your body weight in pounds to get a "strength per pound of body weight" (str/lb/body wt.) score for each of the two exercises.
9. Finally determine your strength rating for your upper body strength (bench press) and lower body (leg press) using chart 9.2.

Chart 9.1 Predicted 1 RM Based on Reps-to-Fatigue

Wt	Repetitions										Wt	Repetitions									
	1	2	3	4	5	6	7	8	9	10		1	2	3	4	5	6	7	8	9	10
30	30	31	32	33	34	35	36	37	38	39	170	170	175	180	185	191	197	204	211	219	227
35	35	37	38	39	40	41	42	43	44	45	175	175	180	185	191	197	203	210	217	225	233
40	40	41	42	44	46	47	49	50	51	53	180	180	185	191	196	202	209	216	223	231	240
45	45	46	48	49	51	52	54	56	58	60	185	185	190	196	202	208	215	222	230	238	247
50	50	51	53	55	56	58	60	62	64	67	190	190	195	201	207	214	221	228	236	244	253
55	55	57	58	60	62	64	66	68	71	73	195	195	201	206	213	219	226	234	242	251	260
60	60	62	64	65	67	70	72	74	77	80	200	200	206	212	218	225	232	240	248	257	267
65	65	67	69	71	73	75	78	81	84	87	205	205	211	217	224	231	238	246	254	264	273
70	70	72	74	76	79	81	84	87	90	93	210	210	216	222	229	236	244	252	261	270	280
75	75	77	79	82	84	87	90	93	96	100	215	215	221	228	235	242	250	258	267	276	287
80	80	82	85	87	90	93	96	99	103	107	220	220	226	233	240	247	255	264	273	283	293
85	85	87	90	93	96	99	102	106	109	113	225	225	231	238	245	253	261	270	279	289	300
90	90	93	95	98	101	105	108	112	116	120	230	230	237	244	251	259	267	276	286	296	307
95	95	98	101	104	107	110	114	118	122	127	235	235	242	249	256	264	273	282	292	302	313
100	100	103	106	109	112	116	120	124	129	133	240	240	247	254	262	270	279	288	298	309	320
105	105	108	111	115	118	122	126	130	135	140	245	245	252	259	267	276	285	294	304	315	327
110	110	113	116	120	124	128	132	137	141	147	250	250	257	265	273	281	290	300	310	321	333
115	115	118	122	125	129	134	138	143	148	153	255	255	262	270	278	287	296	306	317	328	340
120	120	123	127	131	135	139	144	149	154	160	260	260	267	275	284	292	302	312	323	334	347
125	125	129	132	136	141	145	150	155	161	167	265	265	273	281	289	298	308	318	329	341	353
130	130	134	138	142	146	151	156	161	167	173	270	270	278	286	295	304	314	324	335	347	360
135	135	139	143	147	152	157	162	168	174	180	275	275	283	291	300	309	319	330	341	354	367
140	140	144	148	153	157	163	168	174	180	187	280	280	288	296	305	315	325	336	348	360	373
145	145	149	154	158	163	168	174	180	186	193	285	285	293	302	311	321	331	342	354	366	380
150	150	154	159	164	169	174	180	186	193	200	290	290	298	307	316	326	337	348	360	373	387
155	155	159	164	169	174	180	186	192	199	207	295	295	303	312	322	332	343	354	366	379	393
160	160	165	169	175	180	186	192	199	206	213	300	300	309	318	327	337	348	360	372	386	400
165	165	170	175	180	186	192	198	205	212	220	305	305	314	323	333	343	354	366	379	392	407

This chart is used as modified with permission from the *Journal of Physical Education, Recreation & Dance,* January, 1993, p. 89. *JOPERD* is a publication of the American Alliance for Health, Physical Education, Recreation and Dance, 1900 Association Drive, Reston, VA 22091.

Evaluating Isometric Strength

Test

Grip Strength

Adjust a hand dynamometer to fit your hand size. Squeeze it as hard as possible. You may bend or straighten the arm, but do not touch the body with your hand, elbow, or arm. Perform with both right and left hands. *Note:* When not being tested, perform the isometric strength exercises in concept 11, or try to squeeze and indent a new tennis ball (*after* completing the dynamometer test).

Evaluating Leg Muscle Power

Test

Long Jump

Lie on a mat and have your partner mark your body length (height) from head to toe on the mat. Perform a standing long jump the distance of your body height if possible. Make two jumps and measure the better of the two.

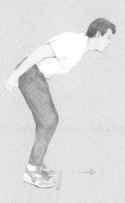

Evaluating Isotonic Strength (Body Weight Test)

Directions: Within each group of exercises, start with the one that you believe is the most difficult one that you can perform. If you can pass it, try the next most difficult one. You receive points for the most difficult exercise that you can perform for each type. *Note:* M = point values for males and F = point values for females.

I. Push-Up: Tests pectorals, triceps, abdominals, and other muscles. (It is a failure if the hips pike or sag.)

Tests	Point values
1. One bent-knee push-up, keeping your body straight and rigid. Bend elbows until chest or nose touches floor.	M=0 F=3

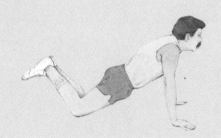

	Point values
2. One straight-leg push-up, keeping your body rigid.	M=3 F=6

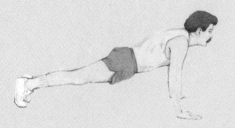

	Point values
3. One declined push-up (straight-leg push-up), keep your body rigid and your feet on the bench.	M=6 F=8

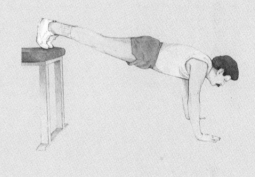

	Point values
4. One partner push-up. Same as no. 2 except have partner do a push-up on back of your shoulders at the same time.	M=8 F=10

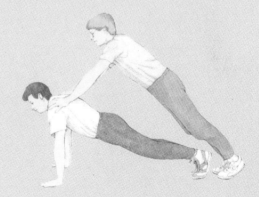

5. One one-arm push-up. Same as no. 2, except use only one arm.

Point values

M=10

F=12

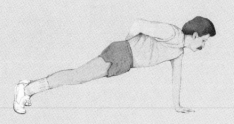

II. Pull-up: Tests biceps, latissimus, rhomboids, trapezius, and other muscles.

Tests

1. One inclined pull-up.
  a. Hang from a bar placed at the height of the lower end of your sternum.
  b. Body should be inclined at a forty-five degree angle.
  c. Have partner brace your feet or brace against bench or wall.
  d. Pull up until your chin or chest touches the bar.

Point values

M=1

F=3

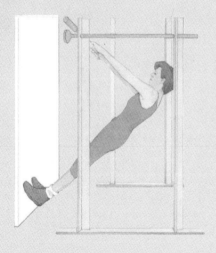

2. One bent-arm hang.

Stand on a chair and assume a position with palms facing body, elbows bent, and chin over bar.
  a. Assistant remove chair.
  b. Slowly lower yourself, taking eight seconds to extend the elbows.

Point values

M=3

F=6

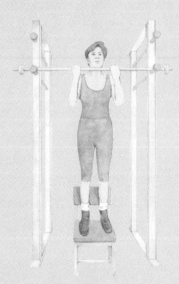

3. One standard pull-up.

Pull-up from a hanging position with palms facing your body.

Point values

M=6

F=8

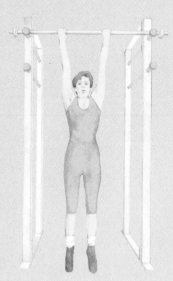

4. One weighted pull-up. Same as no. 3 except two bleach bottles filled with water (2 lbs. each) are suspended on the ends of a short rope across the back of your neck. (A towel may be used to pad the neck to prevent discomfort caused by the rope.)

Point values

M=8

F=10

5. Climb a rope to a height of ten feet above your head, using arms only (no leg use). *Caution:* Use a mat and spotters for safety.

Point values

M=10

F=12

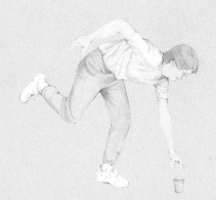

III. One-Leg Squat: Tests hip and knee extensors (quadriceps, gluteals, hamstrings, etc.).

Test

1. One one-leg squat and pick up a paper cup with one hand; return to a stand. Keep the back erect and maintain balance.
   a.   Use one leg only.
   b.   Use right leg only, then use left only.

Point values

M/F=3

M/F=6

IV. Trunk Lift: Tests the strength of the upper back and neck muscles.

Test

1. One trunk lift. Lie prone. Lift your upper trunk until the sternum leaves the floor (do not lift higher than 12 inches). Keep your feet on the floor (partner may hold feet if necessary).
   a.   Place the hands under the thighs.

Point values

M/F=3

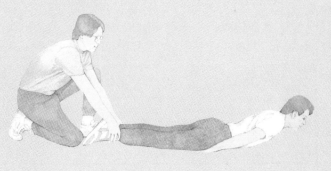

   b.   Same as "a," except clasp the hands behind the neck.

Point values

M/F=6

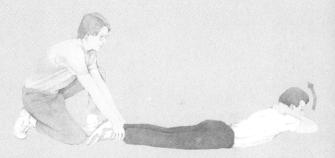

   c.   Same as "a," except extend both arms forward and clamp them against the ears.

Point values

M/F=8

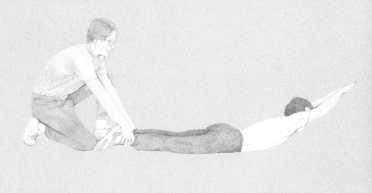

Chart 9.2 Strength Per Pound of Body Weight Ratings

Men

Rating Age	Leg Press 30 or Less	31–50	51+	Bench Press 30 or Less	31–50	51+
High Performance	2.06+	1.81+	1.61+	1.26+	1.01+	.86+
Good Fitness	1.96–2.05	1.66–1.80	1.51–1.60	1.11–1.25	.91–1.00	.76–.85
Marginal	1.76–1.95	1.51–1.65	1.41–1.50	.96–1.10	.86–.90	.66–.75
Low Fitness	1.75 or less	1.50 or less	1.40 or less	.96 or less	.80 or less.	.65 or less

Women

Rating Age	Leg Press 30 or Less	31–50	51+	Bench Press 30 or Less	31–50	51+
High Performance	1.61+	1.36+	1.16+	.75+	.61+	.51+
Good Fitness	1.46–1.60	1.21–1.35	1.06–1.15	.65–.75	.56–.60	.46–.50
Marginal	1.31–1.45	1.11–1.20	.96–1.05	.56–.65	.51–.55	.41–.45
Low Fitness	1.30 or less	1.10 or less	.95 or less	.55 or less	.50 or less	.40 or less

Chart 9.3 Isotonic Strength *Rating Scale* (Men and Women)

Classification	Age 17–26	27–39	40–49	50–59	60+
High Performance zone	31+	28+	28+	26+	24+
Good fitness zone	24–30	22–27	22–27	20–25	19–23
Marginal zone	19–23	17–21	15–21	14–19	12–18
Low Zone	<19	<17	<15	<14	<12

Chart 9.4 Isometric Strength *Rating Scale* for Men (Pounds)

Classification	Left Grip	Right Grip	Total Score
High performance zone	125+	135+	260+
Good fitness zone	100–124	110–134	210–259
Marginal zone	90–99	95–109	185–209
Low zone	<90	<95	<185

Chart 9.5 Isometric Strength *Rating Scale* for Women (Pounds)

Classification	Left Grip	Right Grip	Total Score
High performance zone	75+	85+	160+
Good fitness zone	60–74	70–84	130–159
Marginal zone	45–59	50–69	95–129
Low zone	<>45	<>50	<>95

Charts 2 and 3 are suitable for use by young adults between 18 and 30 years of age. After 30, an adjustment of 0.5 of 1 percent per year is appropriate because some loss of muscle tissue typically occurs as you grow older.

Chart 9.6 *Rating Scale* of Leg Power (Men)

Age	17–26	27–39	40–49	50–59	60+
CLASSIFICATION	Length of Jump (by height)				
High performance zone	ht.+	ht.+	¾ fht.+	¾ fht.+	½ dht.+
Good performance zone	¾ fht.	¾ fht.	½ dht.	½ dht.	½ dht.
Marginal zone	½ dht.	½ dht.	⅓ hht.	⅓ hht.	⅓ hht.
Low zone	<½ dht.	<½ dht.	<⅓ iht.	<⅓ hht.	<⅓ hht.

*Because power is a skill-related fitness component and relates more to performance than to health, "good performance zone" is used rather than "good fitness zone."

Chart 9.7 *Rating Scale* of Leg Power (Women)

Age	17–26	27–39	40–49	50–59	60+
Classification	Length of Jump (by height)				
High performance zone	¾ fht.+	¾ fht.+	¾ fht.+	⅔ iht.+	½ dht.+
Good performance zone	⅔ iht.	⅔ iht.	½ dht.	½ dht.	⅓ hht.
Marginal zone	½ dht.	½ dht.	⅓ hht.	⅓ hht.	¼ bht.
Low zone	<½ dht.	<½ dht.	<⅓ hht.	<⅓ hht.	<¼ bht.

*Because power is a skill-related fitness component and relates more to performance than to health, "good performance zone" is used rather than "good fitness zone."

CONCEPT ·10·

Muscular Endurance

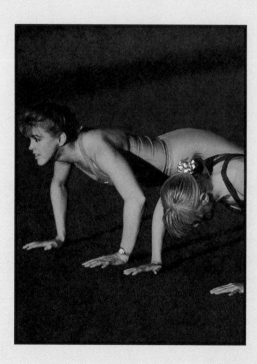

Concept 10

Muscular endurance is an important health-related component of physical fitness.

Introduction

When considering training programs, it is difficult to isolate **muscular endurance,** strength, and power from one another since a program designed specifically to develop one of these components would also tend to develop the other attributes to some degree. Muscular endurance is often neglected in discussions of fitness programs, and it is usually mentioned only in connection with strength, as if they were the same thing. Yet, experts agree that muscular endurance is a distinct and separate component of health-related fitness and that it requires a specific training program.

Health Goal for the Year 2000

- Increase the proportion of people who engage in activity to enhance muscular strength, muscular endurance, and flexibility. (<>)

Note: (↑) indicates progress toward goal, (↓) indicates regression from goal, and (< >) indicates either no change or lack of new data since 1990.

Terms

Also see concept 9 terms.

- **Absolute Muscular Endurance (Dynamic type)** Endurance measured by the maximum number of repetitions (muscle contractions) one can perform against a given resistance; for example, the number of times you can lift 50 pounds in a bench press.

- **Dynamic Muscular Endurance** A muscle's ability to contract and relax repeatedly. This is usually measured by the number of times (repetitions) you can perform a body movement in a given time period. It is also called isotonic endurance.

- **Muscular Endurance** Fatigability of the skeletal muscles.

- **Relative Muscular Endurance (Dynamic type)** Endurance measured by the maximum number of repetitions one can perform against a resistance that is a given percentage of one's 1RM; for example, the number of times you can lift 50 percent of your 1RM.

- **Static Muscular Endurance** A muscle's ability to remain contracted for a long period. This is usually measured by the length of time you can hold a body position. It is also called isometric endurance.

Some Facts About Muscular Endurance

Benefits of Muscular Endurance

Muscular endurance is an important health-related component of physical fitness.

Muscular endurance is the capacity of a skeletal muscle or group of muscles to continue contracting over a long period. When you have good muscular endurance, you have the ability to resist fatigue and you can hold a position or carry something for a long period. You also have the ability to repeat a movement without getting tired.

When muscles become fatigued, they do not completely relax between contractions and are more susceptible to injury, and the rate of contraction slows, so less work is done. One's ability to withstand fatigue depends partly upon inheritance, partly upon the ability to tolerate pain and discomfort, and partly upon proper training. In the absence of fatigue, there is greater success and enjoyment in daily work activities and in athletic and recreational endeavors.

Good muscular endurance provides many other benefits.

In addition to providing resistance to fatigue, research has shown that a program (low load, high volume) of sufficient intensity can reduce cardiovascular disease risk by enhancing your blood lipid profile (increasing the HDL and decreasing cholesterol). Good muscular endurance also increases the static strength of bones, ligaments, and tendons. One study indicates it may be even more important than strength in preventing back problems (Holmstrom et al. 1992).

It also increases lean body mass, and produces small changes in body girth and skinfolds. (Noticeable changes in body weight and muscle hypertrophy, however, should *not* be expected.)

This is the type of training that beginning resistance trainers should engage in before using heavy resistance for strength; it is also believed to be safer for pregnant women, adolescents, and the elderly than high-load strength training.

Muscular endurance training tends to develop the slow-twitch fibers in your muscles.

As you train specifically for muscular endurance, the muscles adapt as a result of changes in slow-twitch fibers, including increased activity of aerobic enzymes in the muscle. Strength training, on the other hand, tends to produce changes in fast-twitch fibers, including increased activity of anaerobic enzymes.

Facts About Principles of Training

The overload principle applies to muscular endurance.

Though strength is developed by high resistance overload with low repetitions, **dynamic muscular endurance** requires just the opposite: higher repetitions and lower resistance. The ideal combination for maximum endurance is not known at this time. One study suggests that after progressing to twenty-five repetitions, it may be more effective to increase the resistance and keep the repetitions constant.

To develop **static muscular endurance,** the overload principle is applied by progressively increasing the length of time the muscles remain contracted against an immovable resistance and increasing the number of repetitions.

There is a threshold of training and a target zone for muscular endurance exercises.

There is a level of frequency, intensity, and time at which a training effect will begin to take place (threshold). There is also an optimal range, or target zone, where the most effective and efficient improvement will occur (see table 10.1). We do not know the exact range, but studies suggest that it has wide limits. The intensity, or resistance (load), is less important than the number of repetitions or the length of time a muscle contracts.

A muscular endurance training program should apply the principle of specificity by closely resembling the activity for which the endurance is needed.

Muscular endurance is specific to the muscles being used, the type of muscle contraction (static or dynamic), the speed or cadence of the movement, and the amount of resistance being moved.

For example, if you want endurance in the elbow flexor muscles (e.g., biceps), you must train those muscles. Performing muscular endurance exercise for the elbow extensor (e.g., triceps) or the leg muscles will not improve the muscular endurance of the biceps. Likewise, if you are trying to develop endurance for a dynamic task, you should do isotonic or isokinetic exercises. If you need endurance to hold you in a static position, do isometric exercises. If the activity requires a rapid movement, it is better to train with fast movements. There may be transfer from fast practice to slow movement in a skill, but the reverse is not necessarily true.

Garhammer (1986) believes that athletes wishing to develop muscular endurance for a particular sport may benefit more from performing the sport skill repeatedly than from doing special exercises such as resistance training. If injury or weather prevents practice of the sport, then resistance training for endurance would be an effective alternative.

> Muscular endurance is slightly related to cardiovascular endurance, but it is not the same thing.

Cardiovascular endurance depends primarily upon the efficiency of the heart muscle, circulatory system, and respiratory system. It is developed with activities that stress these systems, such as running, cycling, and swimming. Muscular endurance depends upon the efficiency of the local skeletal muscles and the nerves that control them. You might train for cardiovascular endurance by running, but if the leg muscles lack the muscular endurance to continue contracting for more than five minutes, the cardiovascular system will not be stressed, even if it is in good condition.

> Muscular endurance is related to strength, but is different.

Studies show that the person who is strength-trained will fatigue as much as four times faster than the person who is endurance-trained. However, there is a slight correlation between strength and endurance because the person who trains for strength will develop some endurance, and the person who trains for muscular endurance will develop some strength.

The graph in figure 10.1 illustrates the relationship between strength and **absolute muscular endurance.** In *A,* the training program calls for a high number of repetitions and light resistance. This results in a small gain in strength (the area of the bar to the right of the line), and a large increase in absolute endurance (the area of the bar to the left of the line). In *B,* the training program calls for a moderate number of repetitions (less than in *A*), and a moderate resistance (more than in *A*). This results in slightly less absolute endurance and slightly more strength than in program *A.* Program *C* results in the least gain in endurance and the most gain in strength because it uses high resistance and low repetitions. Thus, if you are primarily interested in muscular endurance, program *A* is your optimal choice.

> Some endurance tests penalize the weaker person.

If you are tested on absolute endurance (the number of times you can move a designated number of pounds), a stronger person has an advantage. However, if you are tested on **relative muscular endurance** (the number of times you can move a designated percentage of your maximum strength), the stronger person does not have an advantage, and men

Table 10.1
Muscular Endurance Threshold of Training and Fitness Target Zone

	Threshold of Training	Target Zone
Dynamic Endurance		
Frequency	• 2 days per week.	• Every other day.
Intensity	• Move 20%–30% of the maximum resistance you can lift.	• Move 40%–70% of the maximum resistance you can lift.
Time	• One set of 9 repetitions of each exercise.	• 2–5 sets of 9–25 repetitions. • Rest 15–60 sec. between sets.
Static Endurance		
Frequency	• 3 days per week.	• Every other day.
Intensity	• Hold a resistance 50%–100% of the weight you ultimately will need to hold in your work or leisure activity.	• Hold a resistance equal to and up to 50% greater than the amount you will need to hold in your work or leisure activity.
Time	• Hold for lengths of time 10%–50% shorter than the time you plan to do the activity. Repeat 10–20 times.	• Hold for lengths of time equal to and up to 20% greater than the time you plan to do the activity. For longer times, use fewer repetitions (5–10).
	• Rest 30 sec. between reps.	• Rest 30–60 sec. between reps.

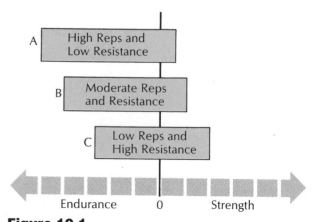

Figure 10.1
Comparison of absolute endurance and strength developed by different exercise regimens

and women can compete more evenly. In fact, on some tasks women have done as well or better than men on endurance. For example, the women at West Point Military Academy do as well as the men on sit-up tests.

> Strength training will not help you improve your relative endurance.

This is illustrated in the research study on which the graph in figure 10.1 was based. When the relative endurance of the three training groups was calculated, it was discovered that although the low rep-high resistance group had a 20 percent increase in absolute endurance, it actually decreased 7 percent in relative endurance (table 10.2).

> Muscular endurance and strength are part of the same continuum.

As mentioned previously, muscular strength and muscular endurance are similar but different. They are part of the same continuum (figure 10.2). This has led some writers to refer to muscular endurance as "strength endurance." "Pure" strength is approached as one nears the end (right) of the continuum, where only one maximum contraction is made. As the number of repetitions increases and the force of the contractions decreases, one nears the other end (left) of the continuum and approaches "pure" endurance. In between the two extremes varying degrees of strength and endurance are combined. The activities listed along the continuum are examples that might represent points along the scale.

Facts About Training Programs

> There are a variety of effective programs for developing muscular endurance.

All methods used in strength development are applicable to endurance development. Resistance training, calisthenics, isometrics, isokinetics, and such activities as running, swimming, circuit training, and aerobic dance can all be designed to increase muscular endurance. Even games, such as rope climbing, tug-of-war, Indian wrestling, and hopping races can contribute to muscular endurance. Figure 10.3 illustrates an isokinetic endurance training device used by swimmers.

> One popular method of training for muscular endurance is Circuit Resistance Training (CRT).

Circuit resistance training for muscular endurance consists of the performance of high repetitions of an exercise with low to moderate resistance, progressing from one

Table 10.2
Absolute versus Relative Endurance: Percentage Change Due to Different Training Regimes

	Absolute Endurance	Relative Endurance
Low resistance/high reps	5%	28%
Medium resistance/medium reps	8%	22%
High resistance/low reps	20%	7%

From T. Anderson and J. T. Kearney, "Effects of Three Resistance Training Programs on Muscular Strength and Absolute and Relative Endurance" in *Research Quarterly for Exercise and Sport*, 53:4, 1982. This article is reproduced with permission from American Alliance for Health, Physical Recreation, and Dance, Reston, VA 22091.

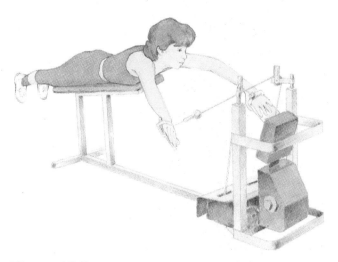

Figure 10.3
Isokinetic training device for swimmers

Repetitive Sub-Maximal Contractions ← | Assembly Line Work | Tournament Tennis | Construction Work | Varsity Wrestling | Olympic Weight Lift | → Single Maximum Contraction

Figure 10.2
Muscular strength-endurance continuum

station to another performing a different exercise at each station. The stations are usually placed in a circle. CRT typically employs about twenty to twenty-five reps against a resistance that is 30 to 40 percent of 1RM for forty-five seconds. Fifteen seconds of rest is provided while changing stations. Approximately ten exercise stations are used, and the participant repeats the circuit two to three times (sets). A sample circuit is included in the Lab Resource Materials.

Circuit training on weight or hydraulic machines has been found to be more effective than standard set weight training for caloric consumption during and after exercise and for improving cardiovascular endurance, although it is not as effective as aerobic exercises such as cycling or bench stepping.

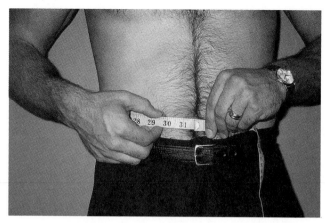

Exercise may help body measurements, but does not spot-reduce body fat.

> High-intensity endurance is best trained by multiple sets rather than by one set of repetitions to exhaustion.

There has been a long-running debate over which is more effective for developing muscular endurance: a single set of exercise to exhaustion, or the traditional method of multiple sets. Recent studies have shown that the traditional method is superior.

> Exercises to slim the figure/physique should be of the muscular endurance type.

Many men and women are interested in exercises designed to decrease girth measurements. High repetition, low resistance exercise is suitable for this because it usually brings about some strengthening and some decrease in skinfold and girth, which in turn, changes body contour. Exercises *do-not* spot-reduce fat. (See concept 22.) Endurance exercises do speed up metabolism so more calories are burned, though if weight or fat reduction is desired, aerobic (cardiovascular) exercises are best. To increase girth, strength exercises such as those power lifters use for hypertrophy and/or a weight gain program are best (see concept 9).

> Endurance training may have a negative effect on strength and power.

Some studies have shown that for athletes who rely primarily on strength and power in their sports event, too much endurance training can cause a loss of strength and power because of modification of different muscle fibers. Strength and power athletes need some endurance training, but not too much, just as endurance athletes need some strength and power training, but not too much.

> Some training methods can interfere with athletic performance.

Some research studies have shown that certain techniques used in training may actually cause a decrease in performance. For example, when distance runners were trained with weighted wristlets, anklets, and belts, they performed worse than runners who did not wear weights in training. In another study, people who were running and bicycling for aerobic endurance six days per week combined those exercises with a strength training program five days per week. The results yielded a decrease in strength development near the upper limits.

> Guidelines for muscular endurance training programs are the same as those for strength development.

The performance guidelines for safety and effectiveness presented in concept 9, should be reviewed before starting a program of exercise. It is particularly important that all muscle groups are exercised. For example, if your program for cardiovascular fitness stresses the muscles of the legs (front and back), then these might be omitted from your muscular endurance program and special attention given to the muscles on the inside and outside of the legs, and the muscles of the trunk and upper extremities.

Suggested Readings

Holmstrom, E., et al. "Trunk Muscle Strength and Back Muscle Endurance in Construction Workers With and Without Low Back Disorders." *Scandinavian Journal of Rehabilitation Medicine* 24(1992):3–10.

Wilmore, J., and D. Costill. *Physiology of Sport and Exercise.* Champaign, IL: Human Kinetics Publishers, 1994.

Work, J. A. "Is Weight Training Safe During Pregnancy?" *Physician and Sports Medicine* 17(1989):257.

LAB RESOURCE MATERIALS

Evaluating Muscular Endurance

1. Curl-Up (Dynamic)

Sit on a mat or carpet with your legs bent more than 90 degrees so your feet remain flat on the floor (about half way between 90 degrees and straight). Make two tape marks four ½ inches apart or lay a four ½ inch strip of paper or cardboard on the floor. Lie with your arms extended at your sides, palms down and the fingers extended so that your finger tips touch one tape mark (or one side of the paper or cardboard strip). Keeping your heels in contact with the floor, curl the head and shoulders forward until your fingers reach four ½ inches (second piece of tape or other side of strip). Lower slowly to beginning position. Repeat one curl-up every three seconds. Continue until you are unable to keep the pace of one curl-up every three seconds.

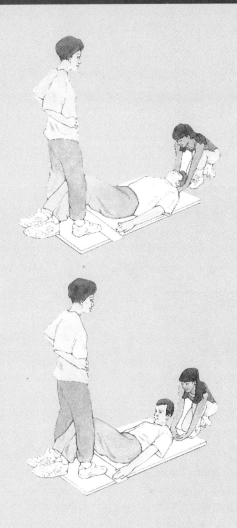

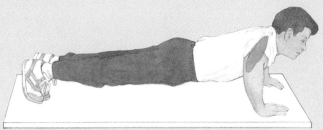

2. Ninety-Degree Push-Up (Dynamic)

Support the body in a push-up position from the toes. The hands should be just outside the shoulders, the back and legs straight, and the toes tucked under. Lower the body until the upper arm is parallel to the floor or the elbow is bent at 90 degrees. The rhythm should be approximately one push-up every three seconds. Repeat as many times as possible up to 35.

3. Flexed-Arm Support (Static)

Women: Support the body in a push-up position from the knees. The hands should be outside the shoulders, and the back and legs straight. Lower the body until the upper arm is parallel to the floor or the elbow is flexed at 90 degrees. *Men:* Use the same procedure as for women except support the push-up position from the toes instead of the knees. (Same position as for 90 degree push-up, see above.) Hold the 90-degree position as long as possible, up to 35 seconds.

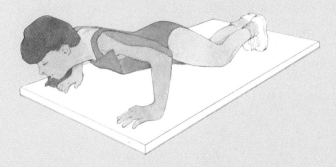

Chart 10.1 Rating Scale for Dynamic Muscular Endurance (Men)

Age	17–26		27–39		40–49		50–59		60+	
Classification	Curl-Up	Push-Ups	Curl-Up	Push-Ups	Curl-Up	Push-Ups	Curl-Up	Push-Ups	Curl-Up	Push-Ups
High performance zone	35+	29+	34+	27+	33+	26+	32+	24+	31+	22+
Good fitness zone	24–34	20–28	23–33	18–26	22–32	17–25	21–31	15–23	20–30	13–21
Marginal zone	15–23	16–19	14–22	15–17	13–21	14–16	12–20	12–14	11–19	10–12
Low zone	<15	<16	<14	<15	<13	<14	<12	<12	<11	<10

Chart 10.2 Rating Scale for Dynamic Muscular Endurance (Women)

Age	17–26		27–39		40–49		50–59		60+	
Classification	Curl-Up	Push-Ups	Curl-Up	Push-Ups	Curl-Up	Push-Ups	Curl-Up	Push-Ups	Curl-Up	Push-Ups
High performance zone	25+	17+	24+	16+	23+	15+	22+	14+	21+	13+
Good fitness zone	18–24	12–16	17–23	11–15	16–22	10–14	15–21	9–13	14–20	8–12
Marginal zone	10–17	8–11	9–16	7–10	8–15	6–9	7–14	5–8	6–13	4–7
Low zone	<10	<8	<9	<7	<8	<6	<7	<5	<6	<4

Chart 10.3 Rating Scale for Static Endurance (Flexed-Arm Support)

Classification	Score In Seconds
High performance zone	30+
Good fitness zone	20–29
Marginal zone	10–19
Low zone	<10

CONCEPT ·11·

Strength and Muscular Endurance Exercises

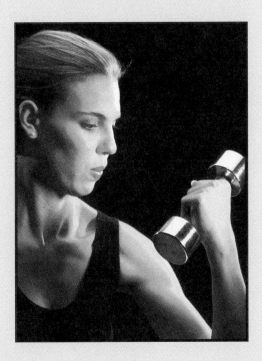

Concept 11

Strength exercises should be performed against a near maximum resistance using only a few repetitions. Endurance exercises require only a moderate resistance, but a high number of repetitions.

Introduction

There are several kinds of strength and endurance exercises. Among the most popular are *isotonic (dynamic) calisthenics,* which require little or no special equipment; *isometric (static) exercises,* which can be done in a small space; and *progressive resistance exercises* (PRE), which can be performed isotonically or isokinetically. The machines pictured in this concept may look different than the machines you will be using but the exercises will probably be very similar.

Health Goal for the Year 2000

— Increase the proportion of people who engage in activity to enhance muscular strength, muscular endurance, and flexibility. (<>)

Note: (↑) indicates progress toward goal, (↓) indicates regression from goal, and (<>) indicates either no change or lack of new data since 1990.

Terms

Refer to the terms in concepts 9 and 10.

The Facts

Calisthenic exercises are among the most popular forms of exercise among adults.

Calisthenics, such as curl-ups and push-ups, are suitable for people of different ability levels, and can be used to improve both strength and muscular endurance. One disadvantage is that this type of exercise does little to increase strength unless more resistance is added. For example, doing a push-up will build strength to a point. However, once you can do several, adding more repetitions will only build muscular endurance but *not* strength. To develop additional strength, you can add more weights to increase the resistance or change the body position so there is a greater gravitational effect or more torque. For example, you can elevate your feet or wear a weighted vest while doing push-ups. Some calisthenics that you can do at home are illustrated on pages 128–132.

Resistance training with "free weights" is a popular form of isotonic progressive resistance exercise.

Free weights are weights that are not attached to a machine or exercise device. Typically, they come in the form of a barbell which can be adjusted as necessary for different exercises to provide optimal resistance or dumbbells which can be held in one hand. Weight training with free weights is very popular because it can be done in the home with inexpensive equipment. Homemade barbell weights can even be constructed from pieces of pipe and plastic bottles filled with water. Elastic tubes or bands may be substituted for the weights. These are available in varying strengths. Some exercises that are good for developing strength and muscular endurance are illustrated on pages 133–136.

Exercise with resistance training machines, pulley exercisers, and isokinetic machines have become more popular and more accessible in recent years.

Resistance training machines can be effective in developing strength and muscular endurance if used properly. They can save time because unlike free weights, the resistance can be changed easily and quickly. They are also safer because you are less likely to drop weights on machines. A disadvantage is that the kinds of exercises that can be done on these machines are more limited than those for free weights. Elastic bands or tubes may be substituted for the pulley device in these exercises. Some good exercises using resistance training machines and pulley exercisers are illustrated on pages 137–140. Isokinetic exercises are also illustrated.

Isometric exercise is an effective and inexpensive way to build strength and muscular endurance.

Isometric exercise is an attractive form of exercise because it is effective in building strength and muscular endurance, and can be done in the home, office, or car, in a limited space and with little or no equipment. All that is necessary to do many isometric exercises is a piece of rope or a towel, and a doorway. It may be hard for some people to motivate themselves when performing isometrics because of the lack of movement involved. Also, isometric exercises may elevate blood pressure, and for that reason, those who have cardiovascular problems should be under the supervision of a physician when involved in them. Recent evidence indicates that for normal, healthy individuals, isometrics do not cause cardiovascular problems. Some good isometric exercises are illustrated on pages 142–147.

Sample Isotonic Exercises for Muscular Endurance and Mild Strengthening

The exercises suggested here should be performed as described until you are able to increase the repetitions to approximately twenty-five. Additional weight should then be added. Muscles depicted in color are those primarily involved in the exercises.

1. Full-Length Push-Ups

Purpose

Develop muscles of the arms, shoulders, and chest.

Position

Take front-leaning rest position, arms straight.

Movement

Lower chest to floor. Press to beginning position in same manner. Repeat. *Caution:* Do not arch back.

Variation

90-degree push-up: From the "up" position, lower until elbows are at a 90-degree angle.

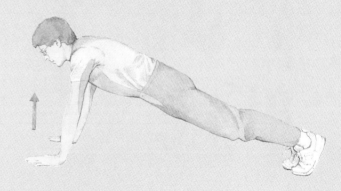

2. Bent-Knee Push-Ups

For those who cannot do full-length push-ups.

Purpose

Develop muscles of the arms, shoulders, and chest.

Position

Assume the push-up position, but rest the weight on the knees, not the feet.

Movement

Lower the body until the chest touches the floor; return to the starting position keeping the body straight. Repeat. *Caution:* Do not arch back. For 90-degree push-up see variation in exercise 1, above.

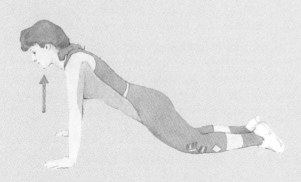

3. Bent-Knee Let-Downs

For those who cannot do bent-knee push-ups.

Purpose

Develop muscles of the arms, shoulders, and chest.

Position

Same as a bent-knee push-up position.

Movement

Slowly lower body to the floor, keeping the body line straight; return to the starting position in any manner. Repeat. *Caution:* Do not arch back.

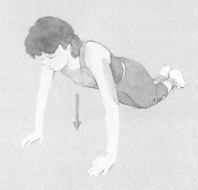

4. Modified Pull-Ups

Purpose

Develop muscles of the arms and shoulders.

Position

Hang (palms forward and shoulder width apart) from a low bar (may be placed across two chairs), heels on floor, with the body straight from feet to head. Bracing the feet against a partner or fixed object is helpful.

Movement

Pull up keeping the body straight, touch the chest to the bar, then lower to the starting position. Stronger persons should perform exercise 5 (pull-up). Repeat.
Note: This exercise is more difficult as the angle of the body approaches horizontal and easier as it approaches the vertical.

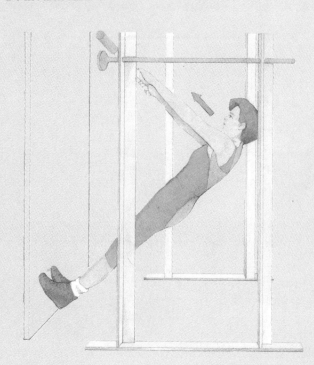

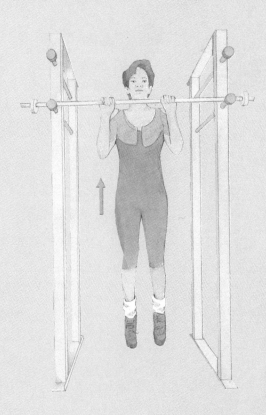

5. Pull-Ups (Chinning)

Purpose

Develop muscles of the arms and shoulders.

Position

Hang from bar, palms forward, body and arms straight.

Movement

Pull up until chin is over bar. Repeat.
Note: When palms are turned away from the face, pull-ups tend to use all the elbow flexors. With palms facing the body, the biceps are emphasized more.

6. Reverse Curl

Purpose

Develop the lower abdominal muscles and correct abdominal ptosis.

Position

Lie on the floor. Bend the knees, place the feet flat on the floor, and place arms at sides.

Movement

Lift the knees to the chest, raising the hips off the floor; do not let the knees go past the shoulders. Return to the starting position. Repeat.

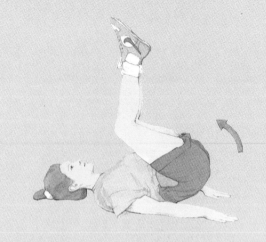

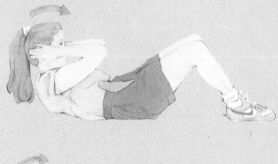

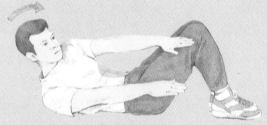

7. Crunch (Curl-Up)

Purpose

Develop the upper abdominal muscles and correct abdominal ptosis.

Position

Assume a hook-lying position with arms extended or crossed with hands on shoulders or palms on ears. If desired, legs may rest on bench to increase difficulty. For less resistance, place hands at side of body (do *not* put hands behind neck). For more resistance, move hands higher.

Movement

Curl up until shoulder blades leave floor, then roll down to the starting position. Repeat. *Note:* Twisting the trunk on the curl-up develops the oblique abdominals.

8. Leg Extension Exercise

Purpose

Develop muscles of the hips.

Position

Assume a knee-chest position, hands on floor with arms extended as far as possible.

Movement

Extend right leg upward in line with trunk, then lower, keeping it straight. Continue repetitions. Repeat with other leg. An ankle weight may be added to increase intensity. *Caution:* Do not allow back to arch, or leg to move higher than a line through the trunk.

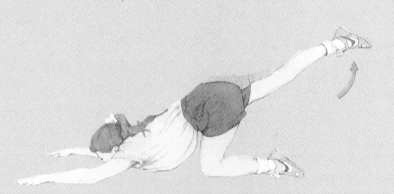

9. Upper Back (Trunk) Lift

Purpose

Develop muscles of the upper back. Correct kyphosis and round shoulders.

Position

Lie prone (face down) with hands clasped behind the neck.

Movement

Pull the shoulder blades together, raising the elbows off the floor. Slowly raise the head and chest off the floor by arching the upper back. Return to the starting position; repeat. For less resistance hands may be placed under thighs. *Caution:* Do not arch the lower back; lift only until the sternum (breast bone) clears the floor.

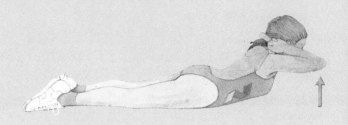

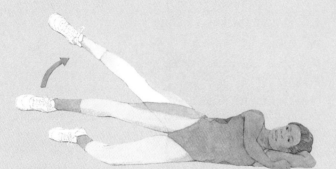

10. Side Leg Raises

Purpose

Develop muscles on the outside of thighs.

Position

Lie on the side. Point knees forward.

Movement

Raise the top leg 45 degrees, then return. Do the same number of repetitions with each leg. *Caution:* Keep knee and toes pointing forward.
Note: Ankle weights may be added for greater resistance.

11. Lower Leg Lift

Purpose

Develop muscles on the inside of thighs.

Position

Lie on the side with the upper leg (foot) supported on a bench. *Note:* If no bench is available, bend top leg and cross it in front of bottom leg for support.

Movement

Raise the lower leg toward the ceiling; repeat. Roll to opposite side and repeat. Keep knees pointed forward.
Note: An ankle weight may be added for greater resistance.

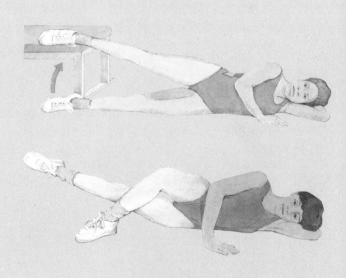

12. Alternate Leg Kneel

Purpose

Develop muscles of the legs and hips.

Position

Stand tall, feet together.

Movement

Take a step forward with the right foot, touching the left knee to the floor. The knees should be bent only to a 90-degree angle. Return to the starting position and step out with the other foot. Repeat, alternating right and left.
Note: Dumbbells may be held in the hands for greater resistance.

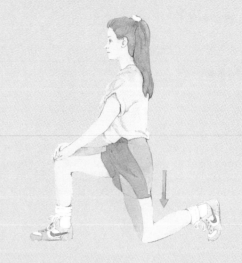

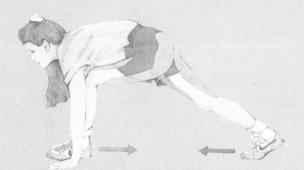

13. Stationary Leg Change

Purpose

Develop muscles of the legs and hips.

Position

Crouch on the floor with weight on hands, left leg bent under the chest, right leg extended behind. Avoid bending front knee beyond 90 degrees.

Movement

Alternate legs; bring right leg up while left leg goes back. Repeat.

14. Knee-to-Nose Touch/Kneeling Leg Extensions

Purpose

Strength or endurance of lumbar and gluteal muscles; stretch low back.

Position

Kneel on all fours.

Movement

Pull knee toward nose, then extend leg horizontally (do not go higher). Repeat. Alternate legs.

Variations:

a. Keep knee extended as leg is raised and lowered.
b. Keep upper back straight and pull knee only to chest.
Note: For greater resistance, an ankle weight may be added.

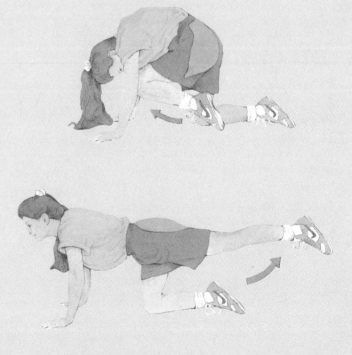

Sample Free Weight Training Exercises

These exercises may be used for strength or for muscular endurance. Muscles depicted in color are those primarily involved in the exercises. Before performing these exercises review resistance training guidelines. (*Note:* Dumbbells, elastic bands or tubes may be substituted for barbells.) Beginners should breathe normally or exhale on the lift and inhale on the return. *Caution:* Spotters should be used for most free weight exercises to (1) place the weight in the lifter's hands (or take it from the lifter after the set) and (2) to be prepared to take the weight if the lifter begins to lose control or balance.

15. Shoulder Shrug

Purpose

Strengthen the muscles of the shoulder girdle.

Position

Stand with palms toward body, bar touching thighs, legs straight, and feet together. *Tighten abdominals and back muscles.*

Movement

Lift shoulders (try to touch ears) then roll shoulders smoothly backward, down, and forward. Repeat. *Caution:* Do not lock knees.
Spotters: usually not needed.

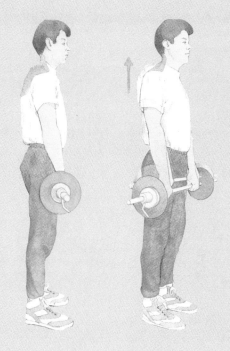

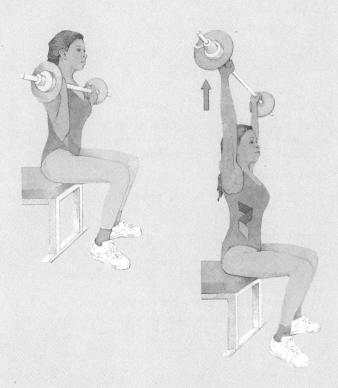

16. Overhead (Military Press)

Purpose

Strengthen the muscles of the shoulders and arms.

Position

Sit erect, bend elbows, palms facing forward at chest level, hands spread (slightly more than shoulder width). Have bar touching chest, spread feet (comfortable distance). *Tighten abdominals and back muscles.*

Movement

Move bar to overhead position (arms straight). Lower to chest position. Repeat. *Caution:* Keep arms perpendicular and do not allow weight to move backwards or wrists to bend backward.
Spotters: are needed.

17. Half-Squat

Purpose

Strengthen the muscles of the thighs and buttocks.

Position

Stand erect, feet turned out 45 degrees. Rest bar behind neck on shoulders. Spread hands in a comfortable position.

Movement

Squat slowly, keeping back straight, eyes ahead. Bend knees to 90 degrees; keep knees over feet. Pause, then stand. Repeat. Spotters: are needed.

Variations:

a. Substitute dumbbell in each hand at sides.
b. Take a lunge step forward and recover backward.

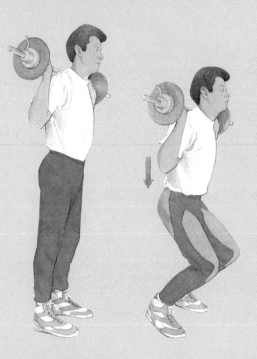

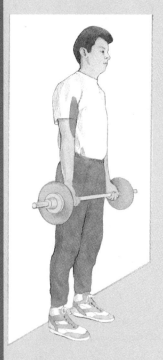

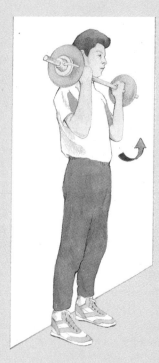

18. Biceps Curl

Purpose

Strengthen the muscles of the upper front part of the arms (biceps).

Position

Stand erect with back against a wall, palms forward; bar touching thighs. Spread feet in comfortable position. Tighten abdominals and back muscles. Do not lock knees.

Movement

Move bar to chin, keeping body straight and elbows near the sides. Lower to original position. Do not allow back to arch. Repeat.
Spotters: are usually not needed.

Variations:

a. Use dumbbell and sit on end of bench with feet in stride position. Work one arm at a time.
b. Hands may be turned palm down or thumb up (with dumbbells) to emphasize other muscles.

19. Triceps Curl

Purpose

Strengthen the muscles on the back of the upper arms (triceps).

Position

Sit erect, elbows and palms facing up. Bar resting behind neck on shoulders, hands near center of bar, feet spread. Tighten abdominals and back muscles.

Movement

Keep upper arms stationary. Raise weight overhead, return bar to original position. Repeat.
Spotters: are needed.

Variation:

Substitute dumbbells (one in each hand, or one held in both hands, or one in one hand at a time).

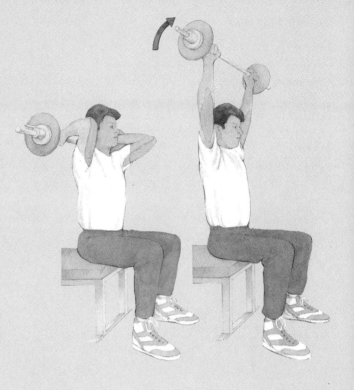

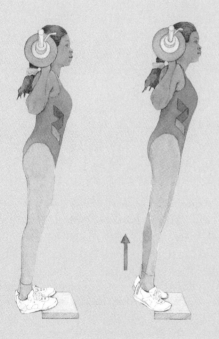

20. Heel Raise

Purpose

Strengthen muscles of the legs (calf).

Position

Stand erect with palms facing forward, hands wider than shoulder width apart, bar resting behind neck on shoulders. Rest balls of feet on two-inch block with heels on floor. Toes together, heels apart.

Movement

Rise on toes quickly, hold for one second. Lower heels to floor. Repeat. Keep toes turned in slightly.
Spotters: are needed.
Note: Some people do this with toes straight ahead or turned out, however this tends to weaken the foot muscles.

21. Upright Row

Purpose

Strengthen muscles of the shoulders and arms.

Position

Stand erect with palms facing body (loose), hands together at center of bar, bar touching thighs, feet spread, head erect, eyes straight ahead. Tighten the abdominals and back muscles.

Movement

Pull bar to chin. Keep bar close to body and elbows well above bar. Lower to extended position. Repeat. Do not arch back or lock knees.
Spotter: usually not needed.

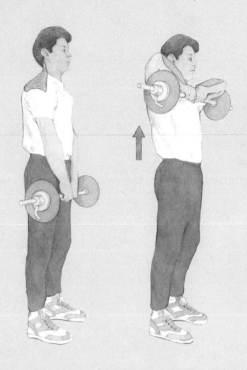

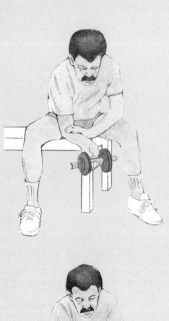

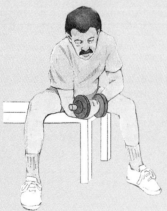

22. Wrist Curl

Purpose

Strengthen the fingers, wrist, and forearm muscles.

Position

Sit astride a bench with the back of one forearm on the bench, wrist and hand hanging over the edge. Hold a dumbbell in the fingers of that hand with the palm facing forward.

Movement

To strengthen the flexors, lift the weight by curling the fingers, then the wrist through a full range of motion. Slowly lower and repeat. To strengthen the extensors, start with the palm down (forearm pronated). Lift the weight by extending the wrist through a full range of motion. Slowly lower and repeat.

Note

Both wrists may be exercised at the same time by substituting a barbell in place of the dumbbell.

Sample Resistance Training Machine/Pulley Exercises

These exercises may be used for strength or for muscular endurance. Before performing these exercises, review resistance training guidelines. Muscles depicted in color are those primarily involved in the exercises.

23. Biceps Curl (Low Pulley)

Purpose

Strengthen the elbow flexor muscles on front of arm.

Position

Stand erect, arms at sides, palms up. *Tighten abdominals and back muscles.* Grasp bar.

Movement

Flex elbows, bringing bar to chest. Keep elbows pressed against sides. Lower; repeat; do not allow back to arch or lock knees.

Variation:

Turn palms down or, if handle permits, thumbs up.

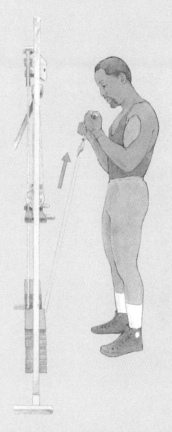

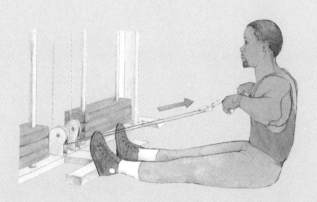

24. Seated Rowing (Low Pulley)

Purpose

Develop the upper arms and back of shoulders.

Position

Sit facing pulley, feet braced and knees slightly bent. Grasp bar, palms down with hands shoulder width apart.

Movement

Pull bar to chest, keeping elbows high and return; repeat.

25. Leg Press

Purpose

Develop the thigh and hip muscles.

Position

Sit on chair with feet on pedals, knees bent to right angle. Grasp handles.

Movement

Extend legs and return; repeat. Do not lock knees when legs straighten. Where two sets of pedals are available, the lower pedal emphasizes thigh muscles, the upper pedal emphasizes hip (gluteal) muscles.

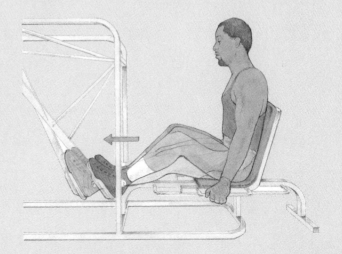

26. Lat Pull-Down (High Pulley)

Purpose

Develop the latissimus ("lats"), biceps, and pectorals ("pecs").

Position

Tailor sit or kneel on both knees or sit on bench. Grasp bar with palms facing away from you, hands shoulder distance apart.

Movement

Pull bar down to chest and return; repeat.

Variations

Turn palms toward face or move hands out to ends of bar, or pull bar behind head.

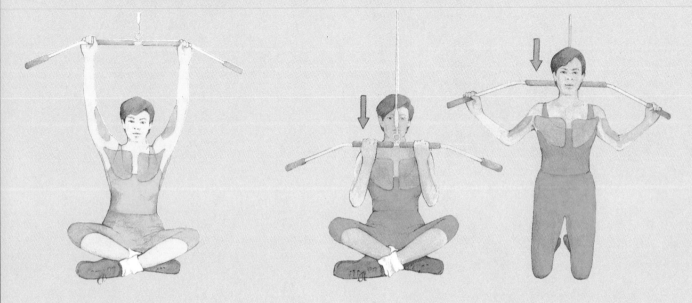

27. Triceps Curl

Purpose

Develop the triceps and other muscles on back of arm.

Position

Stand erect. Grasp bar near center, palms down. Tighten abdominals and back muscles.

Movement

With elbows clamped against sides, pull bar down to thighs and return to chest height without moving elbows. *Caution:* Do not lock knees or arch back; repeat.

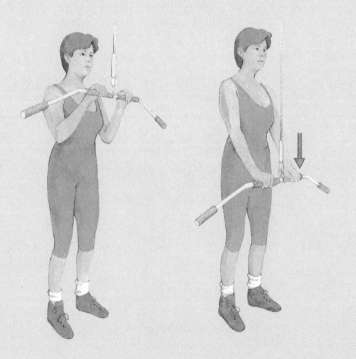

28. Bench Press

Purpose

Develop the chest (pectoral) and triceps muscles.

Position

Lie supine on bench with knees bent and feet flat on bench or flat on floor in stride position. Grasp handles at shoulder level.

Movement

Push bar up until arms are straight. Return; repeat; do not arch lower back.

Note: feet may be placed on floor if lower back can be kept flattened. Do not put feet on bench if unstable.

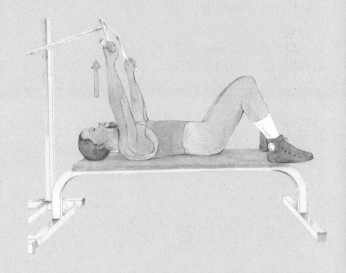

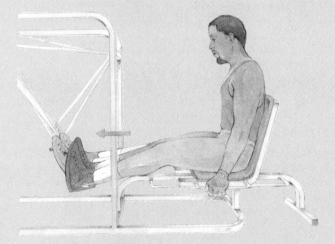

29. Ankle Press

Purpose

Develop the calf muscles.

Position

Sit at leg press station with legs straight. Grasp handles. Put ball of foot at lower edge of pedal.

Movement

Keeping knees straight, point toes by extending (plantar flexing) ankles. Return; repeat.

30. Knee Extension

Purpose

Develop the thigh (quadriceps) muscles.

Position

Sit on end of bench with ankles hooked under padded bar. Grasp edge of table.

Movement

Extend knees. Return; repeat.
Note: This exercise isolates the quadriceps but places greater stress on the structures of the knee than the leg press or half squat. (Signorile, et al 1994)

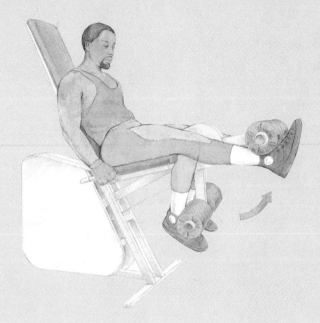

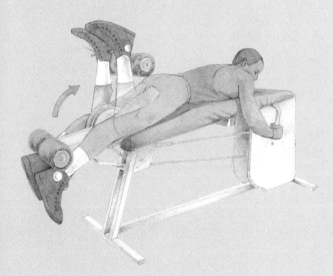

31. Hamstring Curl

Purpose

Develop the hamstrings (muscles on back of thigh) and other knee flexors.

Position

Lie prone on bench with ankles hooked under padded bar. Rest chin on hands or grasp bench.

Movement

Flex knees as far as possible without allowing hips to raise. Return; repeat.
Caution: Do not hyperextend the knees while assuming the starting position. If necessary, ask a partner to raise the pads while you place the heels under the bar.

Strength/Endurance Exercise Circuits

Exercise equipment companies have developed resistance machine circuits which allow you to perform exercises for most of the major muscle groups of the body. A typical exercise circuit is listed below. Exercises are placed in an order that allows you to "rotate" muscle groups to produce optimal benefits. If you do not have a machine or set of machines at your disposal you can create your own circuit using free weights, calisthenics, and other exercises. Some other common circuit exercises are described below the typical circuit.

Typical Circuit

1. **Biceps Curl.** Exercise 23, page 137.
2. **Leg Press.** Exercise 25, page 137.
3. **Bench Press.** Exercise 28, page 139.
4. **Crunch or Curl-Up.** Exercise 7, page 130.
5. **Lat Pull-Down.** Exercise 26, page 138.
6. **Ankle Press.** Exercise 29, page 139.
7. **Seated Rowing.** Exercise 24, page 137.
8. **Wrist Curl.** Exercise 22, page 136.
9. **Triceps Curls.** Exercise 27, page 138.
10. **Upper Back (Trunk) Lift.** Exercise 9, page 131.
11. **Hamstring Curls.** Exercise 31, page 140.

Other Common Circuit Exercises (not included above)

1. **Overhead (Military) Press.** A military press station allows a person to perform an exercise similar to the free weight exercise #16, page 131.
2. **Abdominal (tilt) Board.** The curl-up (see exercise #4 above) in the circuit can be performed on a tilt board to increase resistance. Some machines have special "ab" stations.
3. **Upper Back (Trunk) Lift.** A specialized (trunk lift) bench allows a person to lift the trunk with the feet anchored and the pelvis supported on a pad. This is an advanced form of the trunk lift (see exercise #10 above) and is not for beginners. Care should be taken at this station to avoid back arch and to lift only until the back is parallel to the floor.
4. **Hip Flexion.** A hip flexion station allows a person to support the body weight on the forearms so that the hips are flexed as the legs are lifted (bent or straight). Note: exercises done at such a station may be hazardous to the back. Most people *do not* need to strengthen the hip flexors. Single leg and/or bent knee lifts are less hazardous than double leg lifts.
5. **Dead Lift.** A dead lift station is often the same as the low pulley station. The dead lift is *not* recommended. The Seated Rowing exercise (#7 above) is a good substitute.
6. **Chinning.** A pull-up station can be used to build the same muscles of the arm that are developed by the Biceps Curl and Lat Pull-down station's (see #1 and #5 above). The pull-up exercise is illustrated on page 129.
7. **Dipping.** A dipping station can be used to build the same muscles of the arms that are developed by the Triceps Curl and Bench Press stations (see #3 and #9 above). The various forms of the push-up exercise illustrated on pages 128 build most of the same muscles as dipping.
8. **Wrist Curl.** A wrist exercise station allows development of the wrist flexors and extensors. Exercise #22 on page 136 accomplishes the same purpose.
9. **Hand Grip.** A grip exercise station allows development of the muscles of the hand and forearm to improve grip strength. Squeezing a tennis ball, a hand gripper (available from sporting good stores), or a grip dynamometer will accomplish the same purpose. Exercise #34 on page 140 also builds isometric grip strength.
10. **Neck.** A neck station allows development of the neck muscles. Performing exercise #35 on page 141 and #1 and #5 on page 126 and 127 will accomplish the same purpose.

Note: The authors would like to thank Universal Gym Equipment for their willingness to supply literature and illustrations that were most helpful in the development of this section of the book.

Sample Isometric Exercises

Isometric exercises are intended primarily to develop muscular strength and endurance. Eighteen different exercises for different body parts are presented here. You should select exercises for your program (if you choose isometric exercise) that meet your own personal needs. All of the following exercises should be held for six to eight seconds and should be repeated several times a day. Muscles depicted in red are those primarily involved in the exercises. *Caution:* If you have high blood pressure, see your physician before doing these exercises. To make these exercises isotonic, elastic bands or tubes may be used for resistance.

32. Chest Push

Purpose

Develop muscles of the chest and upper arms.

Position

Place left fist in palm of right hand. Keep hands close to chest, forearms parallel to floor.

Movement

Push hands together with maximum effort.

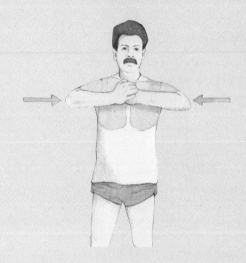

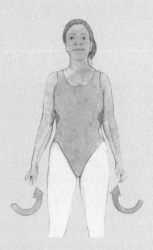

33. Fist Squeeze

Purpose

Develop muscles of the lower arm.

Position

Arms extended at side.

Movement

Clench fists as hard as possible. Repeat.

34. Shoulder Pull

Purpose

Develop muscles of the upper back and arms.

Position

Cup hands and interlock fingers or grasp opposite wrists. Keep hands close to chest, forearms parallel to floor.

Movement

Attempt to pull hands apart with maximum effort.

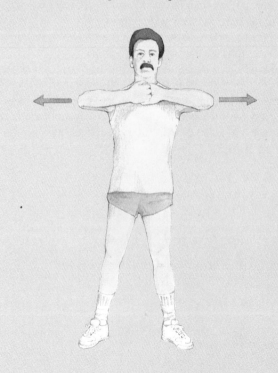

35. Neck Pull

Purpose

Develop muscles of the neck, upper back, and arms.

Position

Interlock fingers behind head, elbows pointing forward; head and neck erect.

Movement

Pull hands forward with maximum effort; resist with neck muscles. Keep chin down.

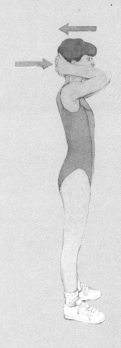

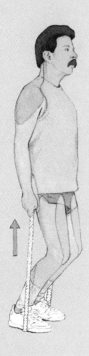

36. Leg Extension

Purpose

Develop muscles of the shoulders, legs, and hips.

Position

Loop rope under feet. Stand on rope (or towel), feet spread shoulder width. Keep back straight. Bend knees, grasp both ends of rope, back erect, arms straight, and buttocks low.

Movement

Try to straighten legs by lifting upward with maximum effort.

37. Overhead Pull

Purpose

Develop muscles of the arms.

Position

Fold rope in a double loop (or grasp towel). Grasp rope overhead, palms outward. Pull hands apart.

Movement

Push outward with maximum force. Repeat with palms turned in.

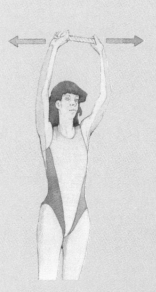

38. Curls

Purpose

Develop muscles on the front of the arms.

Position

Place rope (towel) loop behind thighs while standing in a half-squat position. Grasp loop, palms up, shoulder width apart.

Movement

Lift upward with maximum effort. For reverse curls, repeat, gripping with palms down.

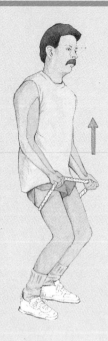

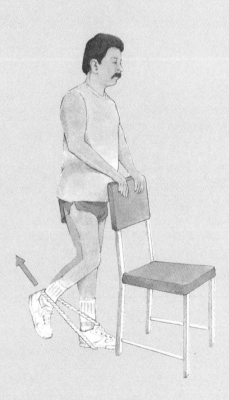

39. Foot Lift

Purpose

Develop muscles on back of legs.

Position

Stand on loop with left foot. Place loop around right ankle. Flex knee until taut.

Movement

Apply maximum force upward. Repeat forward and to side with each foot.

40. Overhead Press in Doorway

Purpose

Develop muscles of the arms and shoulders.

Position

Stand in doorway, face straight ahead, hands shoulder width apart, elbows bent.

Movement

Tighten leg, hip, and back muscles. Push upward as hard as possible.

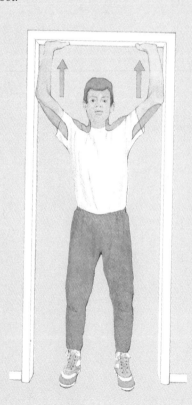

41. Arm Press in Doorway

Purpose

Develop tricep and pectoral muscles.

Position

Stand in doorway, back flat on one side of doorway, hands placed on other side.

Movement

Push with maximum force.

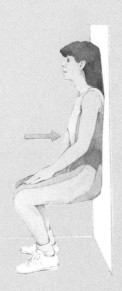

42. Leg Press in Doorway

Purpose

Develop muscles of the legs and hips.

Position

Sit in doorway facing side of door frame. Grasp molding behind head. Keep back flat on side of doorway, feet against other side.

Movement

Push legs with maximum force.

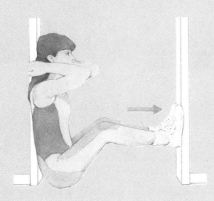

43. Wall Seat

Purpose

Develop muscles of the leg and hips.

Position

Assume half-sit position, back flat against wall, knees bent to 90 degrees.

Movement

Push back against wall with maximum force.

44. Triceps Press

Purpose

Develop muscles on the back of the upper arm (triceps).

Position

Grasp towel (rope) at both ends. Hold left hand at small of back, right hand over shoulder.

Movement

Pull hands apart with maximum force; repeat exercise, reversing position of hands.

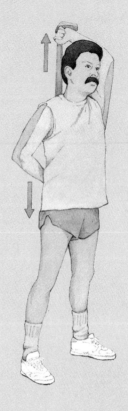

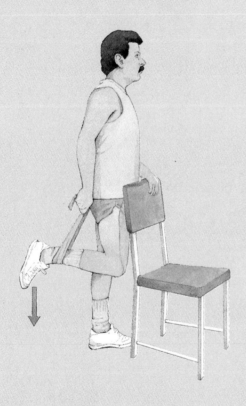

45. Knee Extension

Purpose

Develop muscles on the front of the thigh.

Position

Place towel (rope) around right ankle, knee bent to 90-degree angle. Hold chair with your free hand for balance.

Movement

Grasp towel with both hands behind back, extend leg downward with maximum force. Repeat exercise, changing legs.

46. Waist Pull

Purpose

Develop muscles of the abdomen, chest, and arms.

Position

Grasp ends of towel (rope), palms in, towel around lower back, elbows flexed to right angle.

Movement

Pull forward on towel with maximum force while contracting abdomen and flattening back.

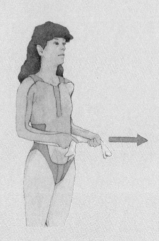

47. Bow Exercise

Purpose

Develop muscles of the shoulders and upper back.

Position

Take archer's position with bow (towel) drawn, left elbow partially extended, right hand at chin, right arm parallel to floor. Tighten abdominals and back muscles.

Movement

Grasp towel and pull arms away from each other. Exchange positions of hands and repeat.

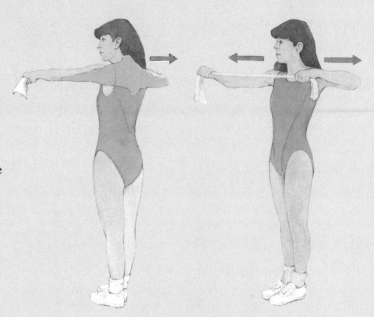

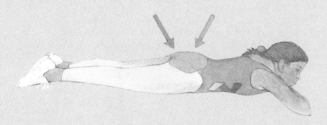

48. Gluteal Pinch

Purpose

Develop muscles of the buttocks.

Position

Lie prone, heels apart and big toes touching.

Movement

Squeeze the buttocks together. Hold several seconds. Slowly relax; repeat several times.

49. Pelvic Tilt

Purpose

Develop muslces of the abdomen and buttocks.

Position

Assume a supine position with the knees bent and slightly apart.

Movement

Press the spine down on the floor and hold for several seconds. Keep abdominals and gluteals tightened.

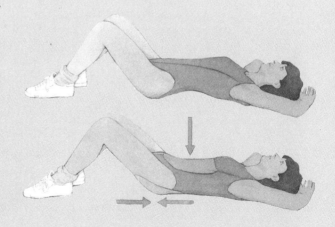

Sample Isokinetic Exercises

Exer-Genie Exercises

Examples of some of the isokinetic exercises that can be performed on the Exer-Genie (see fig. 11.1) are described below:

50. Back Extension

Keep the arms straight and bend the knees and hips until the handle can be grasped. Pull on the rope by extending knees (as in "leg press"), hips, and back, rolling the shoulders backward; strengthens hip, knee, and back extensors.

51. Straight-Leg Position

Stand erect and grasp handles with hands either palm down or palm up; perform "biceps curls" by hugging elbows to the sides while flexing elbows and pulling the handle to the chest; strengthens elbow flexors (biceps).

52. Curling and Abduction Position

Perform an "upright row" exercise by starting as in position B with palms down, then pull the rope upward, bending the elbows out to the side and pulling the shoulders back until the handle reaches chin level; strengthens elbow flexors (including biceps), shoulder rotators, deltoids, and upper back (including trapezius).

53. Press Overhead

Start with the handle at chin level, elbows bent and at the sides of the chest. Push the handle overhead by extending the elbows as in an "overhead press" (military press); strengthens shoulders and arms (including deltoids and triceps).

54. Big Four

All of the muscle groups described here could be strengthened in one exercise by combining movements through the four positions into one continuous movement as shown in the illustration below.

Suggested Readings

Baechle, T., and R. Earle. *Fitness Weight Training.* Champaign, IL: Human Kinetics Publishers, 1995.

Signorile, J. et al. "An Electromyographical Comparison of the Squat and Knee Extension Exercises." *Journal of Strength and Conditioning Research* 8 (1994):178.

Silvester, L. J. *Weight Training for Strength and Fitness.* Boston: Jones & Bartlett Publishers, 1992.

Wescott, W. L. *Strength Fitness: Physiological Principles and Training Techniques.* 4th ed. Dubuque, IA. Brown & Benchmark. 1995.

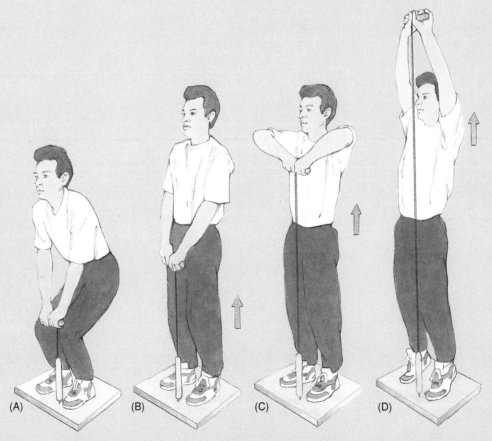

Figure 11.1

Big Four Exer-Genie. (*A*) back-extension position; (*B*) straight-leg position; (*C*) curling and abduction position; (*D*) press overhead position

Source: Big Four Exer-Genie from Exergenie, Inc., Glendale, CA.

CONCEPT ·12·

Questionable Exercises

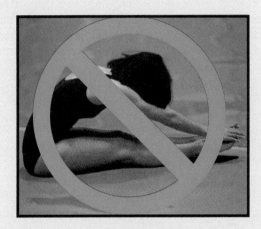

Concept 12

Some exercises should be used with caution or not used at all because they are "high-risk" exercises or because they may cause more harm than good.

Introduction

There are literally thousands of exercises from which one can choose, but they must be chosen carefully because *not all* exercises are good for *all* people. Some exercises should be avoided because there is some risk of injury. We term these exercises "questionable" or "hazardous." Some of these exercises so drastically violate the mechanics of the human frame that they are dangerous and should probably never be used by anyone.

Studies indicate that many commercial enterprises do not employ properly trained instructors. Those most likely to be qualified to advise you about exercise have college degrees and four to eight years of study in such courses as anatomy, physiology, kinesiology, preventive and therapeutic exercise, and physiology of exercise. These qualified individuals are most likely to be physical educators, biomechanists, kinesiotherapists, and physical therapists. On-the-job training, a certificate, a good physique or figure, or good athletic or dancing ability are not sufficient qualifications for teaching or advising about exercise.

If you have had knowledgeable instructors, you may recognize some of these exercises, but others listed here may set off a protest such as: "I've been doing that all my life and it never has hurt me!"

This concept explains the difference between individually prescribed exercise and mass prescription; what is good for you may not be good for me. The difference between microtrauma and acute injury, and the significance of the number of repetitions will also be discussed. Exercises that are believed to be potentially hazardous for most people are presented with the reasons for classifying them as such. Alternative exercises that may be safer are then suggested. The old saying "when in doubt, don't do it" is a good philosophy when choosing exercises, because there are always safe, effective alternative exercises for any specific muscle group.

Health Goal for the Year 2000

▬ Increase the proportion of people who engage in appropriate physical activity for promoting health-related physical fitness. (↑)

Note: (↑) indicates progress toward goal, (↓) indicates regression from goal, and (<>) indicates either no change or lack of new data since 1990.

Terms

▬ **Bursa** Small sac filled with fluid and situated between muscles, or between muscles and bones, to prevent friction.

▬ **Hyperflexion** Bending (flexing) a joint more than normal; excessive bending.

- **Hyperventilation**   "Overbreathing"; forced, rapid, or deep breathing.
- **Microtrauma**   Injury so small it is not detected at the time it occurs.
- **Pyriformis Syndrome**   Muscle spasm and nerve entrapment in the pyriformis muscle of the buttocks region causing pain in the buttock and referred pain down the leg (sciatica).
- **Sciatica**   Pain along the sciatic nerve in the buttock and leg.
- **Shearing Force**   A force tending to make vertebrae or other bones slide on each other parallel to their plane of contact.
- **Spondylolisthesis**   Forward displacement of a vertebra, usually the fourth or fifth lumbar.
- **Spondylolysis**   A stress fracture of a vertebra at the pars interarticularis.
- **Torque**   A twisting or rotating force.
- **Valsalva Maneuver**   Exerting force with the epiglottis closed, thus increasing pressure in the thorax and raising arterial pressure. When released, arterial pressure drops rapidly, blood vessels expand and are then filled, causing a lag in blood flow to the left ventricle. When this occurs, the subject may become dizzy or feel faint. May be caused by holding the breath while exerting force.

The Facts: Rationale

There is a difference between exercises that are good when prescribed for a particular individual and those that are good for everyone (mass prescription).

Individual Prescription

An example of an exercise program in which the exercise is individually prescribed is the clinical setting. A therapist works with one patient and takes a case history, administers tests and measurements to determine which muscles are weak or strong, short or long. A determination of existing limitations that might make any given exercise indicated or contraindicated is made, and then exercises are prescribed for that person. The patient is supervised in the correct execution of the movements.

For example, in a back care program for an individual with lumbar lordosis or lumbar degenerative disk disease and arthritis, back hyperextension exercises might be contraindicated. However, another client might have a flat lumbar spine with limited range of motion, in which case, a set of back hyperextension exercises (McKenzie 1981) would be indicated. Thus, the classification of exercises in this concept does not necessarily apply to the setting where

individual prescription is done by a qualified professional. A qualified professional is one who is expert in applied anatomy, kinesiology, therapeutic exercise, and functional tests as well as being knowledgeable about pathomechanics and other acute and chronic conditions. Typically this includes physical therapists, kinesiotherapists, biomechanists, and physical educators with graduate specialization in corrective/remedial/therapeutic physical education.

Mass Prescription

When a physical educator, aerobics instructor, or coach leads a group of people in exercises, or a book or magazine describes a great exercise to "slim and trim" and all participants in the group or all readers perform the same exercise, this is a *mass prescription*. There is little if any consideration for individual differences except perhaps some allowance made in the number of repetitions or in the amount of weight (resistance) used.

Some of the exercises that would be appropriate for an individual would not be appropriate for all individuals in the group. Since it is not practical to prescribe individually for everyone, it is necessary to consider what the needs of the majority may be and choose the least harmful (but most effective exercises) for the group.

Some exercises can produce microtrauma, and some may cause acute injuries.

Microtrauma refers to "a silent injury"; that is, an injury that results from chronic, repetitive motions such as the ones we use in calisthenics or sports. These injuries also occur in occupations. Other terms which appear frequently in the scientific literature include *repetitive motion syndrome, repetitive strain injury (RSI), cumulative trauma disorder, (CTD)* and *overuse syndrome*. They all refer to injury caused by repetitive movement. We may violate the integrity of our joints by performing, for example, forty backward arm circles with the palms down three days per week for ten or twenty years. The "wear and tear" is usually not noticed by the participant until the friction over time wears down the tendon, ligament, and/or bone, resulting in tendonitis, fascitis, bursitis, arthritis, and nerve compression. The injury may not become apparent until later in life. Chances are, when the injury reaches an acute stage in later life, the cause of the injury is never really identified and it will be attributed to "old age." Because the injury is unseen and unfelt, the participant views the exercise as harmless. Note: Many of the changes in the musculoskeletal system normally attributed to aging are found in *young* athletes. Degenerated disks are not an uncommon finding.

The term *acute injury* as used here refers to the stress, strain, or sprain that produces pain at the time it occurs or within a few hours of performing the exercise. For example, violating the integrity of the knee joint by placing torque on it during a toe touch or knee bend can tear the ligament and cartilage on the inside of the knee so the participant knows immediately that an injury occurred during that exercise. Some of the exercises termed "questionable" in this concept are capable of producing this kind of injury, whereas others in the list are more apt to produce the "silent" microtrauma. Some exercises can produce both types of injury.

Some exercises may be reasonably safe for most people when performed only once, but become hazardous when done repetitively.

An acute exercise injury in any hazardous activity may occur the first time you place yourself at risk, or it may never happen. The odds of performing a hazardous activity safely decrease as the number of repetitions increases. It is like playing Russian roulette! You may have performed bilateral straight leg raises for years and never had a backache but, as the saying goes, "You are living on borrowed time." Microtrauma, on the other hand, occurs with each repetition of an exercise that violates physiologic movements or normal joint mechanics. It is true that we cannot avoid all wear and tear on the body, and it is true that we must "use it or lose it," but we can *reduce* wear and tear by eliminating hazardous activities because *if we do not use it correctly,* then we will also lose it! Some of the exercises that are considered questionable because of microtrauma can probably be performed safely when the number of repetitions is very small and they are rarely used. For example, if it feels comfortable, hyperextending the back in the prone press-up (McKenzie's exercise, p. 212) is probably safe when done once as a static stretch after a series of abdominal strengthening exercises, but repetitive hyperextension exercises, even if comfortable, are hazardous.

The Facts: Questionable Exercises and Safer Alternatives

Common exercises when misused or abused are potentially harmful.

Unless a qualified person evaluates the individual participant and determines one of the exercises listed as questionable in this book to be indicated for that individual, it is prudent to choose a safer exercise to accomplish the same purpose. This concept does not include every possible "questionable" exercise, and space does not permit the inclusion of all good alternative exercises.

Questionable Exercises

1. *Repetitive hyperextension of the lower back* has several objections. First, it stretches the abdominals. These muscles are too long and weak in most people

and should not be further lengthened. Second, it can be harmful to the back, causing an impingement on the nerve, compression, and even herniation of the disk, myofascial "trigger points" and **spondylolysis.** Examples of exercises in which this occurs include: *cobras, back bends, straight leg lifts, straight-leg sit-ups, prone back lifts, donkey kicks, fire hydrants, prone swans, backward trunk circling, weight lifting with the back arched,* and *landing from a jump with the back arched.* One of the back hyperextension exercises commonly seen is the *swan* shown in figure 12.1, used to strengthen the back muscles.

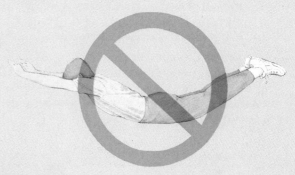

Figure 12.1
Swan

ALTERNATIVE. Lie prone over a roll of blankets or pillows and extend the back to a neutral position (figure 12.2). Or substitute exercise number 9 in concept 11 and exercises 22 and 23 in concept 16.

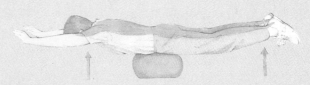

Figure 12.2
Back extension

2. The same hazards are present in the *back-arching abdominal stretch* exercise shown in figure 12.3. This exercise can stretch the hip flexors, quadriceps, and shoulder flexors (such as the pectorals) as well as the abdominals, but it has the additional problem of possibly **hyperflexing** the knee joint, because of the arm pull (see discussion of knee, exercise 11). If your goal is stretching the hip flexors and quadriceps, try substituting the *hip and thigh stretcher* (see figure 12.22). If used for the shoulders, substitute the PNF *pectoral stretch* (see figure 12.4).

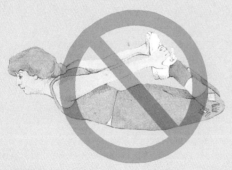

Figure 12.3
Back-arching abdominal stretch

ALTERNATIVE. Stand erect in doorway with arms raised 45 degrees, elbows bent, and hands grasping doorjambs; feet in front-stride position. Press forward on door frame, contracting the arms maximally for several seconds. Relax and shift weight on legs so muscles on front of shoulder joint and chest are stretched; hold. Repeat with arms at 90 degrees and 135 degrees (figure 12.4).

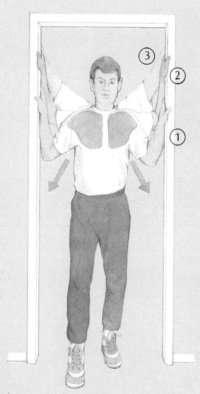

Figure 12.4
Pectoral stretch

3. The *donkey kick* exercise (figure 12.5) is performed for the purpose of developing strength and/or endurance of the buttocks muscles (hip extensors). It may involve touching the nose with the knee, followed by a ballistic backward kick, a lifting of the

head (*neck hyperextension*), and *hyperextension of the lower back*. As discussed earlier, hyperextension of the back is generally undesirable in exercises for the "masses." The same is true for the neck (see exercise 6 for a discussion of the neck). This exercise should be modified as shown in the *knee-to-nose touch* (figure 12.6), so the leg does not lift higher than the hips, and the neck and lower back are not allowed to hyperextend.

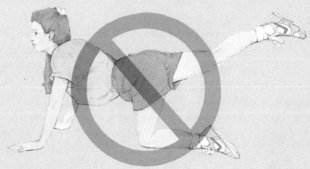

Figure 12.5
Donkey kick

ALTERNATIVE. Kneel on "all fours." Pull knee to nose, then extend leg and head to horizontal (do not go higher). Repeat. Then change legs.

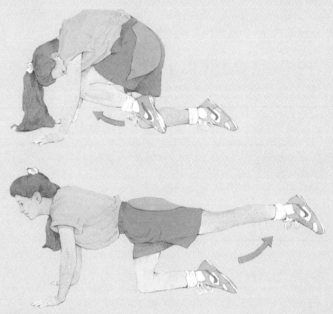

Figure 12.6
Knee-to-nose touch

4. The *double leg lift* (figure 12.7) is usually used with the intent of strengthening the lower abdominals, when in fact it is primarily a hip-flexor (iliopsoas) strengthening exercise. The iliopsoas attaches to the lower back and tilts the pelvis forward, arching the back. Most people have overdeveloped the hip flexors and do not need to further strengthen those muscles. Even if the abdominals are strong enough to contract isometrically to prevent hyperextension of the lower back, the exercise produces excess compression on the disks. The same criticism is true of *straight-leg sit-ups*. These can displace the fifth lumbar vertebra (**spondylolisthesis**). A *bent-knee sit-up*, which is usually used to strengthen the upper abdominals, creates less **shearing force** on the spine, but some recent studies have shown it produces greater compression on the lumbar disks than the straight-leg sit-up. (*Note:* For further discussion of these and other abdominal exercises read Sharpe, Liehmohn, and Snodgrass 1988 and Macfarlane 1993.) An example of a safer and better exercise to strengthen the lower abdominals is the *reverse curl* (figure 12.8).

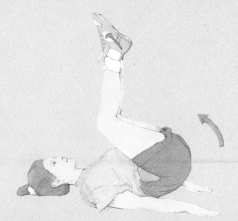

Figure 12.8
Reverse curl

5. The *wind mill* (figure 12.9) is done as follows. Stand, bend, and twist to touch the left toe with the right hand, return to a standing position, then bend and twist to touch the right toe with the left hand. Any exercise in which there is simultaneous rotation and flexion (or extension) of the lower back is contraindicated. Because of the shape of the facet joints in the lumbar spine, these movements violate normal joint mechanics placing tremendous torsional stress on the joint capsule (Saal 1993 and Saudek 1987).

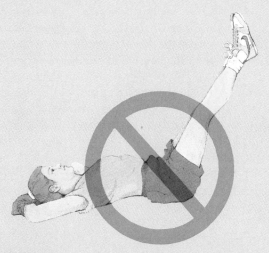

Figure 12.7
Double leg lift

ALTERNATIVE. Lie supine, knees bent, feet flat on floor (hook-lying), arms at side. Lift knees to chest, raising hips off floor. Do not let knees go past the shoulders. Return to starting position and repeat (figure 12.8).

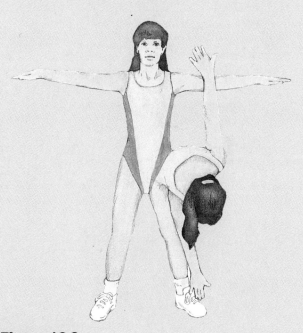

Figure 12.9
Wind Mill

ALTERNATIVE. If the purpose of doing the wind mill is to stretch the hamstrings and back, use the *backsaver hamstring stretch* (figure 12.10).

Sit with one leg extended and one knee bent, foot turned outward and close to buttocks. Place one hand over the other and reach toward the toes. Allow bent knee to move laterally so trunk can move forward. Stretch and hold.

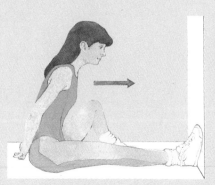

Figure 12.10
Back-saver hamstring stretch

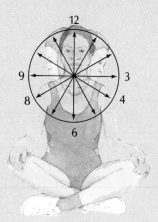

Figure 12.12
Head clock

6. As a general rule, exercises that *hyperextend the neck* should be avoided. Tipping the head backward during an exercise, such as is done in *neck circling* (figure 12.11), can pinch arteries and nerves in the neck and at the base of the skull, grind down the disks, and produce dizziness or myofascial trigger points. In persons with degenerated disks, it can cause dizziness, numbness, or even precipitate strokes. (Beringer 1993). It also aggravates arthritis and degenerated disks. (*Note:* figures 12.1, 12.3, and 12.5 also show improper neck positions.) Another hazardous neck exercise is *bridging* on the head. This places extreme pressure on the cervical disks. If your purpose in doing the exercise is strengthening, try some isometrics keeping your head in good alignment, using your hands as the resistance or use PNF neck-rotation (page 207).

7. As a general rule, exercises that force the *neck and upper back into hyperflexion* should not be used. It has been estimated that 80 percent of the population has forward head and kyphosis (hump back) with accompanying weak muscles. *Hyperflexion of the neck* can be as harmful as hyperextension by causing excessive stretch on the ligaments and nerves. It can also aggravate preexisting thin disks and arthritic conditions. Examples of exercises that tend to promote these conditions include *shoulder stand bicycling* (figure 12.13) and the yoga positions called the *plough* and the *plough shear* (not shown). If the purpose for these exercises is to reduce gravitational effects on the circulatory system or internal organs, try lying on a tilt board with the feet elevated. If the purpose is to warm up the muscles in the legs, try a slow jog in place. If the purpose is to stretch the lower back, try the *leg hug* (figure 12.14) or *single knee-to-chest* exercise (see figure 12.28).

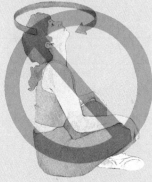

Figure 12.11
Neck circling

ALTERNATIVE. If the purpose of the exercise is relaxation of the neck, substitute the *head clock* in figure 12.12. Pretend your neck is a clock face with the chin at the center when you assume good posture. Flex the neck and point the chin at 6:00, hold, return to the center; repeat pointing at 4:00 and 8:00, then turn the head to 3:00 and 9:00.

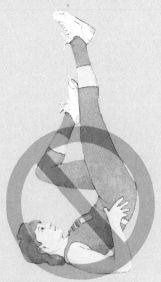

Figure 12.13
Shoulder stand bicycle

ALTERNATIVE. From a hook-lying position, bring both knees to the chest and wrap the arms around the back of the knees. Pull knees to chest and hold (figure 12.14).

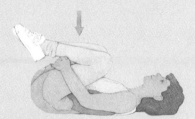

Figure 12.14
Leg hug

8. Placing the *hands behind the neck or head during the sit-up* (figure 12.15) and *crunch* allows the arms to pull the *head and neck into hyperflexion*, stretching the posterior ligaments, as described in exercise 7. If the hands are not placed at the sides or across the chest, then the hands should be placed so the *palms or fists cover the ears* (see figure 12.16) to prevent pulling on the neck. Another alternative is to *cross the hands behind the upper back by reaching* down the spine as far as possible (about the third or fourth thoracic vertebra) and holding this position while *resting* the weight of the head on the arms.

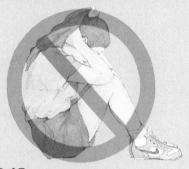

Figure 12.15
Hands-behind-the-head sit-up

ALTERNATIVE. Assume a hook-lying position, with palms of hands lightly covering ears. Curl up until scapulae leave the floor, then roll down to starting position and repeat (figure 12.16).

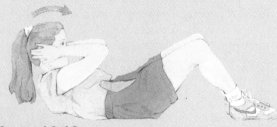

Figure 12.16
Crunch (hands on ears)

9. *The knee joint should not be hyperextended.* This action stretches the ligaments and joint capsule of the knee. Bending the back while the legs are straight may cause back strain, particularly if the movement is done ballistically as in the *standing toe touch* (figure 12.17). Repetitive *bilateral straight-leg toe touches,* whether standing or sitting, may stretch the lower back excessively if the hamstrings are very tight. This can lead to backache and **spondylolisthesis.** If performed only on rare occasions as a test, there is less chance of injury than if incorporated into a regular exercise program. *Standing hamstring stretches with the back flat* have also been condemned (especially when done ballistically) because they can produce degenerative changes at the lumbosacral joint. Safer stretches of the lower back include the *leg hug* (see figure 12.14), and *single knee-to-chest* (see figure 12.28). To stretch the hamstrings, substitute a sitting or lying stretch such as the *back-saver toe touch* (figure 12.18) or the *hamstring stretcher* (see figure 12.26).

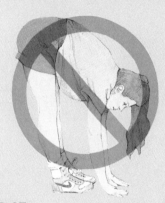

Figure 12.17
Standing toe touch

ALTERNATIVE. Perform the back saver toe touch. See page 36 for description.

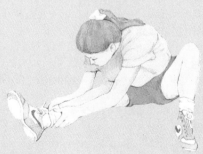

Figure 12.18
Back-saver toe touch

Questionable Exercises **153**

10. *Leg stretches at the ballet bar* (figure 12.19) may be potentially harmful. Some experts have found that where the extended leg is raised 90 degrees or more and the trunk is bent over the leg, it may lead to **sciatica** and **pyriformis syndrome,** especially in the person who has limited flexibility.
ALTERNATIVE. Substitute some of the back and hamstring stretching exercises suggested in figures 12.8, 12.26, and 12.28.

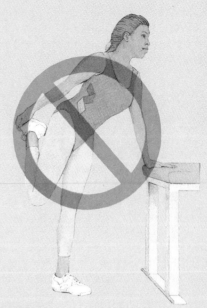

Figure 12.20
Shin and quadriceps stretch

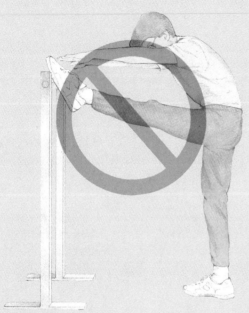

Figure 12.19
Bar stretch

11. When the *knee is hyperflexed* 120 degrees or more, the ligaments and joint capsule are apt to be stretched and the cartilage may be damaged. Among the many exercises that place this type of stress on the knee joint are certain so-called "quadriceps" stretching exercises. *Note:* one of the quadriceps, the rectus femoris, is not stretched by this exercise because it crosses the hip as well as the knee joint. Figure 12.20 illustrates this position and also shows the *shin muscle being stretched.* It is usually not necessary to stretch the shin muscles, since they tend to be weak and elongated; however, if you need to stretch the shin muscles to relieve muscle soreness, try the *shin stretcher* (figure 12.21). To avoid injuring the knee when stretching the quadriceps substitute the *hip and thigh stretcher* (figure 12.22). ALTERNATIVES. Kneel on both knees, turn to right, and press down on right ankle with right hand and hold. Keep hips thrust forward to avoid hyperflexing knees. Do not sit on heels. Repeat on left side (figure 12.21).

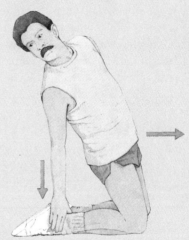

Figure 12.21
Shin stretcher

Kneel with right knee directly above right ankle and stretch left leg backward so knee touches floor. If necessary, place hands on floor for balance. Press pelvis forward and downward and hold stretch for several seconds. Repeat on right side. Do not bend front knee more than 90 degrees. This stretches the rectus femoris and more importantly, the hip flexors (iliopsoas) (figure 12.22).

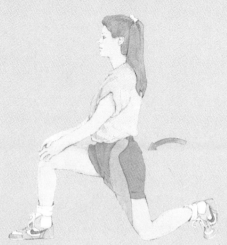

Figure 12.22
Hip and thigh stretcher

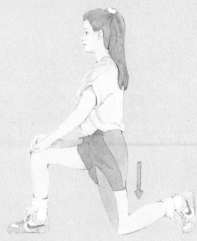

Figure 12.24
Alternate leg kneel (lunge)

12. *Deep squatting exercises* (figure 12.23), with or without weights, placing the knee joint in hyperflexion tends to "wedge it open," stretching the ligaments, irritating the synovial membrane, and possibly damaging the cartilage. There is even greater stress on the joint when the lower leg and foot are not in straight alignment with the knee. If you are performing squats to strengthen the knee and hip extensors, then try substituting the *alternate leg kneel* (figure 12.24) or *half-squat* (also called parallel squat) (knees at right angle) with free weight or leg presses on a resistance machine.

13. The *hero* places the knee in a rotated position with **torque** on the flexed knee, which is apt to stretch the ligaments and capsule, and damage the cartilage. It may also cause strain in the groin muscles and the lower back. If the exercise is used to stretch the quadriceps, refer to exercise 11 regarding quadriceps stretching. The *hurdler's stretch* (not shown) is similar to the hero with one leg turned out rather than two, as shown in the hero (figure 12.25). It produces the same kind of stress on the knee joint. Try substituting the *hamstring stretch* (figure 12.26) or *back-saver hamstring stretch* (figure 12.18).

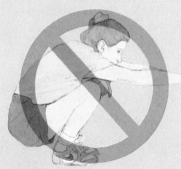

Figure 12.23
Deep knee bends

ALTERNATIVE. From a standing position, with or without a free weight, take a step forward with right foot, touching left knee to floor. The front knee should be bent only to a 90-degree angle. Return to start and lunge forward with other foot. Repeat, alternating right and left (figure 12.24).

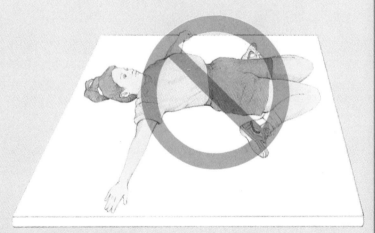

Figure 12.25
The hero

ALTERNATIVE. Lie supine in a hook-lying position. Raise right leg and grasp toes with right hand while pulling on back of thigh with left hand. Push heel toward ceiling and hold. Repeat on other leg (figure 12.26). (You may pull on a rope placed around the ankle of the extended leg, rather than pulling on the toe and thigh.)

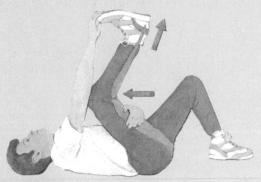

Figure 12.26
Hamstring stretcher

14. *Hyperflexing the knee* by pulling it to the body with the arms or hands placed on top of the shin places undue stress on the knee joint. The *knee pull-down* exercise is one example (figure 12.27). (This position of the knee is also seen in figures 12.20–12.23.) In this case, the exercise is intended to stretch the lower back. The hand position should be changed to hug the thigh rather than the shin to make this a good exercise. Try *single knee-to-chest* (figure 12.28) or *leg hug* (figure 12.14).

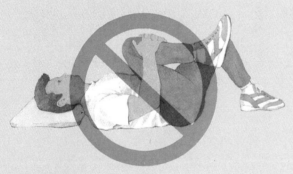

Figure 12.27
Knee pull-down

ALTERNATIVE. From the hook-lying position, draw one knee to the chest by pulling on the thigh with the hands, then extend the knee toward the ceiling; hold. Pull to chest again and return to starting position. Repeat with other leg (figure 12.28).

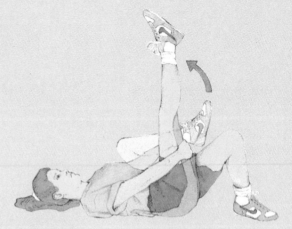

Figure 12.28
Single knee-to-chest

15. *Arm circles with the palms down* (circumduction with the arms straight out to the sides) (figure 12.29) may cause the bony knob near the head of the humerus to impinge upon a shoulder ligament or the lip of the socket, and squeeze some of the muscles and the **bursa** in the shoulder every time the arm is lifted. In addition, if these are done in a forward direction (top of the circle is forward), there is a tendency to emphasize the use of the stronger chest muscles (pectorals) rather than to stretch those muscles and emphasize the weaker upper back muscles. Finally, if they are done while standing, there is a tendency for the head to protrude forward and the low back to arch. This exercise is best done as modified in figure 12.30. To strengthen the upper back muscles, try prone *arm lifts* (page 213) or *seated rowing* (page 137). To stretch the pectorals try *pectoral stretch* (page 93).

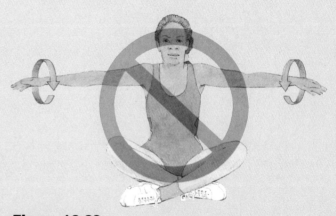

Figure 12.29
Forward arm circles (palms down)

ALTERNATIVE. Sit, turn palms up and pull in chin, contract abdominals. Circle arms backward (figure 12.30).

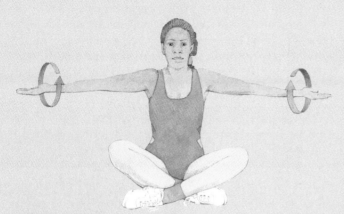

Figure 12.30
Backward arm circles (palms up)

Some Guidelines for Avoiding Hazardous Exercises

Most hazardous exercises can be avoided.

Follow these general guidelines, except where a physician or qualified professional has prescribed otherwise for you.

- Do not hyperflex the knee or neck.
- Do not hyperextend the knee, neck, or lower back.
- Do not apply a twisting or lateral force to the knee.
- Avoid holding your breath during exercise (advanced resistance training is an exception).
- Avoid stretching already long/weak muscles and avoid shortening already short/strong muscles. Most people should:
  a. especially *avoid* aggravation of common postural faults: head forward, "hump back," protruding abdomen, inward rotation of the thigh, and pronation of the foot (see concept 16).
  b. *stretch the chest* muscles, hip flexors, calf, hamstrings, lower back, and medial thigh rotators.
  c. *strengthen* the abdominals, the muscles between the shoulder blades, upper and lower back extensors, the lateral hip rotators, and the shin muscles.
- Avoid overstretching any joint so that ligaments and joint capsules are stretched.
- Be especially careful when using passive stretches by another person (unless it is a therapist). Avoid passive neck stretches and any ballistic passive stretches.
- Avoid movements that place acute compressional forces on spinal disks, such as extending and rotating the spine simultaneously, trunk and neck circling, and double leg lifts (see concept 16 for specific neck and back cautions).
- Avoid movements that cause joint impingements or cartilage damage, such as arm circles in palm-down position. (See discussion of microtrauma in this concept.)
- If the nature of your sport regularly requires the violation of good mechanics (such as the need for a baseball catcher to assume a deep squat position or a gymnast to perform double leg raises), make certain that the muscles and joints are as fit as possible to endure the stress.
- Avoid fast, forceful hyperextension and flexion of the spine.

Other Important Facts

Manual stretching of the shoulders as done by some competitive swimmers has been found to create instability in the shoulder joint.

The practice of some athletes of using the passive assistance of a partner can cause excessive stretch. Examples of such exercises are pulling the arms backward at shoulder level until they cross each other behind the back; or pulling the bent elbows together making them touch while the hands are on the back of the head. Competitive swimmers sometimes begin such practices while they are in children's swimming programs and continue them through their competitive years. Such overstretching has resulted in painful shoulders and disability.

Repeatedly rising on the toes and heels may weaken the long arches of the feet.

Tiptoeing exercises will develop the calf muscles, but at the same time, they will stretch the muscles and ligaments that help support the long arch of the foot. "Heel walking" may have the same effect; that is, it may develop strong shin muscles while further weakening the arch. The potential harm is lessened if these exercises are performed with the toes turned in slightly.

Isometric exercises may be harmful to some people.

Isometric exercises have advantages (see concept 9), but they may be more dangerous to heart patients than isotonic exercises, because they cause a marked rise in blood pressure and may produce irregular heartbeats. People with high blood pressure or heart trouble should not perform isometrics. Isometric exercise (as well as heavy weight training) for adolescents is also questionable because the bones of adolescents have not matured and growth may be affected.

> Jogging and aerobic dance exercises are excellent for cardiovascular conditioning, weight control, and improvement of a variety of conditions; however, reasonable caution should be observed.

Jogging has been used successfully in rehabilitating cardiac patients and those with pulmonary emphysema; in weight reduction of diabetics; in relaxing insomniacs, the emotionally disturbed, and migraine patients; and in reducing the discomfort accompanying arthritis in the legs and back. Like many other exercises, jogging should not be done without a physician's approval for those with arthritis, osteoporosis, and heart and circulatory diseases. It is *not* harmful to women, although some women may need to wear a special bra as a comfort measure. Jogging can cause shin splints, blisters, and foot, ankle, knee, and hip problems. Using the proper footwear and learning how to jog correctly will minimize these hazards. If you have poor leg or foot alignment, you would be wise to jog only three or four days per week because studies show that the risk of injury is greatest for those who jog every day. Or you should choose another activity such as cycling or swimming. The same fitness levels will result with less risk of injury.

Aerobic dance exercise has some of the same hazards as jogging; these include the overstress syndromes from too many hours of high impact landings on the floor. The most common problems are shin splints, Achilles tendon injuries, arch strains, and pain under the knee cap. Most of these problems can be prevented by warming up and stretching properly before exercising, by using low impact movements, and by avoiding hazardous exercises such as those described in this concept. More recently there have been increasing reports of dizziness, hearing loss, and impaired balance—in pupils and in teachers. Loud music can cause hearing loss, and high impact landings may cause inner ear damage, but the causes are not now understood (JOPERD 1990).

> Equipment that can be hazardous for some people is the "gravity inversion boot" and similar devices designed to allow a person to hang upside down.

These devices are supposed to be effective for the treatment of backache. However, studies have shown that during hanging (inactively or while oscillating), significant increases occur in systemic blood pressure; intraocular and retinal arterial pressure (in the eye) doubles; and pulse and other heart irregularities occur. Therefore, this type of equipment is potentially dangerous to the elderly and medically compromised, and to people with high blood pressure, glaucoma, diabetes, and heart abnormalities.

> Exercise can alter the effect of drugs in the body, as well as the effect of certain disorders.

The effect of drugs used to treat thyroid disease may be altered by exercise. Likewise, patients taking certain medicine for asthma and collagen diseases may not be able to perform exercises that require moderate or heavy exertion in a normal fashion. Exercise alters the effect of nonsteroidal analgesics and anti-inflammatory drugs (like aspirin). During exercise, these drugs can cause increased oxygen consumption and increased carbon dioxide production, as well as promote sweating and dehydration. Muscle relaxants may cause depression and hinder coordination. (See concept 9 for discussion of steroids and growth hormones.)

> The **valsalva maneuver** should be avoided when exerting great force in weight lifting, calisthenics, and isometrics.

Dizziness, blackouts, and inguinal hernias may result from the valsalva maneuver. This can be prevented in heavy weight lifting by avoiding **hyperventilation**, squatting as briefly as possible, and raising the weight as rapidly as possible to a position where it can be supported while breathing normally. In all other activities, breathe normally! Do *not* hold your breath during exercise.

Suggested Readings

"Aerobicizers Getting More Than They Asked For." *Journal of Physical Education, Recreation and Dance* 62(1991):16.

Almkinders, L. C., et al. "An In Vitro Investigation Into the Effects of Repetitive Motion and Nonsteroidal Antiinflammatory Medication on Human Tendon Fibroblasts." *American Journal of Sports Medicine,* 23(1995):119.

Beringer, G. B., et al. "Beauty Parlor Stroke: When a Beautician Becomes a Physician." (Letter to the Editor) *Journal of the American Medical Association* 270 (1993):1198.

Friden, J., & R. Lieber. "Structural and Mechanical Basis of Exercise Induced Muscle Injury." *Medicine and Science in Sports and Exercise* 5(1992): 521.

Gunn, C. C. "Fibromyalgia—What Have We Created?" (Letter to the Editor) *Pain* 60 March 1995.

Kelleher, S. "R.S.I.: Treating Repetitive Motion Injuries is Fledgling Science." *Orange County Register* March 1, 1995.

Liehmohn, W. "Choosing the Safe Exercise." *Certified News* 2 (1991):1.

Liemohn, W. S., et al. "Unresolved Controversies in Back Management." *Journal of Orthopaedic and Sports Physical Therapy* 9 (1988):239.

Lindsey, R., and C. Corbin. "Questionable Exercise—Some Alternatives." *Journal of Physical Education, Recreation and Dance* 60 (1989):26.

Macfarlane, P. "Out With the Sit-up, in With the Curl-up!" *Journal of Physical Education, Recreation and Dance* August, 1993:62.

McKenzie, R. *The Lumbar Spine: Mechanical Diagnosis and Therapy.* Upper Hutt, New Zealand: Spinal Publications, Ltd., 1981.

Physical Medicine Research Foundation. "Seventh International Symposium on Repetitive Strain Injuries, Fibromyalgia and Chronic Fatigue Syndrome." Vancouver, B. C. Canada. June 10–12, 1994.

Saal, J. A. "Rehabilitation of Football Players With Lumbar Injuries." *Physician and Sports Medicine,* 16:9, 10 Sept., Oct. (1988).

Safrit, M., et al. "The Difficulty of Sit-up Tests: An Empirical Investigation." *Research Quarterly for Exercise and Sport* 63 (1992):277.

Saudek, C. E., & K. A. Palmer. "Back Pain Revisited." *Journal of Orthopaedic and Sports Physical Therapy* 8 (1987):556.

Sharpe, G. L., et al. "Exercise Prescription and the Low Back." *Journal of Physical Education, Recreation and Dance* 59 (1988):74.

Signorile, J., et al. "An Electromyographical Comparison of the Squat and Knee Extension Exercises." *Journal of Strength and Conditioning Research* 8 (1994):178.

CONCEPT

·13·

Body Composition

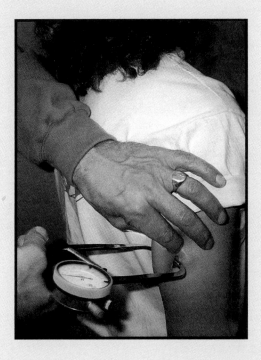

Concept 13

Possessing an optimal amount of body fat contributes to health, wellness, and good appearance.

Introduction

Body composition refers to the relative percentage of muscle, fat, bone, and other tissue of which the body is composed. Of primary concern, because of its association with various health problems, is body fatness. Being overfat or underfat can result in health concerns.

Our national health goals were designed to encourage a decrease in the prevalence of obesity yet recent statistics indicate that we have been ineffective in meeting this goal. Today 33.4 percent of adults are overweight, an increase of 8 percent in the past decade. More women (36 percent) than men (31 percent) are classified as obese. Health statistics also indicate that even the most conservative figures indicate that twice as many children are now overweight than in the 1960s. Since eating disorders such as anorexia nervosa and bulimia are also a significant health concern, especially among teens, the national goal is to keep the percentage of overfat teens from increasing while at the same time reducing the incidence of those who have too little fat associated with eating disorders.

Health Goals for the Year 2000

- Reduce overfatness to no more than 20 percent of people aged 20 or more. (↓)
- Reduce overfatness to no more than 15 percent of people aged 12–19. (↓)
- Increase to 50 percent the proportion of overfat people who have adopted physical activity and sound nutrition to attain desirable body fatness. (< >)

Note: (↑) indicates progress toward goal, (↓) indicates regression from goal, and (<>) indicates either no change or lack of new data since 1990.

Terms

- **Amenorrhea**   Absence of, or infrequent, menstruation.
- **Basal Metabolic Rate (BMR)**   Basal Metabolic Rate refers to your energy expenditure in a basic or rested state.
- **Body Mass Index (BMI)**   A measure of body composition using a height-weight formula. It relates to disease risk.
- **Caloric Balance**   Consuming Calories in amounts equal to the number of Calories expended.
- **Calorie**   A unit of energy supplied by food; the quantity of heat necessary to raise the temperature of a kilogram of water one degree centigrade (actually a kilocalorie but usually called a Calorie for weight control purposes).
- **Diet**   The usual food and drink for a person or animal.

- **Essential Fat**   The minimum amount of fat in the body necessary to maintain healthful living.
- **MET**   METs are multiples of the amount of energy expended at rest, or approximately 3.5 millimeters of oxygen per kilogram (2.2 pounds) of body weight per minute.
- **Nonessential Fat**   Extra fat or fat reserves stored in the body.
- **Obesity**   Extreme overfatness.
- **Overfat**   Too much of the body weight composed of fat; for men, having more than 25 percent fat; for women, having more than 32 percent fat.
- **Overweight**   Weight in excess of normal; not harmful unless it is accompanied by overfatness.
- **Percent Body Fat**   The percentage of total body weight that is comprised of fat.
- **Somatotype**   Inherent body build; ectomorph (thin), mesomorph (muscular), and endomorph (fat).
- **Underfat**   Too little of the body weight composed of fat; for men, having less than 5 percent fat; for women, having less than 8 percent fat.

The Facts: The Meaning and Measurement of Fatness

There are standards that can be used to determine how much body fat an individual should possess.

Every person should possess at least a minimal amount of body fat for good health. This fat is called **essential fat** and is necessary for temperature regulation, shock absorption, and regulation of essential body nutrients, including vitamins A, D, E, and K. **Nonessential fat** accumulates when you take in more Calories than you expend. When nonessential fat accumulates in excessive amounts, overfatness or even **obesity** can occur. For good health, an individual should not allow body fat levels to drop too low or to become too high. There is a desirable range of fatness for good health, different from the range suggested for those who have optimal performance in athletic events as a goal. Even for athletes, especially low levels of body fatness are not desirable. Research has shown that attempts to attain and maintain too low a body fat level are associated with eating disorders such as anorexia nervosa and bulimia. Also, there is evidence that excessive fat loss may result in **amenorrhea** in girls and women. Table 13.1 provides standards of body fatness for both men and women.

Table 13.1
Standards for Fatness (Percent Body Fat)

Classification	Men	Women
Essential fat	no less than 5%	no less than 8%
Borderline	5%–8%	8%–11%
Desirable fatness for good performance	8%–9%	12%–15%
Desirable fatness for good health	10%–20%	16%–26%
Marginal Zone	21%–25%	27%–32%
Overfatness	more than 25%	more than 32%

When using height and weight to assess overweight, the body mass index (BMI) is considered to be a better measure than height-weight charts.

Individuals who are interested in controlling their weight often consult height-weight tables to determine their "desirable" weight. Being 20 percent or more above the recommended table weight is one commonly used indicator of obesity. The usefulness of these tables has been limited in the past because older tables allowed people to become heavier as they grew older. New tables adopted by the federal government no longer allow such weight gains (see chart 13.6). Even the new "healthy weight range tables" have limitations because they do not give an accurate estimate of the amount of fat a person has. A person who has a large muscle mass as a result of regular exercise could appear to be "overweight" using a height-weight table.

The **body mass index (BMI)** is probably the best way to use height and weight to assess fatness. The BMI is calculated using a special formula and has a higher correlation with true body fatness than weights determined from height-weight tables. You may wish to calculate your BMI (see lab resource materials).

Overfat is more important than **overweight** in determining health and wellness.

Though height-weight tables and the BMI can provide guidelines for body fatness, neither is a true measure of body fatness. Because the amount of body fat, not the amount of weight, is the important factor in living a healthy life, it is better to determine the percentage of your body weight that is body fat (**percent body fat**).

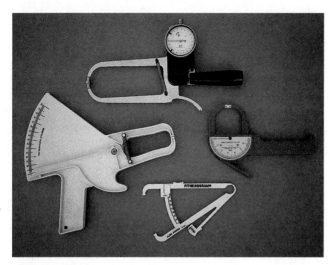

Figure 13.1
Skin-fold calipers

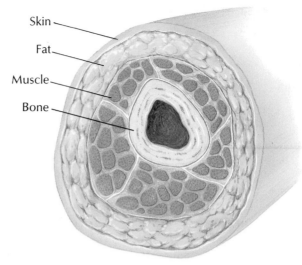

Figure 13.2
Location of body fat

There are many ways to assess body fatness and leanness.

Underwater weighing, also referred to as "hydrostatic weighing," is considered the gold standard for assessing body fatness. In this laboratory procedure, a person is weighed underwater and out of the water. Corrections are made for the amount of air in the lungs when the underwater weight is measured. Using Archimedes principle, the body's density can be determined. Because the density of various body tissues is known, the amount of the total body fat can be determined. Body fatness is usually expressed in terms of a percentage of the total body weight. Because this procedure takes considerable time, equipment, and specialized training, it is not practical for use except in well-equipped laboratories.

Other ways of measuring body fatness are X-rays, ultrasound, impedance measurements, body girths, and skinfold measurements. Not all of these have been shown to be reliable and valid. Skinfold measurements are often used because they are relatively easy to do. They are not nearly as costly as underwater weighing or X-rays. A set of calipers is used to make the measurements. The better, more accurate calipers cost several hundred dollars. However, considerably less expensive calipers are now available. When used by a trained person, these calipers give a good estimate of fatness. An expert's estimate of your body fatness determined by skinfold measurements is informative. It will also be useful for you to learn to use calipers correctly.

Body fat is distributed throughout the body. About one-half of the body's fat is located around the various body organs and in the muscles. The other half of the

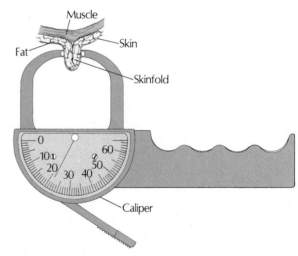

Figure 13.3
Measuring body fat

body's fat is located just under the skin, or in skinfolds (figure 13.2). A skinfold is two thicknesses of skin and the amount of fat that lies just under the skin. At certain locations in the body, the thickness of the skinfolds can be used to obtain a good estimate of total body fatness (figure 13.3). In general, the more skinfolds measured, the more accurate the body fatness estimate. However, measurements with three skinfolds have been shown to be reasonably accurate and can be done in a relatively short period.

Body girth measurements, especially those using only one or two body points, are less accurate than skinfolds but they are easy to do. As the sole measure of fatness, they should be used with caution. They can provide a useful second or third source of information about body fatness, however.

The Facts About Body Composition and Health

> Overfatness or obesity can contribute to degenerative diseases, health problems, and even shortened life.

Some diseases and health problems are associated with overfatness and obesity. In addition to the higher incidence of certain diseases and health problems, there is evidence that people who are moderately overfat have a 40 percent higher than normal risk of shortening their lifespan. More severe obesity results in a 70 percent higher than normal death rate. This is evidenced by the exorbitant life insurance premiums paid by obese individuals.

Recent statistics indicating that underweight people had a higher than normal risk of premature death are very deceptive. Many people included in the data were underweight because of terminal illnesses. Most experts agree that those people who are free from disease and who have lower than average amounts of body fat have a lower than average risk of premature death.

> Excessive abdominal fat and excessive fatness of the upper body can increase the risk of various diseases.

Several research studies have shown that a relationship exists between the amount of abdominal fat and various health problems. For this reason it is important to keep both your total body fat and abdominal fat levels low, especially as you grow older. Other studies have shown that upper body fatness (from the waist up) produces a greater health risk than lower body fatness (from the waist down). Skinfold measures of abdominal fatness could be used to help you monitor abdominal and upper body fatness. Another useful measurement that can be done at home is called the "waist-to-hip circumference ratio." This ratio is calculated using waist and hip circumference measurements. A high ratio has been shown to be correlated with a high incidence of heart attack, stroke, chest pain, breast cancer, and death. Recent evidence indicates that people who exercise regularly accumulate less fat in the upper central regions of the body as they get older. This suggests that regular exercise throughout life will result in a smaller waist-to-hip ratio and a reduced risk of various lifestyle diseases.

> Excessive desire to be thin or low in body **underfat** can result in health problems.

In Western society the near obsession with thinness has been, at least in part, responsible for health conditions now referred to as eating disorders. Eating disorders, or altered eating habits, involve extreme restriction of food intake and/or regurgitation of food to avoid digestion. The most common disorders are anorexia nervosa, bulimia, and anorexia athletica. All of these disorders are most common among highly achievement-oriented girls and young women, although they affect virtually all segments of the population.

Anorexia nervosa is the most severe of the three disorders. In fact, if not treated, it is life threatening. Anorexics restrict food intake so severely that the body becomes emaciated. Among the many characteristics of the anorexic are fear of maturity and inaccurate body image. The anorexic starves herself/himself and may exercise compulsively or use laxatives to prevent the digestion of food in an attempt to attain excessive leanness. The anorexic's image of self is one of being "too fat" even when the person is too lean for good health. Assessing body fatness using procedures such as skinfolds and observation of the eating habits may help identify those with anorexia. Among anorexic girls and women, development of an adult figure is often feared. It is important that people with this disorder obtain medical and psychological help immediately, as the consequences are severe. Those with anorexia may also have some of the characteristics of the bulimic.

Bulimics may or may not be anorexic. It may not be possible to identify the bulimic with measures of body fatness, as they may be lean, normal, or excessively fat. The most common characteristics of bulimia are binging and purging. Bingeing means the periodic eating of large amounts of food at one time. A "binge" might occur after a relatively long period of dieting and often consists of junk foods containing empty Calories. After a binge, the bulimic "purges" the body of the food by forced regurgitation. The bulimic may also use laxatives to purge. Another form of bulimia is bingeing on one day and starving on the next. The consequences of bulimia are not as severe as anorexia, but can result in serious mental and dental problems.

Anorexia athletica is a recently identified eating disorder that appears to be related to participation in sports and activities, such as ballet, that emphasize excessive body leanness. Studies show that participants in sports such as gymnastics, wrestling, body building, and activities such as ballet and cheerleading are most likely to develop anorexia athletica. This disorder has many of the symptoms of anorexia nervosa, but not of the same severity. In some cases, anorexia athletica can lead to anorexia nervosa.

Fear of obesity is a newly discovered condition that is not as severe as anorexia nervosa, but it can still have negative health consequences. This condition is most common among achievement-oriented teenagers who impose a self-restriction on caloric intake because they fear obesity. Consequences include stunting of growth, delayed puberty and sexual development, and decreased physical attractiveness. It is important to avoid excessive eating and inactivity to prevent the problems associated with overfatness and obesity; however, an overconcern for leanness can result in serious health problems, too.

Society can help reduce the incidence of eating disorders by changing its image of "attractiveness" especially among young women. Many of the models and movie stars who convey the "ideal" image are anorexic or are exceptionally thin. Teachers and athletic coaches can help by educating people about these disorders, by not placing too much emphasis on leanness, and by screening students with procedures such as skinfolds and body mass index. Parents and friends can help by looking for excessive changes in body weight and lack of eating. Once an eating disorder is identified, it is important to help the individual obtain treatment for the problem.

Conflicting news reports should not deter efforts to maintain a healthy body fat level.

One recent headline said "Excess pounds deadly." One week later the headline read "It may be better to be a little fat." Sometimes people read these conflicting headlines and adopt a defeatist attitude. It is important *not* to let one headline influence your overall plan of fat control. There will be a continuing debate in the years ahead as to just how much you should weigh or how much fat you should have for your good health and wellness. In the meantime the message is clear! If possible, meet current standards of fatness (see charts in lab resource materials). For some people meeting these standards may be difficult. It is far better to be close to the standard than to say "I can't meet the standard, so I won't even try." Some experts feel that many people are overfat because they have repeatedly failed to meet unrealistic body fatness or weight goals. Adopting a realistic personal standard of fatness is very important.

The Facts About the Origin of Overfatness

Heredity plays a role in overfatness.

Some people have suggested that every individual is born with a predetermined weight (sometimes called your setpoint). This implies that you have little control over your weight or body fat levels. In fact, you do have considerable control over your weight and level of fatness as evidenced by the fact that Calories taken in (diet) and Calories expended (activity) are the two most important factors associated with fat control. Nevertheless, research suggests that people are born with a predisposition toward fatness or leanness. For years, some scholars have suggested that your body type, or **somatotype,** is inherited. Clearly some people will have more difficulty than others controlling fatness because of their body types and because they come from families with a history of obesity. In fact, very recent research by a well-respected team of scholars indicates that the body has a "natural" fatness range which is influenced

by heredity. If you deviate more than 10 to 15 percent from this range, your body may actually alter its metabolism in an attempt to maintain your "natural" fatness level. But even these changes are temporary. If you continue the behavior that caused the weight gain (eating more or exercising less), after a period of time your body accepts your new weight as your "natural" level. Scientists caution people not to overgeneralize the importance of heredity to body fatness. Such overgeneralizations could lead to incorrect conclusions about regulation of body fat levels.

Recently the "ob-gene" (or gene responsible for obesity) was discovered. It is true that this is an important scientific discovery but it is unlikely that it will result in a "cure" for overfatness in the near future. In the meantime, more conventional methods of fat control must be used. Even if you come from a family with a history of obesity, *you should not conclude that nothing can be done to prevent obesity.* Virtually all people have a natural fatness below obese levels. Those with a predisposition to high fatness will have a harder time having a low body fatness level, but with healthy lifestyles, even these people can maintain body fat levels within normal ranges. Research shows that regular physical activity is especially effective in the control of genetically determined predisposition to fatness.

Glandular disorders can play a role in overfatness.

Glandular disorders can cause or contribute to overfatness. For example, thyroid problems can cause a low metabolic rate that results in fat gain. However, most experts suggest that only one to two percent of all overfatness is directly caused by problems of this type. Medical treatment is necessary for people suffering with these problems.

Fatness early in life leads to adult fatness.

Retention of baby fat is not a sign of good health. On the contrary, excess body fat in the early years is a health problem of considerable concern. There is evidence that childhood overfatness results in hyperplasia, or an increased number of fat cells. People who have these extra fat cells are thought to have a greater tendency to become overfat. It was previously thought that only adult obesity was related to health problems. We now know that teens (ages 13–18) who are too fat are at greater risk of heart problems and cancer than their lean peers.

Changes in **basal metabolic rate** can be the cause of overfatness.

Basal Metabolic Rate (BMR) is highest during the growing years. The amount of food eaten increases to support this increased energy expenditure. When growing ceases, if eating does not decrease or activity level increase, fatness can

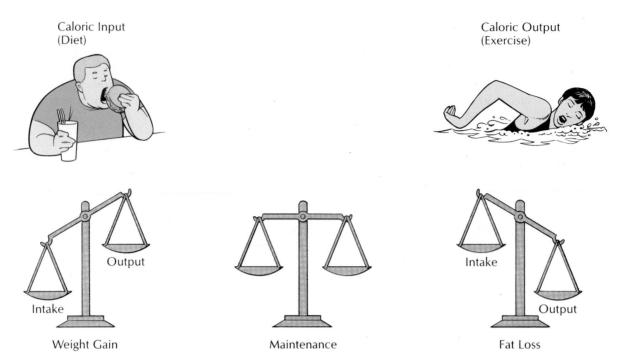

Caloric Input
(Diet)

Caloric Output
(Exercise)

Output

Intake

Intake

Output

Weight Gain

Maintenance

Fat Loss

Figure 13.4
Balancing Calorie input and output

result. Basal metabolism also decreases gradually as you grow older. One major reason for this is the loss of muscle mass associated with inactivity. Regular physical activity throughout life helps keep the muscle mass higher, resulting in a higher BMR. Very recent evidence suggests that regular exercise can contribute in other ways to increased BMR. The higher BMR of active people helps them prevent overfatness, particularly in later life.

"Creeping obesity" is a problem as you grow older.

When people become less active and their BMR gradually decreases with age, even when eating habits remain the same, body fat increases. This is commonly referred to as "creeping obesity" because the increase in fatness is gradual. For a typical person, creeping obesity could result in one-half to one pound of fat gain per year. People who stay active can keep muscle mass high and delay changes in BMR. For those who are not active, it is suggested that caloric intake decrease by 3 percent each decade after twenty-five so that by age sixty-five, caloric intake is at least 10 percent less than it was at age twenty-five. The decrease in Calorie intake for active people need not be as great.

The principal cause of most overfatness is the intake of more calories than are expended.

Though fatness may be associated with any of the factors mentioned previously, and overfatness is no doubt the result of multiple causes, excessive food (Calorie) intake and/or lack of energy expenditure (physical activity) are responsible

for most overfatness. (See figure 13.4.) Thresholds of training and target zones for body fat reduction, including information for both exercise and **diet** are presented in table 13.2.

Excess caloric intake or Calorie expenditure results in an increase in fat cell size.

Overfatness can result in an increase in the number of fat cells among children. For adults, overfatness is a result of the increase in size of fat cells (*hypertrophy*). When fat cells become excessively large, they can cause dimples or lumps under the skin. Some people refer to these large fat cells as *cellulite*. Quacks try to create the impression that this type of fat is different from other types of fat and is removed from the body in different ways than regular fat. This is not true. All fatness among adults is a result of enlarged fat cells. All fat is lost as a result of reduction in fat cell size.

The Facts About Diet, Physical Activity, and Fatness

A combination of regular physical activity and dietary restriction is the most effective means of losing body fat.

Studies indicate that regular physical activity combined with dietary restriction is the *most* effective method of losing fat. One study of adult women indicated that diet alone resulted in loss of weight, but much of this loss was lean body tissue. Those studied who were dieting as well as

Table 13.2
Threshold of Training and Target Zones for Body Fat Reduction

	Threshold of Training*		Target Zones*	
	EXERCISE	**DIET**	**EXERCISE**	**DIET**
FREQUENCY	• To be effective, exercise must be regular, preferably daily, though fat can be lost over the long term with almost any frequency that results in increased caloric expenditure.	• It is best to reduce caloric intake consistently and daily. To restrict Calories only on certain days is *not* best, though fat can be lost over a period of time by reducing caloric intake at any time.	• Daily moderate exercise is recommended. For those who do regular vigorous activity, 5 or 6 days per week may be best.	• It is best to diet consistently and daily.
INTENSITY	• To lose 1 pound of fat, you must expend 3500 Calories more than you normally expend.	• To lose 1 pound of fat, you must eat 3500 Calories fewer than you normally eat.	• Slow, low-intensity aerobic exercise that results in no more than 1–2 pounds of fat loss per week is best.	• Modest caloric restriction resulting in no more than 1–2 pounds of fat loss per week is best.
TIME	• To be effective, exercise must be sustained long enough to expend a considerable number of Calories. At least 15 minutes per exercise bout are necessary to result in consistent fat loss.	• Eating moderate meals is best. Do not skip meals.	• Exercise durations similar to those for achieving aerobic cardiovascular fitness seem best. An exercise duration of 30–60 minutes is recommended.	• Eating moderate meals is best. Skipping meals or fasting is *not* most effective.

*Note: It is best to combine exercise and diet to achieve the 3500 caloric imbalance necessary to lose a pound of fat. Using both exercise and diet in the target zone is most effective.

exercising experienced similar weight losses, but this loss included more body fat. On the basis of this research, all weight loss programs should combine a lower caloric intake with a good physical exercise program.

Good physical activity and diet habits can be useful in maintaining desirable body composition.

Table 13.2 illustrates how fat can be lost through regular physical activity and proper dieting. However, not all people want to lose fat. For those who wish to maintain their current body composition, a **caloric balance** between intake and output is effective. For those who want to increase their lean body weight, increased caloric intake with increased exercise can result in the desired changes.

Physical activity is one effective means of controlling body fat.

Though physical activity or exercise will not result in immediate and large decreases in body fat levels, there is increasing evidence that fat loss resulting from physical activity may be more lasting than fat loss from dieting. Vigorous exercise can increase the resting energy expenditure up to thirteen times (13 **METs**).

Inactivity is more often the cause of childhood obesity than overeating. Many fat children eat less but are considerably less active than their nonfat peers. Excessive television watching may be one reason for inactivity among children if the television viewing is done during daytime hours when children are normally most active. Studies show that adults who watch more than three hours of television per day are twice as likely to be obese as those who view television for less than one hour per day.

If you exercise moderately for an extra fifteen minutes a day, you will lose up to ten pounds in a year's time. Regular walking, jogging, swimming, or any type of sustained exercise can be effective in producing losses in body fat.

Physical activity that can be sustained for relatively long periods is probably the most effective for losing body fat.

Physical activities from virtually any level of the physical activity pyramid can be effective in controlling body fatness because all physical activities expend Calories. Among the most effective activities are those in the aerobic activity section of the pyramid because they can be done for relatively long periods of time. Lifestyle activities are also effective, if performed regularly for extended periods of time. Table 13.3 shows the caloric expenditures for one

Table 13.3
Calories Expended per Hour in Various Physical Activities (Performed at a Recreational Level)*

	Calories Used per Hour				
ACTIVITY	100 LBS (146 KGS.)	120 LBS (55 KGS.)	150 LBS (68 KGS.)	180 LBS (82 KGS.)	200 LBS (91 KGS.)
Archery	180	204	240	276	300
Backpacking (40-lb. pack)	307	348	410	472	513
Badminton	255	289	340	391	425
Baseball	210	238	280	322	350
Basketball (half court)	225	255	300	345	375
Bicycling (normal speed)	157	178	210	242	263
Bowling	155	176	208	240	261
Canoeing (4 mph)	276	344	414	504	558
Circuit training	247	280	330	380	413
Dance, aerobics	315	357	420	483	525
Dance, ballet (choreographed)	240	300	360	432	480
Dance, modern (choreographed)	240	300	360	432	480
Dance, social	174	222	264	318	348
Fencing	225	255	300	345	375
Fitness calisthenics	232	263	310	357	388
Football	225	255	300	345	375
Golf (walking)	187	212	250	288	313
Gymnastics	232	263	310	357	388
Handball	450	510	600	690	750
Hiking	225	255	300	345	375
Horseback riding	180	204	240	276	300
Interval training	487	552	650	748	833
Jogging (5½ mph)	487	552	650	748	833
Judo/karate	232	263	310	357	388
Mountain climbing	450	510	600	690	750
Pool; billiards	97	110	130	150	163
Racquetball; paddleball	450	510	600	690	750
Rope jumping (continuous)	525	595	700	805	875
Rowing, crew	615	697	820	943	1025
Running (10 mph)	625	765	900	1035	1125
Sailing (pleasure)	135	153	180	207	225
Skating, ice	262	297	350	403	438
Skating, roller/inline	262	297	350	403	438
Skiing, cross-country	525	595	700	805	875
Skiing, downhill	450	510	600	690	750
Soccer	405	459	540	621	775
Softball (fast pitch)	210	238	280	322	350
Softball (slow pitch)	217	246	290	334	363
Surfing	416	467	550	633	684
Swimming (fast laps)	420	530	630	768	846
Swimming (slow laps)	240	272	320	368	400
Table tennis	180	204	240	276	300
Tennis	315	357	420	483	525
Volleyball	262	297	350	403	483
Walking	204	258	318	372	426
Waterskiing	306	390	468	564	636
Weight training	352	399	470	541	558

*Note: Locate your weight to determine the Calories expended per hour in each of the activities shown in the table based on recreational involvement. More vigorous activity, as occurs in competitive athletics, may result in greater caloric expenditures.

From *Fitness for Life*, updated 3rd edition by Charles B. Corbin and Ruth Lindsey. Copyright ©1993 by Scott Foresman and Company, a division of Addison-Wesley Educational Publishers Inc. Reprinted by permission.

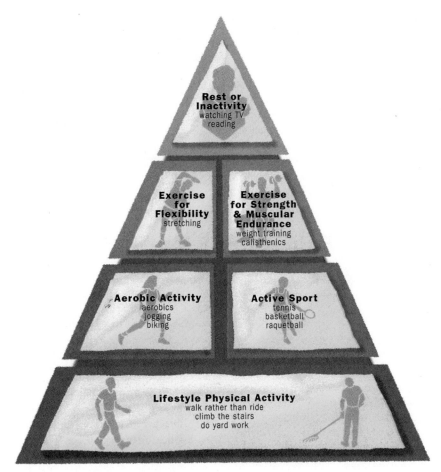

Activities from the lower level of the pyramid are especially effective in fat control.

hour of involvement in various physical activities. Heavier people expend more **Calories** than lighter people because more work is required to move larger bodies.

Popular books have recently claimed that vigorous activities are not effective in helping with body fat loss. Those making these claims say that vigorous activities burn less fat than less intense activities. While this is true in theory, it has little practical meaning for most people. It is the total Calories expended in your activity that counts. If you run for the same period of time that you walk, you will expend more Calories in running.

Even though vigorous activity *can* be effective, it will not work if you do not do it regularly. For this reason more vigorous activity may not be as effective as some less vigorous activities for certain people. For example, running at ten miles per hour (a six-minute mile) will cause a 150-pound person to expend 900 Calories in one hour. Jogging about half as fast, or at five and one-half miles per hour (approximately an eleven-minute mile), will result in an expenditure of about 650 Calories in the same amount of time. At first glance, the more vigorous exercise seems to be a better choice. But how many people can continue to run at a ten-mile-per-hour pace for a full hour? Each mile

run at ten miles per hour results in an expenditure of 90 Calories, while each mile run at five and one-half miles per hour results in an expenditure of 118 Calories. Per mile, you expend more Calories in slow running. It takes longer to run a mile, but by the same token, you can also persist longer. The key is to expend as many Calories as possible during each regular exercise period. Doing less vigorous activity for longer periods is better for fat control than doing very vigorous activities that can be done only for short periods. Nevertheless, vigorous activity can be very effective for some people.

Strength training can be effective in maintaining a desirable body composition.

Performing exercises from the strength and muscular endurance level of the physical activity pyramid can be effective in maintaining desirable body fat levels. People who do strength training increase their muscle mass (lean body mass). This extra muscle mass expends extra Calories at rest resulting in a higher metabolic rate. Also, people with more muscle mass expend more Calories when doing physical activity.

Appetite is not necessarily increased through exercise.

The human animal was intended to be an active animal. For this reason, the human "appetite thermostat" (called the "appestat" by some) is set as if all people are active. Those who are inactive do not have a decreased appetite. Likewise, if a person is sedentary and then begins regular exercise, the appetite does not necessarily increase because this "appetite thermostat" expects activity. Very vigorous activity does not necessarily cause an appetite increase that is proportional to the calories expended in the vigorous exercise.

Suggested Readings

Avery, C. "Abdominal Obesity: Scaling Down This Deadly Risk." *Physician and Sportsmedicine* 19(1991):113.

Foreyt, J. "Factors Common to Successful Therapy for the Obese Patient." *Medicine and Science in Sports and Exercise* 23(1991):292.

People Magazine, "Impossible Mission," 45(June 3, 1996):65.

University of California at Berkeley Wellness Letter, "Weight, Fate, Set Point and Counterpoint." University of California at Berkeley Wellness Letter, 11(1995):1.

Williams, M. H. *Nutrition for Fitness and Sport.* 4th ed. Dubuque, IA: Wm. C. Brown Publishers, 1995.

Wilmore, J. "Exercise, Obesity, and Weight Control." *Physical Activity and Fitness Research Digest* 1(1994):1.

LAB RESOURCE MATERIALS

Evaluating Body Fatness

Skinfold Measurements

Skinfold measurements are made with skinfold calipers. Some of the more accurate and expensive calipers are the Harpenden, the Lange, and the Lafayette calipers. Some of the less expensive calipers include the Slimguide, the Fat-O-Meter, and the Adipometer. Regardless of the type employed, it is important to use a consistent procedure for "drawing up" or "pinching up" a skinfold and making the measurement with the caliper. The following procedures should be used for each skinfold site.

1. Lay the caliper down on a nearby table. Use the thumbs and index fingers of both hands to "draw up" a skinfold or layer of skin and fat. The fingers and thumbs of the two hands should be about one inch apart, or half an inch on either side of the location where the measurement is to be made.

2. The skinfolds are normally "drawn up" in a vertical line rather than a horizontal line. However, if the natural tendency of the skin aligns itself less than vertical, the measurement should be done on the natural line of the skinfold, rather than on the vertical.

3. Do not "pinch" the skinfold too hard. Draw it up so that your thumbs and fingers are not compressing the skinfold.

4. Once the skinfold is "drawn up," let go with your right hand and pick up the caliper. Open the jaws of the caliper and place them over the location of the skinfold to be measured and one-half inch from your left index finger and thumb. Allow the tips, or jaw faces, of the caliper to close on the skinfold at a level about where the skin would be normally.

5. Let the reading on the caliper "settle" for two or three seconds, then note the thickness of the skinfold in millimeters.

6. Three measurements should be taken at each location. Use the middle of the three values to determine your measurement. For example, if you had values of 10, 11, and 9, your measurement for that location would be 10. If the three measures vary by more than 3 millimeters from the lowest to the highest, you may want to take additional measurements.

Skinfold Locations for Women

A. Triceps Skinfold—Make a mark on the back of the right arm, one-half the distance between the tip of the shoulder and the tip of the elbow. Make the measurement at this location.

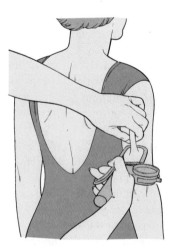

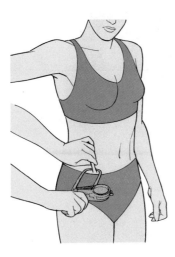

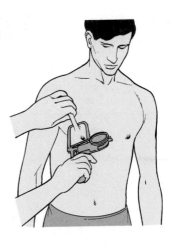

B. Iliac Crest Skinfold—Make a mark at the top front of the iliac crest. This skinfold is taken slightly diagonally because of the natural line of the skin.

B. Chest Skinfold—Make a mark above and to the right of the right nipple (one-half the distance from the midline of the side and the nipple). The measurement at this location is often done on the diagonal because of the natural line of the skin.

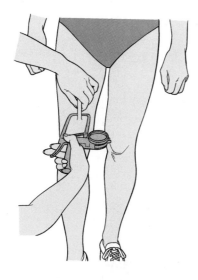

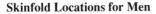

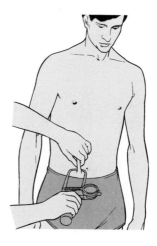

C. Thigh Skinfold—Make a mark on the front of the thigh midway between the hip and the knee. Make the measurement vertically at this location.

Skinfold Locations for Men

A. Thigh Skinfold—Make a mark on the front of the thigh midway between the hip and the knee. Make a vertical measurement at this location (same as for women above).

C. Abdominal Skinfold—Make a mark on the skin approximately one inch to the right of the navel. Make a vertical measurement at that location.

Calculating Fatness from Skinfolds

1. Sum the three skinfolds (triceps, iliac crest, and thigh for women; chest, abdominal, and thigh for men).

2. Use the skinfold sum and your age to determine your percent fat using chart 13.1 for men and chart 13.2 for women. Locate your sum of skinfold in the left column and your age at the top of the chart. Your estimated body fat percentage is located where the values intersect.

3. Use the Fatness Rating Scale (chart 13.3) to determine your fatness rating.

Chart 13.1 Percent Fat Estimates for Men, Sum of Chest, Abdominal, and Thigh Skinfolds*

Sum of Skinfolds (mm)	Age to the Last Year								
	22 and Under	23 to 27	28 to 32	33 to 37	38 to 42	43 to 47	48 to 52	53 to 57	Over 58
8–10	1.3	1.8	2.3	2.9	3.4	3.9	4.5	5.0	5.5
11–13	2.2	2.8	3.3	3.9	4.4	4.9	5.5	6.0	6.5
14–16	3.2	3.8	4.3	4.8	5.4	5.9	6.4	7.0	7.5
17–19	4.2	4.7	5.3	5.8	6.3	6.9	7.4	8.0	8.5
20–22	5.1	5.7	6.2	6.8	7.3	7.9	8.4	8.9	9.5
23–25	6.1	6.6	7.2	7.7	8.3	8.8	9.4	9.9	10.5
26–28	7.0	7.6	8.1	8.7	9.2	9.8	10.3	10.9	11.4
29–31	8.0	8.5	9.1	9.6	10.2	10.7	11.3	11.8	12.4
32–34	8.9	9.4	10.0	10.5	11.1	11.6	12.2	12.8	13.3
35–37	9.8	10.4	10.9	11.5	12.0	12.6	13.1	13.7	14.3
38–40	10.7	11.3	11.8	12.4	12.9	13.5	14.1	14.6	15.2
41–43	11.6	12.2	12.7	13.3	13.8	14.4	15.0	15.5	16.1
44–46	12.5	13.1	13.6	14.2	14.7	15.3	15.9	16.4	17.0
47–49	13.4	13.9	14.5	15.1	15.6	16.2	16.8	17.3	17.9
50–52	14.3	14.8	15.4	15.9	16.5	17.1	17.6	18.1	18.8
53–55	15.1	15.7	16.2	16.8	17.4	17.9	18.5	18.2	19.7
56–58	16.0	16.5	17.1	17.7	18.2	18.8	19.4	20.0	20.5
59–61	16.9	17.4	17.9	18.5	19.1	19.7	20.2	20.8	21.4
62–64	17.6	18.2	18.8	19.4	19.9	20.5	21.1	21.7	22.2
65–67	18.5	19.0	19.6	20.2	20.8	21.3	21.9	22.5	23.1
68–70	19.3	19.9	20.4	21.0	21.6	22.2	22.7	23.3	23.9
71–73	20.1	20.7	21.2	21.8	22.4	23.0	23.6	24.1	24.7
74–76	20.9	21.5	22.0	22.6	23.2	23.8	24.4	25.0	25.5
77–79	21.7	22.2	22.8	23.4	24.0	24.6	25.2	25.8	26.3
80–82	22.4	23.0	23.6	24.2	24.8	25.4	25.9	26.5	27.1
83–85	23.2	23.8	24.4	25.0	25.5	26.1	26.7	27.3	27.9
86–88	24.0	24.5	25.1	25.5	26.3	26.9	27.5	28.1	28.7
89–91	24.7	25.3	25.9	25.7	27.1	27.6	28.2	28.8	29.4
92–94	25.4	26.0	26.6	27.2	27.8	28.4	29.0	29.6	30.2
95–97	26.1	26.7	27.3	27.9	28.5	29.1	29.7	30.3	30.9
98–100	26.9	27.4	28.0	28.6	29.2	29.8	30.4	31.0	31.6
101–103	27.5	28.1	28.7	29.3	29.9	30.5	31.1	31.7	32.3
104–106	28.2	28.8	29.4	30.0	30.6	31.2	31.8	32.4	33.0
107–109	28.9	29.5	30.1	30.7	31.3	31.9	32.5	33.1	33.7
110–112	29.6	30.2	30.8	31.4	32.0	32.6	33.2	33.8	34.4
113–115	30.2	30.8	31.4	32.0	32.6	33.2	33.8	34.5	35.1
116–118	30.9	31.5	32.1	32.7	33.3	33.9	34.5	35.1	35.7
119–121	31.5	32.1	32.7	33.3	33.9	34.5	35.1	35.7	36.4
122–124	32.1	32.7	33.3	33.9	34.5	35.1	35.8	36.4	37.0
125–127	32.7	33.3	33.9	34.5	35.1	35.8	36.4	37.0	37.6

*Percent fat calculated by the formula by Siri. Percent fat = $[(4.95/BD) - 4.5] \times 100$, where BD = body density.

Chart 13.2 Percent Fat Estimates for Women, Sum of Triceps, Iliac Crest, and Thigh Skinfolds*

Sum of Skinfolds (MM)	Age to the Last Year								
	22 and Under	23 to 27	28 to 32	33 to 37	38 to 42	43 to 47	48 to 52	53 to 57	Over 58
23–25	9.7	9.9	10.2	10.4	10.7	10.9	11.2	11.4	11.7
26–28	11.0	11.2	11.5	11.7	12.0	12.3	12.5	12.7	13.0
29–31	12.3	12.5	12.8	13.0	13.3	13.5	13.8	14.0	14.3
32–34	13.6	13.8	14.0	14.3	14.5	14.8	15.0	15.3	15.5
35–37	14.8	15.0	15.3	15.5	15.8	16.0	16.3	16.5	16.8
38–40	16.0	16.3	16.5	16.7	17.0	17.2	17.5	17.7	18.0
41–43	17.2	17.4	17.7	17.9	18.2	18.4	18.7	18.9	19.2
44–46	18.3	18.6	18.8	19.1	19.3	19.6	19.8	20.1	20.3
47–49	19.5	19.7	20.0	20.2	20.5	20.7	21.0	21.2	21.5
50–52	20.6	20.8	21.1	21.3	21.6	21.8	22.1	22.3	22.6
53–55	21.7	21.9	22.1	22.4	22.6	22.9	23.1	23.4	23.6
56–58	22.7	23.0	23.2	23.4	23.7	23.9	24.2	24.4	24.7
59–61	23.7	24.0	24.2	24.5	24.7	25.0	25.2	25.5	25.7
62–64	24.7	25.0	25.2	25.5	25.7	26.0	26.7	26.4	26.7
65–67	25.7	25.9	26.2	26.4	26.7	26.9	27.2	27.4	27.7
68–70	26.6	26.9	27.1	27.4	27.6	27.9	28.1	28.4	28.6
71–73	27.5	27.8	28.0	28.3	28.5	28.8	28.0	29.3	29.5
74–76	28.4	28.7	28.9	29.2	29.4	29.7	29.9	30.2	30.4
77–79	29.3	29.5	29.8	30.0	30.3	30.5	30.8	31.0	31.3
80–82	30.1	30.4	30.6	30.9	31.1	31.4	31.6	31.9	32.1
83–85	30.9	31.2	31.4	31.7	31.9	32.2	32.4	32.7	32.9
86–88	31.7	32.0	32.2	32.5	32.7	32.9	33.2	33.4	33.7
89–91	32.5	32.7	33.0	33.2	33.5	33.7	33.9	34.2	34.4
92–94	33.2	33.4	33.7	33.9	34.2	34.4	34.7	34.9	35.2
95–97	33.9	34.1	34.4	34.6	34.9	35.1	35.4	35.6	35.9
98–100	34.6	34.8	35.1	35.3	35.5	35.8	36.0	36.3	36.5
101–103	35.3	35.4	35.7	35.9	36.2	36.4	36.7	36.9	37.2
104–106	35.8	36.1	36.3	36.6	36.8	37.1	37.3	37.5	37.8
107–109	36.4	36.7	36.9	37.1	37.4	37.6	37.9	38.1	38.4
110–112	37.0	37.2	37.5	37.7	38.0	38.2	38.5	38.7	38.9
113–115	37.5	37.8	38.0	38.2	38.5	38.7	39.0	39.2	39.5
116–118	38.0	38.3	38.5	38.8	39.0	39.3	39.5	39.7	40.0
119–121	38.5	38.7	39.0	39.2	39.5	39.7	40.0	40.2	40.5
122–124	39.0	39.2	39.4	39.7	39.9	40.2	40.4	40.7	40.9
125–127	39.4	39.6	39.9	40.1	40.4	40.6	40.9	41.1	41.4
128–130	39.8	40.0	40.3	40.5	40.8	41.0	41.3	41.5	41.8

*Percent fat calculated by the formula by Siri. Percent fat = $[(4.95/BD) - 4.5] \times 100$, where BD = body density.
From Ted A. Baumgartner and Andrew S. Jackson, *Measurement for Evaluation,* 5th edition. Copyright © 1995 Times Mirror Higher Education Group, Inc., Dubuque, Iowa. All rights reserved. Reprinted by permission.

Chart 13.3 Standards for Fatness (Percent Body Fat)

Classification	Men	Women
Essential fat	no less than 5%	no less than 8%
Borderline	5%–8%	8%–11%
Desirable fatness for good performance	8%–9%	12%–15%
Desirable fatness for good health	10%–20%	16%–26%
Marginal Zone	21%–25%	27%–32%
Overfatness	more than 25%	more than 32%

Chart 13.4 Waist to Hip Ratio Nomogram

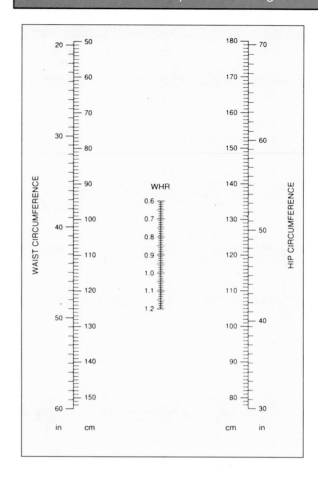

Determining the Waist-to-Hip Circumference Ratio

The Waist-to-Hip Circumference Ratio is recommended as the best available index for determining risk and disease associated with fat and weight distribution. Disease and death risk are associated with abdominal and upper body fatness. When a person has both high fatness and a high waist-to-hip ratio, additional risks exist. The following steps should be taken in making measurements and calculating the waist-to-hip ratio.

1. Both measurements should be done with a nonelastic tape. Make the measurements while standing with the feet together and the arms at the sides, elevated only high enough to allow the measurements. Be sure that the tape is horizontal and around the entire circumference. Record scores to the nearest millimeter or ¹⁄₁₆th of an inch. Use the same units of measure for both circumferences (millimeters or ¹⁄₁₆th of an inch). The tape should be pulled snugly but not to the point of causing an indentation in the skin.

2. *Waist Measurement.* Measure at the natural waist (smallest waist circumference). If there is no natural waist, the measurement should be made at the level of the umbilicus. Measure at the end of a normal inspiration.

3. *Hip Measurement.* Measure at the maximum circumference of the buttocks. It is recommended that the measurement be made in briefs that do not add significantly to the measurement.

4. Divide the hip measurement into the waist measurement or use the waist to hip nomogram (chart 13.4) to determine your waist-to-hip ratio.

5. Use the Waist-to-Hip Ratio Rating Scale (chart 13.5) to determine your rating for the waist-to-hip ratio.

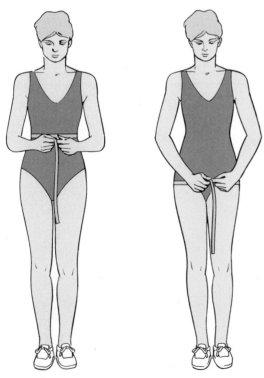

Waist Circumference   Hip Circumference

Chart 13.5 Waist-to-Hip Ratio *Rating Scale*

Classification	Men	Women
High risk	>1.0	>.85
Moderately high risk	.90–1.0	.80–.85
Lower risk	<.90	<.80

Source: Data from Van Stallie, 1988.

Chart 13.6 Frame Size Determined from Height (ft. and in.) and Elbow Breadth (mm)

		Frame Size	
Height	Small	Medium	Large
Males			
5′ 2½″ or less	<64	64–72	>72
5′ 3″–5′ 6½″	<67	67–74	>74
5′ 7″–5′ 10½″	<69	69–76	>76
5′ 11″–6′ 2½″	<71	71–78	>78
6′ 3″ or less	<74	74–81	>81
Females			
4′ 10½″ or less	<56	56–64	>64
4′ 11″–5′ 2½″	<58	58–65	>65
5′ 3″–5′ 6½″	<59	59–66	>66
5′ 7″–5′ 10½″	<61	61–68	>69
5′ 11″ or less	<62	62–69	>69

Height is given including one-inch heels.
Courtesy of the Metropolitan Life Insurance Company.

Chart 13.7 Healthy Weight Ranges for Adult Women and Men

Classification					
Women			Men		
Height Feet	Inches	Pounds	Height Feet	Inches	Pounds
4	10	91–119	5	9	129–169
4	11	94–124	5	10	132–174
5	0	97–128	5	11	136–179
5	1	101–132	6	0	140–184
5	2	104–137	6	1	144–189
5	3	107–141	6	2	148–195
5	4	111–146	6	3	152–200
5	5	114–150	6	4	156–205
5	6	118–155	6	5	160–211
5	7	121–160	6	6	164–216
5	8	125–164			

Source: Data from 1995 Dietary Guidelines U.S. Department of Agriculture and Department of Health and Human Services.

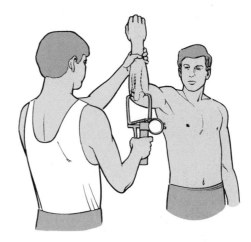

Height-Weight Measurements

1. *Height*. Measure your height in inches or centimeters. Take the measurement without shoes, but add 2.5 centimeters or 1 inch to measurements, as the charts are based on heels of this height.

2. *Weight*. Measure your weight in pounds or kilograms without clothes. Add 3 pounds or 1.4 kilograms because charts are based on clothes of this weight. If weight must be taken with clothes on, wear indoor clothing of 3 pounds or 1.4 kilograms in weight.

3. Determine your frame size using the elbow breadth. The measurement is most accurate when done with a broad-faced sliding caliper. However, it can be done using a skinfold caliper or can be estimated with a metric ruler. The right arm is measured when is is elevated with the elbow bent at 90 degrees and the upper arm horizontal. The back of the hand should face the person making the measurement. Using the caliper, measure the distance between the epicondyles of the humerus (inside and outside bony points of the elbow). Measure to the nearest millimeter (¹/₁₀ of a centimeter). If a caliper is not available, place the thumb and the index finger of the left hand on the epicondyles of the humerus and measure the distance between the fingers with a metric ruler. Use your height and elbow breadth in centimeters to determine your frame size using chart 13.6. Once you have determined your frame size, you need not repeat this procedure each time you use a height-weight chart.

4. Use chart 13.7 to determine your healthy weight range. The new healthy weight range charts do not account for frame size. However, you may want to consider frame size when determining a personal weight within the health weight range. Those with a larger frame size typically can carry more weight within the range than those with a smaller frame size.

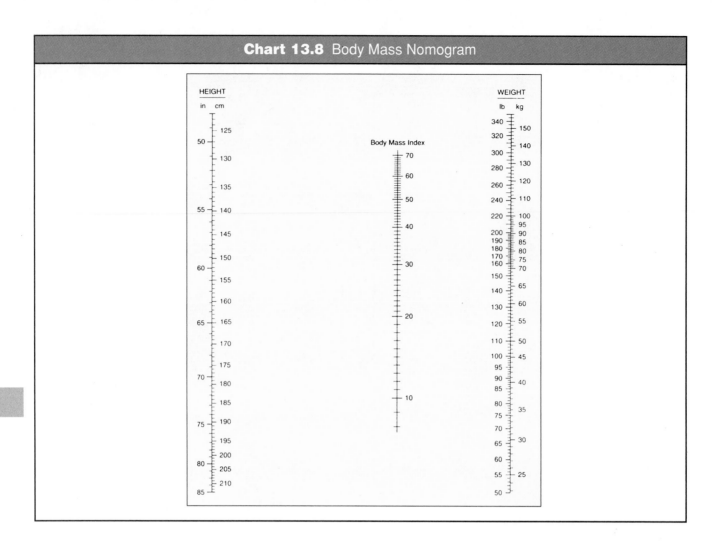

Chart 13.8 Body Mass Nomogram

Body Mass Index (BMI)

Use the steps listed below or use chart 13.8 to calculate your BMI.

1. Divide your weight in pounds by 2.2 to determine your weight in kilograms.

2. Multiply your height in inches by .0254 to determine your height in meters.

3. Square your height in meters (multiply your height in meters by your height in meters).

4. Divide the value you obtain in step 3 (square of height in meters) into the value you obtain in step 1 (weight in kilograms).

5. Use the Rating Scale for Body Mass Index (chart 13.9) to obtain a rating for your BMI.

Chart 13.9 *Rating Scale* for Body Mass Index

Classification	Men	Women
High risk	27.8	27.3
Marginal	25.0–27.7	24.5–27.2
Good fitness zone	19.0–24.9	18.0–24.4
Low	17.9–18.9	15.0–17.9

Note: An excessively low BMI is not desirable. Low BMI values can be indicative of eating disorders and other health problems.

Chart 13.10 Determination of Desirable Body Weight for Men (based on 10 to 20% fat)

Weight	<10%	10%	12%	14%	16%	18%	20%	>20%	22%	24%	26%	28%	30%
				Current Estimated Body Fatness									
240 lbs		240-270	235-264	229-258	224-252	219-246	213-240		208-234	203-228	197-222	192-216	187-210
235 lbs	B	235-264	230-259	225-253	219-247	214-241	209-235	A	204-229	198-223	193-217	188-212	183-206
225 lbs	E	225-253	220-248	215-242	210-236	205-231	200-225	B	195-219	190-214	185-208	180-203	175-197
220 lbs	L	220-248	215-242	210-237	205-231	200-226	196-220	O	191-215	186-209	181-204	176-198	171-193
215 lbs	O	215-242	210-237	205-231	201-226	196-220	191-215	V	186-210	182-204	177-199	172-194	167-188
210 lbs	W	210-236	205-231	201-226	196-221	191-215	187-210	E	182-205	177-200	173-194	168-189	163-184
205 lbs		205-231	200-226	196-220	191-215	187-210	182-205		178-200	173-195	169-190	164-185	159-179
200 lbs	G	200-225	196-220	191-215	187-210	182-205	178-200	G	173-195	169-190	164-185	160-180	156-175
195 lbs	O	195-219	191-215	186-210	182-205	178-200	173-195	O	169-190	165-185	160-180	156-176	152-171
190 lbs	O	190-214	186-209	182-204	177-200	173-195	169-190	O	165-185	160-181	156-176	152-171	148-166
185 lbs	D	185-208	181-204	177-199	173-194	169-190	164-185	D	160-180	156-176	152-171	148-167	144-162
180 lbs		180-203	176-198	172-194	168-189	164-185	160-180		156-176	152-171	148-167	144-162	140-158
175 lbs	F	175-197	171-193	167-188	163-184	159-179	156-175	F	152-171	148-166	144-162	140-158	136-153
170 lbs	I	170-191	166-187	162-183	159-179	155-174	151-170	I	147-166	144-162	140-157	136-153	132-149
165 lbs	T	165-186	161-182	158-177	154-173	150-169	147-165	T	143-161	139-157	136-153	132-149	128-144
160 lbs	N	160-180	156-176	153-172	149-168	146-164	142-160	N	139-156	135-152	132-148	128-144	124-140
155 lbs	E	155-174	152-171	148-167	145-163	141-159	138-155	E	134-151	131-147	127-143	124-140	121-136
150 lbs	S	150-169	147-165	143-161	140-158	137-154	133-150	S	130-146	127-143	123-139	120-135	117-131
145 lbs	S	145-163	142-160	139-156	135-152	132-149	129-145	S	126-141	122-138	119-134	116-131	113-127
140 lbs		140-158	137-154	134-151	131-147	128-144	124-140		121-137	118-133	115-130	112-126	109-123
135 lbs	Z	135-152	132-149	129-145	126-142	123-138	120-135	Z	117-132	114-128	111-125	108-122	105-118
130 lbs	O	130-146	127-143	124-140	121-137	118-133	116-130	O	113-127	110-124	107-120	104-117	101-114
125 lbs	N	125-141	122-138	119-134	117-131	114-128	111-125	N	108-122	106-119	103-116	100-113	97-109
120 lbs	E	120-135	117-132	115-129	112-126	109-123	107-120	E	104-117	101-114	99-111	96-108	93-105
115 lbs		115-129	112-127	110-124	107-121	105-118	102-115		100-112	97-109	95-106	92-104	89-101
110 lbs		110-124	108-121	105-118	103-116	100-113	98-110		95-107	93-105	90-102	88-99	86-96
105 lbs		105-118	103-116	100-113	98-110	96-108	93-105		91-102	89-100	86-97	84-95	82-92
100 lbs		100-113	98-110	96-108	93-105	91-103	89-100		87-98	84-95	82-93	80-90	78-88
95 lbs		95-107	93-105	91-102	89-100	87-97	84-95		82-92	80-90	78-88	76-86	74-83
90 lbs		90-101	88-99	86-97	84-95	82-93	80-90		78-88	76-86	74-83	72-81	70-79

Along the side, locate your current body weight. Across the top, locate your estimated percent fat. The intersection of the two entries represents weights that correspond to 10 to 20% fat (the good fitness zone). For example, if you weigh 180 pounds and are now 14% fat the lines intersect at 172–194 pounds. You are already in the good fitness zone. The 172 represents the weight you would need to reach to be 10% fat and the 194 represents the weight you would be at 20% fat. These values help you decide what you would weigh for different fat levels in the good fitness zone. Fat levels below 10% are not calculated because they are below the good fitness zone. For those with fat levels above 20% the weight ranges represent the weight you would have to attain to be between 10 and 20% fat. For example a person who weight 210 pounds and is 30% fat would have to weigh 163 to be 10% fat and 184 to be 20% fat. Credit to Ron Hager for his assistance in developing this chart.

To make a metric conversion, see Appendix A.

Chart 13.11 Determination of Desirable Body Weight for Women (based on 16 to 26% fat)

Weight	<16%	16%	18%	20%	22%	24%	26%	>26%	28%	30%	32%	34%	36%
		Current Estimated Body Fatness											
200 lbs	B	240-270	235-264	229-258	224-252	219-246	213-240	A	208-234	203-228	197-222	192-216	187-210
195 lbs	E	195-219	191-215	186-210	182-205	178-200	173-195	B	169-190	165-185	160-180	156-176	152-171
190 lbs	L	190-214	186-209	182-204	177-200	173-195	169-190	O	165-185	160-181	156-176	152-171	148-166
185 lbs	O	185-208	181-204	177-199	173-194	169-190	164-185	V	160-180	156-176	152-171	148-167	144-162
180 lbs	W	180-203	176-198	172-194	168-189	164-185	160-180	E	156-176	152-171	148-167	144-162	140-158
175 lbs		175-197	171-193	167-188	163-184	159-179	156-175		152-171	148-166	144-162	140-158	136-153
170 lbs	G	170-191	166-187	162-183	159-179	155-174	151-170	G	147-166	144-162	140-157	136-153	132-149
165 lbs	O	165-186	161-182	158-177	154-173	150-169	147-165	O	143-161	139-157	136-153	132-149	128-144
160 lbs	O	160-180	156-176	153-172	149-168	146-164	142-160	O	139-156	135-152	132-148	128-144	124-140
155 lbs	D	155-174	152-171	148-167	145-163	141-159	138-155	D	134-151	131-147	127-143	124-140	121-136
150 lbs		150-169	147-165	143-161	140-158	137-154	133-150		130-146	127-143	123-139	120-135	117-131
145 lbs	F	145-163	142-160	139-156	135-152	132-149	129-145	F	126-141	122-138	119-134	116-131	113-127
140 lbs	I	140-158	137-154	134-151	131-147	128-144	124-140	I	121-137	118-133	115-130	112-126	109-123
135 lbs	T	135-152	132-149	129-145	126-142	123-138	120-135	T	117-132	114-128	111-125	108-122	105-118
130 lbs	N	130-146	127-143	124-140	121-137	118-133	116-130	N	113-127	110-124	107-120	104-117	101-114
125 lbs	E	125-141	122-138	119-134	117-131	114-128	111-125	E	108-122	106-119	103-116	100-113	97-109
120 lbs	S	120-135	117-132	115-129	112-126	109-123	107-120	S	104-117	101-114	99-111	96-108	93-105
115 lbs	S	115-129	112-127	110-124	107-121	105-118	102-115	S	100-112	97-109	95-106	92-104	89-101
110 lbs		110-124	108-121	105-118	103-116	100-113	98-110		95-107	93-105	90-102	88-99	86-96
105 lbs	Z	105-118	103-116	100-113	98-110	96-108	93-105	Z	91-102	89-100	86-97	84-95	82-92
100 lbs	O	100-113	98-110	96-108	93-105	91-103	89-100	O	87-98	84-95	82-93	80-90	78-88
95 lbs	N	95-107	93-105	91-102	89-100	87-97	84-95	N	82-93	80-90	78-88	76-86	74-83
90 lbs	E	90-101	88-99	86-97	84-95	82-92	80-90	E	78-88	76-86	74-83	72-81	70-79
85 lbs		85-96	83-94	81-92	79-90	77-88	75-86		72-84	72-82	70-79	68-77	66-75

Along the side, locate your current body weight. Across the top, locate your estimated percent fat. The intersection of the two entries represents weights that correspond to 16 to 26% fat (the good fitness zone). For example, if you weigh 120 pounds and are now 20% fat the lines intersect at 115–129 pounds. You are already in the good fitness zone. The 115 represents the weight you would need to reach to be 16% fat and the 129 represents the weight you would be at 26% fat. These values help you decide what you would weigh for different fat levels in the good fitness zone. Fat levels below 16% are not calculated because they are below the good fitness zone. For those with fat levels above 26% the weight ranges represent the weight you would have to attain to be between 16 and 26% fat. For example a person who weight 160 pounds and is 30% fat would have to weigh 135 to be 16% fat and 152 to be 26% fat. Credit to Ron Hager for his assistance in developing this chart.

To make a metric conversion, see Appendix A.

CONCEPT ·14·

Controlling Body Fatness

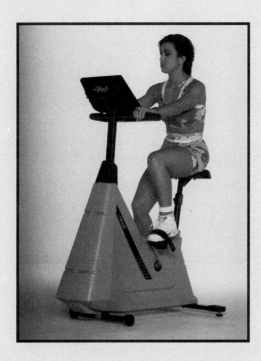

Concept 14

There are various strategies for eating and performing physical activity that can be useful in fat (weight) control.

Introduction

Estimates indicating that 33.4 percent of adults are overfat is cause for concern, especially since it represents a dramatic increase in recent years. However, it is important to keep the concern about fat and weight control in perspective. A recent poll indicated that 96 percent of all adult males and 99 percent of all adult females would change something about their physical appearance. The leading concern was weight loss. In fact, 66.5 percent of all Americans want to lose weight in the upcoming year (see figure 14.1). Experts suggest that movies, television, and magazines have created an obsession with weight loss among many teens and adults. In many cases the concern is with losing weight rather than fat, and with appearance rather than good health. Caution is necessary so that we do not create more problems than we solve.

Because of the misplaced concern with weight loss among large numbers of people, the emphasis of this concept will be on fat loss for good health. When properly done, fat control can be safe and effective. This concept will make suggestions for losing, maintaining, and gaining body fat.

Health Goals for the Year 2000

- Reduce overfatness to no more than 20 percent of people aged 20 or more. (↓)
- Reduce overfatness to no more than 15 percent of people aged 12 to 19. (↓)
- Increase to 50 percent the proportion of overfat people who have adopted physical activity and sound nutrition to attain desirable body fatness. (<>)

Note: (↑) indicates progress toward goal, (↓) indicates regression from goal, and (<>) indicates either no change or lack of new data since 1990.

Terms

- **Behavioral Goal**   A statement of intent to perform a specific behavior (changing a lifestyle) for a specific period of time. An example would be, "I will reduce the fat in my diet to 30 percent or less of my total calories."
- **Empty Calories**   Calories in foods considered to have little nutritional value.
- **Long-Term Goal**   A statement of intent to change behavior or achieve a specific outcome in a period of months or years.
- **Negative Self-Talk**   Self-defeating discussions with yourself focusing on your failures rather than your successes.
- **Outcome Goal**   A statement of intent to achieve a specific test score or a specific standard associated with good health or wellness. An example would be, "I will lower my body fat level by three percent."

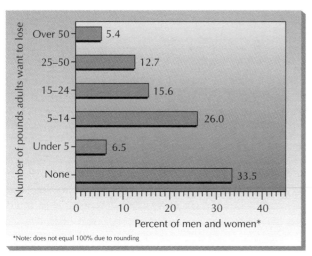

Figure 14.1
Pounds of weight Americans want to lose

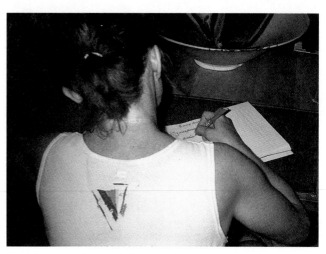

Keeping exercise and dietary records is important.

- **Positive Self-Talk** Telling yourself positive, encouraging things that help you succeed in accomplishing your goals.
- **Short-Term Goal** A statement of intent to change a behavior or outcome in a period of days or weeks.

The Facts: Lifestyles and Fat Control

> The first step in fat control is establishing realistic goals.

Too many teens and adults, both men and women, establish unrealistic goals for their physical appearance. Fat, weight, and body proportions are all factors that can be changed, but people often set standards for themselves that will be difficult, if not impossible, to achieve. It is important that goals be set for fat and weight control that can be accomplished for both the short and the long term. This necessitates developing an understanding of your own body proportions as well as your body fatness. Unrealistic goals may result in eating disorders, failure to meet goals, or the failure to maintain fat loss over time. Measurement procedures can be used to help you establish realistic goals.

> Goals that emphasize the behavior of eating less and exercising more are more effective than those emphasizing a specific outcome such as weight or fat lost (or gained).

Researchers have shown that setting **outcome goals,** or goals that set a specific amount of weight or fat loss (gain), can be discouraging. If a behavioral goal of eating a reasonable number of calories per day and expending a reasonable number of

calories in exercise is met, outcome goals will be achieved. Most experts believe that **behavioral goals** work better than weight or fat loss goals, especially in the short term.

> People who have a large amount of fat to lose may do better setting **short-term** rather than **long-term goals.**

Losing 50 pounds (22.7 kilograms) may seem impossible. Losing 2 pounds (1 kilogram) in a week may seem more achievable. Because your weight can fluctuate with the amount of water lost or retained, daily monitoring of weight can also be discouraging. Weight may drop dramatically one day because of water loss and increase the next. Care must be taken not to worry too much about daily weight or fat losses or gains in the early stages of a program.

> Record keeping is important to meeting fat control goals and making moderation a part of your normal lifestyle.

Studies have shown that it is easy to fool yourself when determining the amount of food you have eaten or the amount of exercise you have done. Once fat control goals have been set, whether for weight loss, maintenance, or gain, it is important to keep records of your behavior. People often underestimate the amount of food they have eaten, particularly the number of calories consumed. They also tend to overestimate the amount of exercise they do. Keeping a diet log and an exercise log can help you monitor your behavior and maintain the lifestyle necessary to meet your goals. A log can also help you monitor changes in weight and body fatness. But remember, care should be taken to avoid too much emphasis on short-term weight changes. A log can be used for record keeping.

> The best way to control body fatness is to establish a healthy lifestyle.

One way to ascertain whether fat control goals are realistic is to determine if they can be maintained for a lifetime. Diets that require severe caloric restriction or exercise programs that require exceptionally large caloric expenditure can be effective in fat loss over a short period, but are seldom maintained for a lifetime. Studies show that extreme programs for fat and weight control, designed to "take it off fast," result in long-term success rates of less than 5 percent. A healthy lifestyle includes a healthy diet and regular exercise. For some people it may be necessary to develop a daily habit of eating several hundred calories less than other people or maintaining an exercise schedule that expends more calories than the normal person if desirable body fat levels are to be maintained. These habits of "moderation" can realistically become part of your normal lifestyle.

Some Facts About Eating and Fat Control

> There are some general guidelines for eating that can help people interested in losing body fat.

- Restrict calories in moderate amounts per day rather than make large reductions in daily caloric intake.
- Eat less fat. Research shows that reduction of the fat in the diet not only results in fewer calories consumed (fats have more than twice the calories per gram as carbohydrates or proteins), but in greater body fat loss as well!
- Severely restrict **empty calories.** Foods with empty calories provide little nutrition and can account for an excessive amount of your daily caloric intake. Examples of these foods are candy (often high in simple sugar) and potato chips (often fried in saturated fat).
- Increase complex carbohydrates. Foods high in fiber, such as fresh fruits and vegetables, contain few calories for their volume. They are nutritious and filling, and are especially good foods for a fat loss program.
- Learn the difference between craving and hunger. Hunger is a physiological phenomenon that is a result of the body's need to supply energy to sustain life. A craving is simply a desire to eat something; sometimes a food that is not particularly liked. When you feel the urge to eat, you may want to ask yourself: is this real hunger or a craving? Hunger is accompanied by growling of the stomach and is most likely to occur after long periods without food. If you have the urge to eat soon after a meal, it is probably from craving, not hunger.

> There are some guidelines about shopping that can help people interested in fat control.

- Shop from a list. This helps you avoid the purchase of foods that contain empty calories and other foods that will tempt you to overeat.
- Shop with a friend. This is another way to help you avoid the purchase of unneeded foods. For this technique to work, the other person must be sensitive to your goals. In some cases, a friend can have a bad, rather than a good, influence.
- Shop on a full stomach to avoid the temptations of snacking on and buying junk food.
- Check the label for contents of foods. If the calories are not listed, be wary of buying them. Many so-called weight reduction foods have caloric contents equal to or in excess of normal foods.
- Consider foods that take some preparation time. If it takes time to prepare food, you may be less likely to eat it on the spur of the moment. It is acceptable to purchase foods prepackaged in small portions and that contain low caloric content, even if they require little preparation.

> There are some guidelines about the way you eat that can be useful in fat loss.

- When you eat, do nothing else but eat. If you watch television, read, or do some other activity while you eat, you may be unaware of what you have eaten. Also, you should enjoy your eating, not share it with some other activity.
- Eat slowly. Taste your food. Pause between bites. Chew slowly. Don't take the next bite until you have swallowed what you have in your mouth. Periodically take a longer pause. Be the last one finished eating.
- Do not eat food you do not want. Some people do not want to waste food so they clean their plate even when they feel full.
- Follow an eating schedule. Eating at regular meal times can help you avoid snacking. If meals are spaced equally throughout the day, it can help reduce appetite.
- Do your eating in designated areas only. Designate areas such as the kitchen and dining room as eating areas.
- Eat meals of equal size. Some people try to restrict calories at one or two meals to save up for a big meal. Eating several *small* meals helps you to avoid hunger (fools the appetite) and helps you keep from losing control at one meal.

- Leave the table after eating and clear dishes early. Clearing the dishes and leaving the table help prevent you from taking extra unwanted bites and servings.
- Avoid second servings. Limit your intake to one moderate serving. If second servings are taken, make them one-half the size of first servings.
- Limit servings of salad dressings and condiments (catsup, etc.). These are often high in fat and calories, and can sometimes amount to greater calorie consumption than the food on which you put them.
- Limit servings of nonbasic parts of the meal. It is easy to consume large numbers of calories on alcohol, soft drinks, breads, and desserts. Limit these items.

There are some guidelines that are useful for controlling the home environment to aid in fat loss.

- Keep busy, especially at high-risk times or times when you are most likely to eat when you do not want to. If you have an urge to eat, exercise, talk to someone, go shopping, drink a glass of water, or find something active to do.
- Store food out of sight. Avoid containers that allow you to see food. It is especially important to limit the accessibility of foods that tempt you and foods with empty calories. "Foods that are out of sight, are out of mouth."
- Avoid serving food to others, especially between meals. Let them prepare their own snacks.
- If you snack, eat foods high in complex carbohydrates and low in fats, such as fresh fruits and carrot sticks.
- Freeze leftovers. Leftover foods are often tempting to eat. Freezing them so that it takes preparation to eat them will help you avoid temptation.

There are some guidelines for controlling the work environment to aid in fat loss.

- Take food from home rather than eating from vending machines or catering trucks. Even snacks should be brought from home, where they can be prepared based on guidelines listed above.
- Avoid snack machines. Most snacks from machines are high in calories and low in nutritional value. Fresh fruit from machines is an exception.
- If you eat out, plan your meal selection ahead of time. Write it down and know its calorie content. Be aware that many fast foods are high in caloric content and fat.
- Do not eat while working.
- Avoid sources of food provided by coworkers; for example, food in work rooms, such as birthday cakes, or candy in jars.

- Do something active during breaks. For example, take a walk.
- Have drinking water or low-calorie drinks available to substitute for snacks.

There are some guidelines about eating on special occasions that can be useful in fat loss.

- Practice ways to refuse food. Practice in front of a mirror or with friends. Know exactly what to say when you plan to refuse food. Do not let yourself be intimidated into eating something you do not want. For example, you might say something as simple as "No thank you." Be wary of persistent hosts. Do not let them make you feel guilty for not eating. Be polite but emphatic; give no indication that you might change your mind.
- In extreme cases, you may wish to avoid situations that create a high risk of overeating.
- Eat before you go out.
- When eating out, order à la carte.
- Do not stand near food sources.
- If you feel the urge to eat, talk to someone or find something else to occupy your thoughts.

Fad diets are not a satisfactory means to long-term weight reduction and may adversely affect your health.

There are hundreds of fad diets and diet books, but dietitians warn that there is no scientific basis for drastic juggling of food constituents. Such diets are usually unbalanced and may result in serious illness or even death, especially for the obese person who is already apt to be suffering from a number of health disorders. Fad diets cannot be maintained for long periods; therefore, the individual usually regains any lost weight. Less than five percent of those who lose weight maintain the loss for more than a year. Constant losing and gaining, known as the "yo-yo syndrome," may be as harmful as the original obese condition.

Total fasting is dangerous, as are crash (fast) diets. Crash diets that bring about weight loss by dehydration of only five percent in forty-eight hours have been shown to reduce the individual's working capacity by as much as forty percent. The practice of making weight in athletics, whether by dehydration, induced vomiting, or starvation diets, is dangerous to health and should be condemned. Much of the weight loss on such fad diets is valuable lean muscle mass.

Pill popping, hormone injections, and powder and liquid diets have little value in long-term weight control programs and present many health hazards. When in doubt, avoid diets that:

- Promise fast, easy solutions.
- Promise to help you achieve ideal weight without mental inspiration and perspiration.

- Favor one food as the answer to weight problems.
- Promise that your fat will melt away.

> Artificial sweeteners and fat substitutes may help, but are not a "sure cure," for body fatness problems.

- Artificial sweeteners have dramatically reduced the calories in some soft drinks and foods. However, since they were introduced the general public has not eaten fewer calories and more people are now overweight than before they were introduced.
- In 1996 "Olestra," a fat substitute, was approved. Olestra is often referred to as "fake fat" and is used as a fat substitute in baking and cooking. It will result in potato chips and other fried foods with less fat and fewer calories and will also result in lower fat and calories in baked goods. If you eat no more food than usual and substitute foods with Olestra you will consume fewer calories and less fat. Experts worry that the tendency will be to eat more "empty calories". For example, a chocolate chip cookie with Olestra has one half the calories of a regular cookie so some may feel that they can now eat two (or more). Olestra passes through the body without being digested and has been shown to remove some vital nutrients (especially fat soluble vitamins) as it passes through the digestive system. In some cases some people it causes gastrointestinal problems including diarrhea.

> Many of the eating guidelines that are useful for fat loss are also valuable in maintaining desirable levels of body fat.

Once a person has achieved a desirable level of body fatness, it is important that this level be maintained throughout life. Many of the eating strategies for losing body fatness listed in the previous sections are also appropriate for maintaining body fat levels at desirable levels. If you follow them, you will develop new and healthier eating patterns that you will retain for the rest of your life.

> Some people need to gain weight and can benefit from a change in their eating patterns.

Most people who want to gain weight want to gain lean body tissue. Only those who have body fat percentages less than what is considered to be essential for good health need to gain body fat. Some eating guidelines for people interested in gaining weight are listed here:

- Increase the calories consumed. Increasing caloric intake by amounts of 500–1000 calories a day will help most people gain weight over time.
- The majority of extra calories should come from complex carbohydrates. Breads, pasta, rice, fruits such

as bananas, and potatoes are good sources. High-protein diets or diet supplements are not particularly effective if you maintain a normal diet. High-fat diets can result in weight gain but may not be best for good health, especially if they are high in saturated fat.
- If extra exercise results in extra calories expended, caloric intake will need to be adjusted to compensate. It may be difficult to eat when you are not hungry. Eating more than three meals per day may help.
- Drink lots of juice and milk. Grape and cranberry juices are good because they are high in calories.
- Eat snacks. Bananas, granola, and nuts are high-calorie, healthy snacks.
- If weight gain does not occur over a period of weeks and months with extra caloric consumption, medical assistance may be necessary.

> More calories are required to maintain weight during the growing years than in adulthood.

Typically, those most likely to have difficulty in gaining weight are age ten to twenty. They have probably been told more than once that they will not have trouble gaining weight when they grow older. This is true for most people, but it is of little consolation to those who want to gain weight now. During adolescence, most people begin to gain weight, including muscle mass that can be enhanced with regular exercise. If they follow the guidelines just listed, they may have success in gaining weight. Excessive eating to gain weight (especially during adolescence) is not without its problems. The body requires more caloric intake during the teen years because the body is growing. A person who develops a habit of high caloric intake during this time may have a difficult time controlling fatness when the demands on the body are less.

Some Facts About Physical Activity and Fat Control

> There are some guidelines for physical activity that can be of value in losing or maintaining desirable body-fat levels.

- Perform regular aerobic exercise. Since aerobic exercise can be maintained for a long period, it allows you to expend large numbers of calories. For this reason, it is the best type of physical activity for fat loss and maintenance.
- Find a time, a place, and a type of physical activity that will permit you to work out regularly. Regularity is the key. Exercise must be regular if it is to be of value.
- Performing strength training can increase muscle mass and result in fat loss without loss in weight. If you follow the guidelines for strength training, you can increase your muscle mass provided calorie intake is constant.

> Two principal guidelines for physical activity are of value in gaining weight, including muscle mass.

- Performing strength training can aid in weight gain. It is the best form of exercise for people interested in gaining weight. Of course, strength training is most effective in weight gain when accompanied by an increase in calorie intake.
- Excessive aerobic exercise may make it difficult to gain weight. Although some regular aerobic exercise is necessary for health and cardiovascular fitness, it may be necessary to limit aerobic exercise if weight gain is the goal. Studies have shown that extensive aerobic training can even cause a reduction in muscle mass. When training to gain weight, aerobic exercise expending no more than 3500 calories per week is probably best.

Some Facts About Social and Psychological Strategies

> The support of family and friends can be of great importance in fat control.

The importance of family and friends to successful exercise adherence can't be overemphasized. Family and friends can also help you in changing and adhering to healthy eating practices. It is known that parents who overeat often have children who eat more than normal. In these cases, it is important for the entire family to participate in a program to control fatness. Family and friends should provide support for the person trying to gain or lose fat by helping them follow the guidelines presented in this concept, rather than tempting the person to eat improperly. Unfortunately there is sometimes a danger of overemphasis on fat loss by a friend or family member. This can have the opposite effect of that intended if it is perceived as an attempt to control one's behavior. Studies have shown that the use of extrinsic rewards such as money or special gifts for achieving goals may be effective in the *short* term, but may result in resentment rather than adherence over the long term. Encouragement and support rather than control of behavior is the key!

> Group support can be one of the best reinforcers of proper eating and exercise behavior.

Group support has been found to be beneficial to many individuals who are attempting to change their behavior. Alcoholics have found that the support of others is critical to their rehabilitation (Alcoholics Anonymous grew as a result of this need). If you want to alter your body composition, especially to lose body fat, group support is important if you are to make permanent lifestyle changes in diet and exercise. Groups such as Overeaters Anonymous and Weight Watchers have been organized to help those who need the support of peers in attaining and maintaining desirable fat levels for a lifetime.

> There are some psychological strategies that can be of assistance in eating and exercising to attain and maintain a desirable level of body fatness.

- Avoid food fantasies. Sometimes the thought of food is what causes overeating. Practice restructuring your thought process to something other than food fantasies. Use mental imagery to create a mind's eye view of something you enjoy other than food. When food fantasies occur, you may want to exercise or engage in some activity that refocuses your attention.
- Avoid weight fantasies. Sometimes the thought of being excessively thin or muscular occurs. By itself, this may not be bad. If, however, it causes you to become discouraged and makes your goals seem unattainable, it is bad. When weight fantasies occur, do some other activity to redirect your focus of attention or imagine something other than the weight fantasy. Altering mental fantasies takes practice.
- Avoid **negative self-talk.** One type of negative self-talk occurs when a person starts self-criticism for not meeting a goal. For example, if a person is determined not to eat more than one serving of food at a party, but fails to meet this goal, he or she might say, "It's no use stopping now; I've already blown it." It is not too late. Failing to meet goals can happen to anyone. Negative self-talk makes it easy to fail in the future. A more appropriate response would involve **positive self-talk** such as, "I'm not going to eat anything else tonight; I can do it."

Suggested Readings

Brownell, K., et al. "Matching Weight Control Programs to Individuals." *The Weight Control Digest* 1(1991):65.

Brownell, K., J. Rodin, and J. Wilmore (Eds.). *Eating, Body Weight, and Performance in Athletes: Disorders of Modern Society.* Philadelphia: Lea & Febiger, 1992.

Clark, N. "How to Gain Weight Healthfully." *Physician and Sportsmedicine* 19(1991):53.

Lemonick, M. D. "Are We Ready for Fat Free Fat?" *Time Magazine* 4(January 22, 1996), 40.

University of California at Berkeley Wellness Letter. "Thin Thighs In A Bottle," *University of California at Berkeley Wellness Letter,* 10(1994):1.

Work, J. "Exercise for the Overweight Patient." *Physician and Sportsmedicine* 18(1990):113.

LAB RESOURCE MATERIALS

Chart 14.1 Diet Log		
Food Eaten and Amount	**Calories**	**Time of Day**
Total Calories	_____	
Daily Calorie Goal	_____	

Chart 14.2 Exercise Log		
Activity	**Time (min.)**	**Calories**
Total Calories	_____	
Daily Calorie Goal	_____	

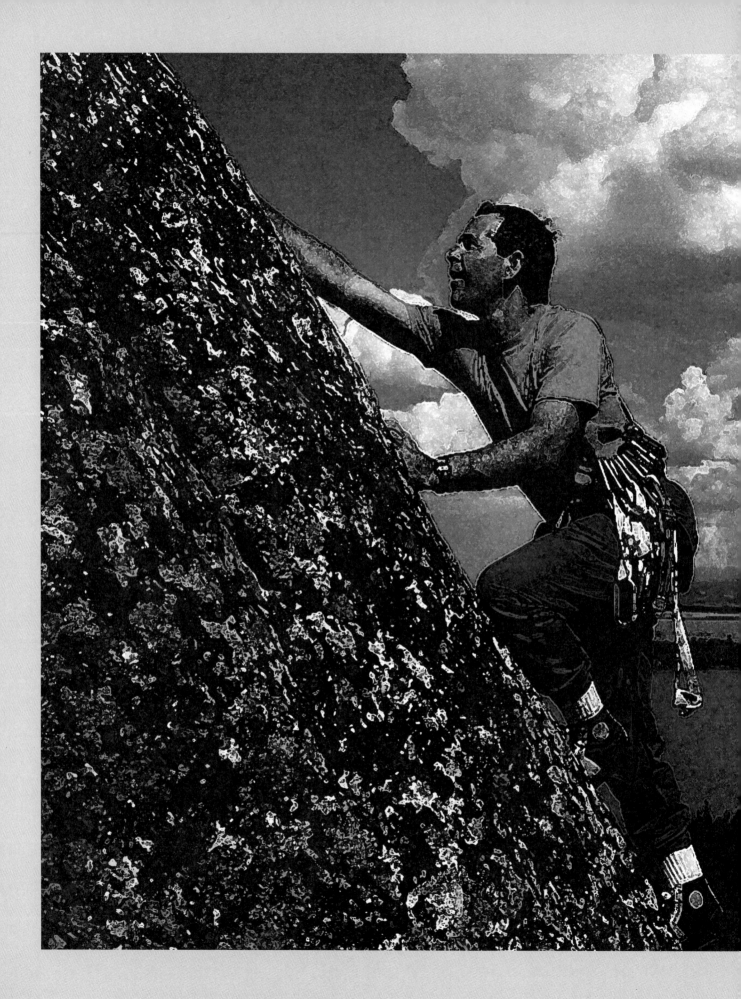

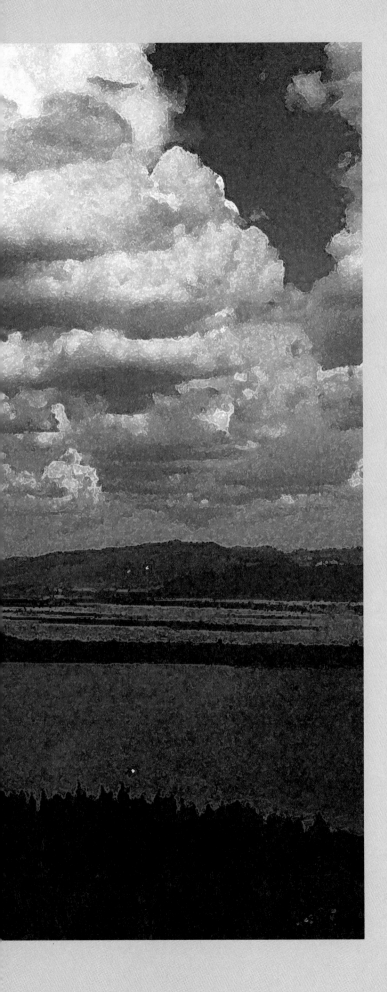

SECTION
·III·

Special Considerations for Physical Activity

CONCEPT ·15·

Sports and Other Physical Activities and Skill-Related Physical Fitness

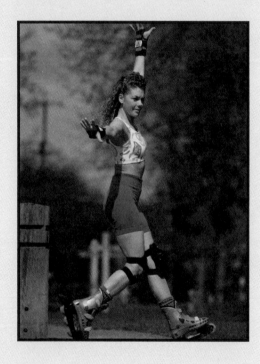

Concept 15

Everyone, regardless of physical ability, can find a sport or physical activity to enjoy for a lifetime.

Introduction

Sports are an important part of Western culture. Virtually all people are involved with sports, either as a spectator or as a participant. Sports can be used as recreational activities for enjoying free time or, if done as a participant, can be a significant part of a personal physical fitness program. In addition to sports, there are other physical activities that are enjoyable as lifetime recreational pursuits. Sports, more than any other type of physical activity, requires skill and skill-related physical fitness. Learning about skilled-related physical fitness can help you select a sport that is well suited for your personal needs, interests, and abilities.

Health Goals for the Year 2000

- Increase the proportion of people who engage in regular physical activity. (↑)
- Reduce the proportion of people who engage in no free-time physical activity. (<>)
- Increase worksite physical activity programs. (↑)

Note: (↑) indicates progress toward goal, (↓) indicates regression from goal, and (<>) indicates either no change or lack of new data since 1990.

Terms

- **Lifetime Sport**   A sport suitable for people of all ages; a sport that can be performed "from the cradle to the grave" (for a lifetime).
- **Motor Fitness**   A term commonly used for skill-related physical fitness.
- **Preplanned Exercise Programs**   Preplanned exercise programs are exercise regimes planned by someone other than the person doing the exercise. Often they are designed for a large group of people rather than for one individual. They are often developed using exercises from the aerobic, strength and muscular endurance, and flexibility areas of the physical activity pyramid.
- **Self-Promoting Activities**   Physical activities in which the performer is not required to have a high level of skill to perform with some degree of success.
- **Sport**   Activity from the second level of the physical activity pyramid that involves competition between teams or individuals in which the goal is to beat the opponent or win the game. Except in the case of ties, there is a winner and a loser. Activities such as swimming, cycling, and jogging/running are classified as sports by some writers; however, in this text they are defined as aerobic activities rather than as sports because most adults do not perform these activities competitively.
- **Sports Fitness**   A term commonly used for skill-related physical fitness.

The Facts About Skill-Related Fitness

There are several components of skill-related physical fitness.

The six components of skill-related physical fitness (agility, coordination, balance, reaction time, speed, and power) were chosen because they are among the most important to sports performance and easiest to measure. There are probably other abilities that also contribute to performing skills. For example, many experts consider various perceptual abilities such as depth and distance perception (ability to judge depth and distances accurately) and visual tracking (ability to visually follow a moving object) to be skill-related parts of physical fitness. Skill-related physical fitness is also sometimes referred to as **motor fitness** or **sports fitness.**

There are subcomponents of each part of skill-related physical fitness.

Most of the six parts of skill-related physical fitness have subcomponents. For example, coordination includes foot-eye coordination and hand-eye coordination, which are measured quite differently. The tests in this concept were chosen to measure some of the skill-related fitness aspects most important to **sports** performance.

An individual might possess ability in one area and not in another. For this reason, "general motor ability" probably does not really exist. Individuals do not have one general capacity for performing. Rather, the ability to play games or sports is determined by combined abilities in each of the separate skill-related components. It is, however, possible and even likely that some performers will be above average in many areas.

Skills are *not* the same thing as skill-related fitness.

Skill-related physical fitness abilities, such as those described above, predispose some people to be better performers than others. But skills can be learned by anyone with practice. Examples of skills are catching or kicking a ball, throwing, hitting a tennis ball, and even running efficiently. Coordination, a component of skill-related fitness, allows you to learn catching and throwing more easily but even people with relatively poor coordination can learn to throw with practice. For most people it is wisest to practice the specific skills you want to perform rather than spending a lot of time trying to improve your skill-related fitness abilities.

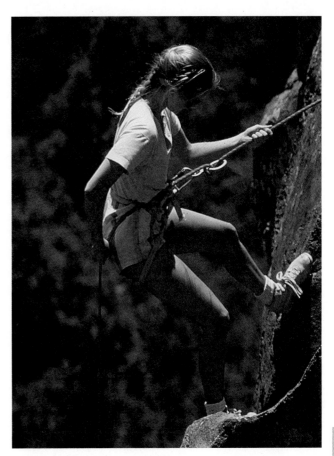

Different activities require different components of skill-related fitness.

Exceptional athletes tend to be outstanding in more than one component of skill-related fitness.

Though people possess skill-related fitness in varying degrees, great athletes are likely to be above average in most, if not all, aspects. Indeed, exceptional athletes must be exceptional in many areas of skill-related fitness. Different sports require different skills, each of which requires varying degrees of the six components of skill-related fitness.

Excellence in one skill-related fitness component may compensate for a lack in another.

Each individual possesses a specific level of each skill-related fitness aspect. The performer should learn his or her other strengths and weaknesses in order to produce optimal performances. For example, a tennis player may use good coordination to compensate for lack of speed.

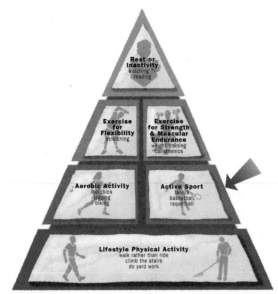

Figure 15.1
Sports require high levels of skill-related fitness and skill.

Excellence in skill-related fitness may compensate for a lack of health-related fitness when playing sports and games.

As you grow older, health-related fitness potential declines much more rapidly than many components of skill-related fitness. You may use superior skill-related fitness to compensate. For example, a baseball pitcher who lacks the strength and power to dominate hitters may rely on a pitch such as a knuckleball, which is more dependent on coordination than on power.

Health-related fitness is important in playing sports and games.

Health-related fitness is not a substitute for skill-related fitness when it comes to performing successfully in sports. However, good health-related fitness is critical to exceptional performances of many kinds. For example, a gymnast with coordination, balance, and agility must have strength and flexibility to excel, and a football player with power and coordination must have cardiovascular fitness and muscular endurance to perform at optimal levels.

Activities from the sports category of the physical activity pyramid require more skill-related fitness and skills than activities from other categories of activities from the pyramid.

Most sports require relatively high levels of skill-related fitness and also require specific skills of the game. If you plan to do these activities later in life you must practice the skills of these activities. Activities from other areas of the pyramid (see figure 15.1) require less skill-related fitness and skill. You can learn to assess your own skill-related fitness using some simple tests provided in the Lab Resource Materials. When you have completed the tests use table 15.1 to help you determine which activities best match your skill-related fitness abilities. You will have the easiest time learning and performing those activities that require the parts of skill-related fitness in which you score well. No matter what your skill-related fitness or skill level there is some activity in which you can succeed.

The Facts About Sports

Sports can be a good form of leisure.

True leisure is a state of mind associated with a feeling of freedom and being able to enjoy yourself. Sports receive the highest ratings of all daily activities in terms of perceived feelings of freedom. Sport is rated as "something I want to do" more often than other work or free-time activities, such as cultural activities and home leisure.

The most popular participation sports are not the same as the most popular spectator sports.

Team sports are the most popular spectator sports, with football leading the list. Other popular spectator sports, as well as the most popular participation sports among adults, are listed in table 15.2. The sports that adults enjoy watching are not the same as the ones they enjoy playing.

The most popular sports share characteristics that contribute to their popularity.

The most popular sports are often considered to be **lifetime sports** because they can be done at any age. The characteristics that make these sports appropriate for lifelong participation probably contribute significantly to their popularity. Six of the top ten are individual sports that do not require a large group of people to play them. Often the popular sports are adapted so that people without exceptional skill can play them. For example, bowling uses a "handicap system" to allow people with a wide range of abilities to compete. Slow pitch softball is much more popular than fast pitch because it allows people of all abilities to play successfully.

Sports are most enjoyable when the challenge is optimal.

One of the primary reasons sports participation is so popular is that sports provide a challenge. For the greatest enjoyment, the challenge of the activity should be balanced by

Table 15.1
Skill-Related Benefits of Sports and Other Activities

Activity	Balance	Coordination	Reaction Time	Agility	Power	Speed
Archery	Good	Excellent	Poor	Poor	Poor	Poor
Backpacking	Fair	Fair	Poor	Fair	Fair	Poor
Badminton	Fair	Excellent	Good	Good	Fair	Good
Baseball	Good	Excellent	Excellent	Good	Excellent	Good
Basketball	Good	Excellent	Excellent	Excellent	Excellent	Good
Bicycling	Excellent	Fair	Fair	Poor	Fair	Fair
Bowling	Good	Excellent	Poor	Fair	Fair	Fair
Canoeing	Good	Good	Fair	Poor	Good	Poor
Circuit training	Fair	Fair	Poor	Fair	Good	Fair
Dance, aerobic	Fair	Excellent	Fair	Good	Poor	Poor
Dance, ballet	Excellent	Excellent	Fair	Excellent	Good	Poor
Dance, disco	Fair	Good	Fair	Excellent	Poor	Fair
Dance, modern	Excellent	Excellent	Fair	Excellent	Good	Poor
Dance, social	Fair	Good	Fair	Good	Poor	Fair
Fencing	Good	Excellent	Excellent	Good	Good	Excellent
Fitness calisthenics	Fair	Fair	Poor	Good	Fair	Poor
Football	Good	Good	Excellent	Excellent	Excellent	Excellent
Golf (walking)	Fair	Excellent	Poor	Fair	Good	Poor
Gymnastics	Excellent	Excellent	Good	Excellent	Excellent	Fair
Handball	Fair	Excellent	Good	Excellent	Good	Good
Hiking	Fair	Fair	Poor	Fair	Fair	Poor
Horseback riding	Good	Good	Fair	Good	Poor	Poor
Interval training	Fair	Fair	Poor	Poor	Poor	Fair
Jogging	Fair	Fair	Poor	Poor	Poor	Poor
Judo	Good	Excellent	Excellent	Excellent	Excellent	Excellent
Karate	Good	Excellent	Excellent	Excellent	Excellent	Excellent
Mountain climbing	Excellent	Excellent	Fair	Good	Good	Poor
Pool; billiards	Fair	Good	Poor	Fair	Fair	Poor
Racquetball; paddleball	Fair	Excellent	Good	Excellent	Fair	Good
Rope jumping	Fair	Good	Fair	Good	Fair	Poor
Rowing, crew	Fair	Excellent	Poor	Good	Excellent	Fair
Sailing	Good	Good	Good	Good	Fair	Poor
Skating, ice	Excellent	Good	Fair	Good	Fair	Good
Skating, roller	Excellent	Good	Poor	Good	Fair	Good
Skiing, cross-country	Fair	Excellent	Poor	Good	Excellent	Fair
Skiing, downhill	Excellent	Excellent	Good	Excellent	Good	Poor
Soccer	Fair	Excellent	Good	Excellent	Good	Good
Softball (fast pitch)	Fair	Excellent	Excellent	Good	Good	Good
Softball (slow pitch)	Fair	Excellent	Good	Fair	Good	Good
Surfing	Excellent	Excellent	Good	Excellent	Good	Poor
Swimming (laps)	Fair	Good	Poor	Good	Fair	Poor
Table tennis	Fair	Good	Good	Fair	Fair	Fair
Tennis	Fair	Excellent	Good	Good	Good	Good
Volleyball	Fair	Excellent	Good	Good	Fair	Fair
Walking	Fair	Fair	Poor	Poor	Poor	Poor
Waterskiing	Good	Good	Poor	Good	Fair	Poor
Weight training	Fair	Fair	Poor	Poor	Fair	Poor

From *Fitness for Life,* updated 3rd edition, by Charles B. Corbin and Ruth Lindsey, Copyright © 1993 Scott Foresman and Company, a division of Addison-Wesley Educational Publishers Inc. Reprinted by permission.

Table 15.2
Popular Sports

Sport	Participation Rank	Spectator Rank
Bowling	1	9 (tie)
Pool/billiards	2	*
Race cycling	3	*
Softball	4	*
Volleyball	5	*
Golf	6	5 (tie)
Basketball	7	3
Table tennis	8	*
Baseball	9	2
Tennis	10	4
Football	*	1
Ice hockey	*	5 (tie)
Boxing	*	9 (tie)
Ice Skating	*	7 (tie)
Wrestling	*	9 (tie)
Auto Racing	*	7 (tie)
Gymnastics	*	9 (tie)

*Not in top ten sports.
Source: Data from the Gallup Poll.

the person's skill in the sport. If you choose to play against one of lesser skill, you will not be challenged. On the other hand, if you lack skill or your opponent has considerably more skill, the activity will be frustrating. For optimal challenge and enjoyment, the skills of a given sport should be learned before participation. Likewise, an opponent of similar skill level should be chosen.

In many cases, a person needs to exercise to get fit for sports rather than play sports to get fit.

Many sports require a considerable amount of fitness, especially those involving vigorous competition, yet the sport may do relatively little to develop fitness. For example, you need considerable strength, muscular endurance, and flexibility to play football. However, football is not a particularly good activity for developing these aspects of fitness.

Sports are activities that can be enjoyed by virtually all people.

It is true that sports are most popular among younger people. Yet sports are enjoyed by people of all ages and abilities.

The senior olympics and masters sports programs have expanded participation for people of all ages. In some locations, softball leagues for people age 75 and older have been formed. Though research evidence suggests that most skills are learned early in life, this does not mean that "old dogs cannot learn new tricks." It does suggest a need to teach skills to children at an early age.

Many people with physical disabilities now participate in a wide variety of sports, including wheelchair basketball and beep-beep softball for the blind. The Special Olympics, and other similar programs, have provided many sports opportunities for people with special physical needs and those with learning difficulties.

Some Facts About Sports, Skills, Fitness, and Wellness

Participation in sports can contribute to good health-related physical fitness.

The health-related fitness benefits of participation in the ten most popular sports are presented in table 15.3. Several of the top participation sports, such as softball and pool/billiards, are *not* particularly good activities for building health-related physical fitness. However, experts now agree that regular participation of some kind is better than no participation at all. Individuals who possess good skills in sports and games have the potential to succeed in sports. Research shows that people who make an effort to learn activities involving skills are more likely to be active in sports and games for a lifetime. Remember that anyone can learn skills with practice.

There are benefits to both watching and participating in sports.

Active involvement in sports can have many physical, social, and personal benefits. Though watching sports will not build physical fitness, it does have other benefits. According to recent research, watching sports "almost always" makes people feel happy when their team wins and gives them a feeling of accomplishment and pride, even though they did not participate. On the downside, when the favorite team loses, feelings of depression and lack of accomplishment may occur. In extreme cases, displays of poor sportsmanship and even violence have occurred.

Skill can improve your ability to work efficiently.

In manual labor, skillful performance improves efficiency. For example, a ditchdigger with great ditchdigging skills

Table 15.3
Achieving Fitness through Sports

Sport	Rank	Cardiovascular Fitness	Muscular Endurance	Strength	Flexibility	Fat Control
Bowling	1	*	*	-	-	*
Pool/billiards	2	-	-	-	-	-
Race cycling	3	***	***	**	*	***
Softball	4	*	*	-	-	*
Volleyball	5	**	**	*	*	**
Golf (walking)	6	**	**	*	*	**
Basketball	7	***	**	*	-	***
Table tennis	8	*	*	-	*	*
Baseball	9	*	*	-	-	*
Tennis	10	**	**	*	*	**

***Very Good   **Good   *Minimum-Low

uses less energy than one who has not mastered the skill. Seemingly simple skills are often quite complex but even those with relatively low skill-related fitness scores can learn skills with practice.

Skills and skill-related fitness can improve your ability to meet emergencies.

Good agility would enable you to dodge an oncoming car; good balance would lessen the likelihood of a fall; and good reaction time would decrease the chances of being hit by a flying object. Each aspect of skill-related fitness contributes in its own way to your ability to avoid injury and meet emergencies.

Skills are beneficial to carrying out normal daily routines and enjoying your leisure time.

Walking, sitting, climbing, pushing, pulling, and other such tasks are essential to effective normal daily functioning. Accordingly, improved skills resulting from regular practice may improve efficiency in performing daily activities and in enjoying leisure or recreational time.

The Facts About Nonsport Activities

Nonsport fitness activities are more popular for participation than most sports.

The most popular participation activities among adults are listed in table 15.4. Only three of the top lifetime activities

Table 15.4
Rankings of the Most Popular Lifetime Physical Activities

Activity	Rank	Activity	Rank
Swimming	1	Softball	11
Fishing	2	Volleyball	12
Bicycling	3	Motorboating	13
Bowling	4	Dance Exercise	14
Camping	5	Golf	15
Hiking	6	Basketball	16
Pool/billiards	7	Darts	17
Running/jogging	8	Table Tennis	18
Weight Training	9	Calisthenics	19
Bicycle Touring	10	Hunting	20

Source: Data from the Gallup Poll.

are sports. Four are fitness activities, including swimming, bicycling, running/jogging, and weight training, which come from a part of the physical activity pyramid different from sports. These fitness activities, according to recent statistics, are not only among the most popular, they are also ones in which participants are most likely to perform on a regular basis throughout the year. The remaining three in the top ten are outdoor activities, one of which—hiking—has significant health-related fitness benefits. *Note:* swimming, bicycling, and running/jogging are not classified as sports because most participants in these activities do not compete on a regular basis. Race cycling, as

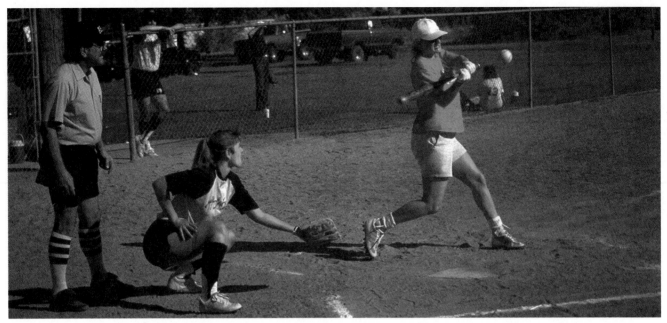
Softball is fun, but does little for health-related fitness components such as cardiovascular fitness.

opposed to bicycling, is classified as a sport. It should also be pointed out that walking is probably the most often performed activity but is not considered by many to be a leisure time pursuit.

Close scrutiny of the most popular lifetime fitness and outdoor activities indicates that they can be done, like popular lifetime sports, without the need for large groups of people, and they do not require a high degree of skill. Activities with these characteristics are considered to be **self-promoting activities** because they make the performer feel good. Some people avoid activities that require a high degree of skill because they often result in failure rather than success. Failure causes self-criticism rather than self-promotion. People who have had little previous success in organized sports should consider individualized skill instruction if they want to participate. An alternative would be to choose participation in self-promoting activities such as swimming, bicycling, jogging, weight training, or dance exercise.

Because self-promoting activities allow you to set your own standards of success and can be done individually or in small groups, they are especially suited to people with special needs. Wheelchair distance events, weight training, and aquatics are a few examples of these activities.

Among the twenty most popular types of physical activities are weight training, dance exercise, and calisthenics. All of these are programs that are frequently done in the home. Programs of this type are often preplanned and published as a booklet or in video format. You may like **preplanned exercise programs** because someone else directs your program.

Because preplanned exercise programs are planned by one person (or group) for individuals of many different levels of fitness, they may not be equally effective for all people who use them.

When selecting a preplanned exercise program, the following suggestions may be useful.

- Find out who wrote the program. Is the person(s) an expert? What makes the person an expert? Look for a program written by someone with a good educational background in physical education, exercise physiology, or sports medicine. Programs written by movie stars and television celebrities are rarely sound.
- Choose a program with more than one level of exercise. A good program will have exercises for beginning, intermediate, and advanced levels of fitness. This

allows you to select a program appropriate to your needs. Be skeptical of programs that include one set of exercises for all people.

- Make certain that all exercises are "good" exercises. Some exercises are contraindicated or "questionable." Avoid programs that include these exercises.
- Choose a program that meets your needs. Because physical fitness has many components, you need a program that includes exercises and activities for the fitness areas in which you need improvement.
- Choose a program that you enjoy enough to continue on a regular basis. No matter how good a program is, if you don't do it, it won't work.
- Choose a program that can be adapted to your need as your fitness improves.

> Preplanned programs that are not well designed but provide motivation to exercise can be adapted to make them safe and effective programs.

Some preplanned exercise programs, especially those prepared by celebrities with little exercise expertise, can be modified to improve them. Exercise programs on videotape and television can provide motivation to do regular exercise. Well-informed people can adapt these programs to make them safe and effective. You may want to use table 15.5 as a guide to making the necessary modifications.

Table 15.5
Guidelines for Adapting Preplanned Exercise Programs

1. If the program contains contraindicated or "bad" exercises, don't do them or substitute safe exercises.

2. Determine if the program gets you to exercise in the target zone for all parts of fitness. If not, supplement it with appropriate exercises. Many programs emphasize one component of fitness while neglecting others.

3. If the program is too difficult, don't continue. Modify with easier exercises that are more suited to your needs. For cardiovascular exercises, you may slow the speed of the exercise or eliminate arm movements to make them easier. Don't feel that you need to keep up with the instructor.

4. If you experience pain, stop exercising or reduce the intensity of the exercise. The "no pain, no gain" idea is a misconception!

5. If the program is too easy, supplement it with additional exercises.

6. Rotate programs regularly to keep your interest level high.

Suggested Readings

Gallup, G. and Newport, F. Football Remains America's Number One Spectator Sport, *Gallup Poll Monthly,* 325, 36(1992).

Gallup, G. and Newport, F. Gallup Leisure Audit. *The Gallup Poll Monthly,* 295, 27(1990).

Haywood, K. *Lifespan Motor Development.* 2nd ed. Champaign, IL: Human Kinetics Publishers, 1993.

Magill, R. A. *Motor Learning: Concepts and Applications.* 4th ed. Dubuque, IA: Wm. C. Brown Publishers, 1993.

LAB RESOURCE MATERIALS

Important Note: Because skill-related physical fitness does not relate to good health, the rating charts used in this section differ from those used for health-related fitness. The rating charts that follow can be used to compare your scores to those of other people. You *do not* need exceptional scores on skill-related fitness to be able to enjoy sports and other types of physical activity. After the age of thirty, you should adjust ratings by 1 percent per year.

Evaluating Skill-Related Physical Fitness

I. Evaluating agility: The Illinois agility run [1]

An agility course using four chairs ten feet apart, and a thirty-foot running area will be set up as depicted in this illustration. The test is performed as follows:

1. Lie prone with your hands by your shoulders and your head at the starting line. On the signal to begin, get on your feet and run the course as fast as possible.

2. Your score is the time required to complete the course.

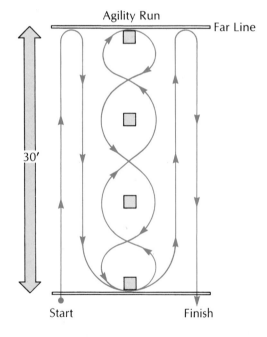

II. Evaluating balance: The Bass test of dynamic balance

Eleven circles (9½-inch) are drawn on the floor as shown in the illustration. The test is performed as follows:

1. Stand on the right foot in circle X. *Leap* forward to circle one, then circles two through ten, alternating feet with each leap.

2. The feet must leave the floor on each leap and the heel may not touch. Only the ball of the foot and toes may land on the floor.

3. Remain in each circle for five seconds before leaping to the next circle. (A count of five will be made for you aloud.)

4. Practice trials are allowed.

5. The score is fifty, plus the number of seconds taken to complete the test, minus the number of errors.

6. For every error, deduct three points each. Errors include touching the heel, moving the supporting foot, touching outside a circle, or touching any body part to the floor other than the supporting foot.

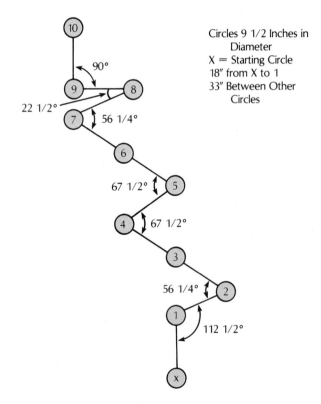

Circles 9 1/2 Inches in Diameter
X = Starting Circle
18″ from X to 1
33″ Between Other Circles

Chart 15.1 Agility *Rating Scale*		
Classification	**Men**	**Women**
Excellent	15.8 or faster	17.4 or faster
Very good	16.7–15.9	18.6–17.5
Good	18.6–16.8	22.3–18.7
Fair	18.8–18.7	23.4–22.4
Poor	18.9 or slower	23.5 or slower

[1]Source: Data from Adams, et al., *Foundations of Physical Activity,* 1965, p. 111.

Chart 15.2 Balance Test *Rating Scale*	
Rating	**Score**
Excellent	90–100
Very good	80–89
Good	60–79
Fair	30–59
Poor	0–29

Chart 15.3 Coordination *Rating Scale*		
Classification	**Men**	**Women**
Excellent	14–15	13–15
Very good	11–13	10–12
Good	5–10	4–9
Fair	3–4	2–3
Poor	0–2	0–1

III. Evaluating coordination: The stick test of coordination

The stick test of coordination requires you to juggle three wooden wands. The wands are used to perform a one-half flip and a full flip as shown in the illustrations.

1. *One-Half Flip*—Hold two twenty-four-inch (one-half inch in diameter) dowel rods, one in each hand. Support a third rod of the same size across the other two. Toss the supported rod in the air so that it makes a half turn. Catch the thrown rod with the two held rods.

2. *Full Flip*—Perform the preceding task, letting the supported rod turn a full flip.

The test is performed as follows:

1. Practice the half-flip and full flip several times before taking the test.

2. When you are ready, attempt a half-flip five times. Score one point for each successful attempt.

3. When you are ready, attempt the full flip five times. Score two points for each successful attempt.

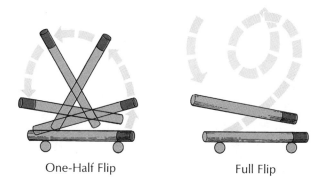

One-Half Flip   Full Flip

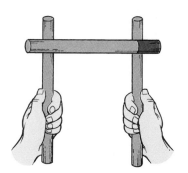

Hand Position

IV. Evaluating power: The vertical jump test

The test is performed as follows:

1. Hold a piece of chalk so its end is even with your fingertips.

2. Stand with both feet on the floor and your side to the wall and reach and mark as high as possible.

3. Jump upward with both feet as high as possible. Swing arms upward and make a chalk mark on a 5′ × 1′ wall chart marked off in half-inch horizontal lines placed six feet from the floor.

4. Measure the distance between the reaching height and the jumping height.

5. Your score is the best of three jumps.

Chart 15.4 Power *Rating Scale*		
Classification	**Men**	**Women**
Excellent	25½″ or more	23½″ or more
Very good	21″–25″	19″–23″
Good	16½″–20½″	14½″–18½″
Fair	12½″–16″	10½″–14″
Poor	12″ or less	10″ or less

Metric conversions for this chart appear in Appendix B.

V. Evaluating reaction time: The stick drop test

To perform the stick drop test of reaction time, you will need a yardstick, a table, a chair, and a partner to help with the test. To perform the test, follow these procedures:

1. Sit in the chair next to the table so that your elbow and lower arm rest on the table comfortably. The heel of your hand should rest on the table so that only your fingers and thumb extend beyond the edge of the table.

2. Your partner holds a yardstick at the very top, allowing it to dangle between your thumb and fingers.

3. The yardstick should be held so that the 24-inch-mark is even with your thumb and index finger. No part of your hand should touch the yardstick.

4. Without warning, your partner will drop the stick and you will catch it with your thumb and index finger.

5. Your score is the number of inches read on the yardstick just above the thumb and index finger after you catch the yardstick.

6. Try the test three times. Your partner should be careful not to drop the stick at predictable time intervals so that you cannot guess when it will be dropped. It is important that you react to the dropping of the stick only.

7. Use the middle of your three scores (example: if your scores are 21, 18, and 19, your middle score is 19). The higher your score, the faster your reaction time.

Chart 15.5 Reaction Time *Rating Scale*

Classification	Score in Inches
Excellent	More than 21
Very good	19–21
Good	16–18¾
Fair	13–15¾
Poor	Below 13

Metric conversions for this chart appear in Appendix B.

VI.   Evaluating speed: Running test of speed

To perform the running test of speed, it will be necessary to have a specially marked running course, a stopwatch, a whistle, and a partner to help you with the test. To perform the test, follow this procedure:

1. Mark a running course on a hard surface so that there is a starting line and a series of nine additional lines, each two yards apart, the first marked at a distance ten yards from the starting line.

2. From a distance one or two yards behind the starting line, begin to run as fast as you can. As you cross the starting line, your partner starts a stopwatch.

3. Run as fast as you can until you hear the whistle that your partner will blow exactly three seconds after the stopwatch was started. Your partner marks your location at the time when the whistle was blown.

4. Your score is the distance you were able to cover in three seconds. You may practice the test and take more than one trial if time allows. Use the better of your distances on the last two trials as your score.

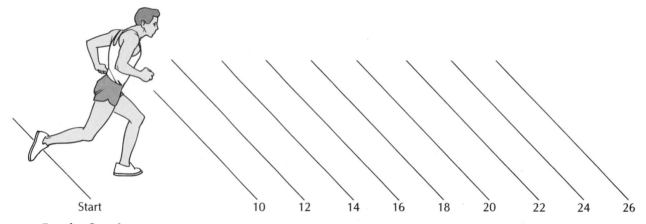

Start   10 12 14 16 18 20 22 24 26

Running Speed

Chart 15.6 Speed *Rating Scale*

Classification	Men	Women
Excellent	24–26 yards	22–26 yards
Very good	22–23 yards	20–21 yards
Good	18–21 yards	16–19 yards
Fair	16–17 yards	14–15 yards
Poor	Less than 16 yards	Less than 14 yards

Metric conversions for this chart appear in Appendix B.

CONCEPT ·16·

Body Mechanics: Posture and Care of the Back and Neck

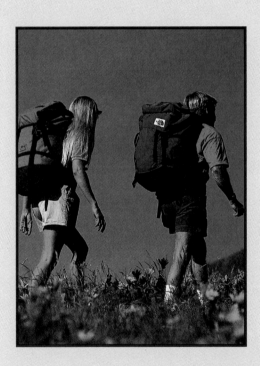

Concept 16

Because the human body is a system of weights and levers, its efficiency and effectiveness at rest or in motion can be improved by the application of sound mechanical and anatomical principles.

Introduction

"Body mechanics" is the application of physical laws to the human body. The bones of the body act as levers or simple machines, with the muscles supplying the force to move them. Therefore, mechanical laws can be applied to the body to aid in performing more and better work with less energy while avoiding strain or injury.

This concept focuses on four aspects of body mechanics. The first part of the concept discusses the mechanics of body alignment while sitting or standing (*static postures*). The second part of the concept emphasizes the *prevention of low back and neck pain* through proper body mechanics. The third section of the concept stresses *dynamic postures* for activities of daily living. The fourth section includes *exercises that are effective in correcting postural problems* and removing the cause of neck and back pain.

Health Goal for the Year 2000

▬ Reduce activity limitations due to chronic back conditions. (<>)

Note: (↑) indicates progress toward goal, (↓) indicates regression from goal, and (<>) indicates either no change or lack of new data since 1990.

Terms

▬ **Center of Gravity**   The center of the mass of an object.

▬ **Cervical Lordosis**   Excessive hyperextension in the neck region ("swayback of the neck").

▬ **Effectiveness**   The degree to which the purpose is accomplished.

▬ **Head Forward**   The head is thrust forward in front of the gravity line; also called "poke neck."

▬ **Herniated Disk**   The soft nucleus of the spinal disk protrudes through a small tear in the surrounding tissue; also called prolapse.

▬ **Hyperextended Knees**   The knees are thrust backward in a locked position.

▬ **Intervertebral Disk**   Spinal disk (disc); a cushion of cartilage between the bodies of the vertebrae. Each disk consists of a fibrous outer ring (annulus fibrosus) and a pulpy center (nucleus pulposus).

▬ **Kyphosis**   Increased curvature (flexion) in the upper back; called "hump back" or "dorsal kyphosis." In the lower back it is called "flat back" or "lumbar kyphosis."

▬ **Linear Motion**   Movement in a straight line.

- **Lumbar Lordosis**   Increased curvature (hyperextension) in the lower back (lumbar region), with a forward pelvic tilt; commonly known as "swayback."
- **Posture**   The relationship of body parts, whether standing, lying, sitting, or moving. Good posture is the relationship of body parts that allows you to function most effectively, with the least expenditure of energy and with a minimum amount of strain on muscles, tendons, ligaments, and joints.
- **Ptosis (Abdominal)**   Sagging, protruding abdomen.
- **Referred Pain**   Pain that appears to be located in one area, while in reality it originates in another area.
- **Round Shoulders**   The tips of the shoulders are drawn forward in front of the line of gravity.
- **Sciatica**   Pain radiating down the sciatic nerve in the back of the hip and leg.
- **Scoliosis**   A lateral curvature with some rotation of the spine; the most serious and deforming of all postural deviations.
- **Trigger Point**   An especially irritable spot, usually a tight band or knot in a muscle or fascia. This often refers pain to another area of the body. For example, a trigger point in the shoulder might cause a headache. This condition is referred to as "myofascial pain syndrome" and is often caused by muscle tension, fatigue, or strain.

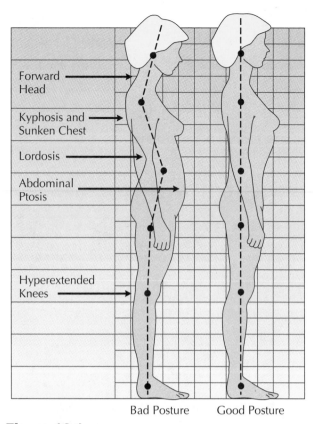

Figure 16.1
Comparison of bad and good posture

The Facts About Static Postures

Good posture has aesthetic benefits.

The first impression one person makes on another is usually a visual one. Good **posture** can help convey an impression of alertness, confidence, and attractiveness.

There is probably no one best posture for all individuals, because body build affects the balance of body parts. In general, certain relationships are desirable, however.

In the standing position, the head should be centered over the trunk, the shoulders should be down and back, but relaxed, with the chest high and the abdomen flat. The spine should have gentle curves when viewed from the side, but should be straight as seen from the back. When the pelvis is tilted properly, the pubis falls directly underneath the lower tip of the sternum. The knees should be relaxed, with the kneecaps pointed straight ahead. The feet should point straight ahead and the weight should be borne over the heel, on the outside border of the sole, and across the ball of the foot and toes (see figure 16.1).

Clinical evidence cited by physicians and opinions of educators indicate that poor posture can cause a number of health problems.

Some examples of health problems include:

- Protruding abdomen and **lumbar lordosis** may contribute to painful menstruation, back injury, and low back syndrome.
- A forward position of the head can result in headache, dizziness, and neck, shoulder, and arm pain.
- **Round shoulders** may impair respiratory capacity.
- **Hyperextended knees** may predispose a person to knee injury and cause the pelvis to tilt forward, producing lumbar lordosis.
- Unbalanced postural lines can cause excessive tension in muscle groups, produce joint strain, stretch ligaments, damage joint cartilage leading to its degeneration, and become a factor in arthritic changes.
- Poor posture creates mechanical stresses that perpetuate myofascial **trigger points.**

If one part of the body is out of line, other parts must move out of line to balance it, thus increasing the strain on muscles, ligaments, and joints.

The body is made in segments that are held balanced in a vertical column by muscles and ligaments. If gravity or a short muscle pulls one segment out of line, other portions of the body will move out of alignment to compensate, producing worse posture, more stress and strain, and possible deformity of the musculoskeletal system.

Approximately 80 percent of the adult population suffers from acquired foot defects.

Most foot defects are acquired and are preventable. They are most often caused by improperly fitting shoes and socks; excessive hard use (such as in athletics); long standing or walking on hard surfaces; obesity or rapid weight gain (as in pregnancy); and improper bearing of weight through poor foot and leg alignment.

There are many causes of poor posture, including hereditary, congenital, and disease conditions, as well as certain environmental factors.

Some environmental factors that may contribute to poor posture include ill-fitting clothing and shoes, chronic fatigue, improperly fitting furniture (including poor chairs, beds, and mattresses), emotional and personality problems, poor work habits, lack of physical fitness due to inactivity, and lack of knowledge relating to good posture. Some posture problems, especially **scoliosis,** may be congenital, hereditary, or acquired, but can often be corrected with exercise, braces, and/or other medical procedures. Early detection is critical in treating these problems.

Lordosis usually results from weak abdominals and short hip flexor muscles.

As can be seen in figure 16.1, the lower part of the back normally has a slight inward curvature. If the lower back curve is too great, the muscles of the low back are more easily fatigued, more likely to suffer muscle spasms, and more prone to injury.

The best way to prevent lordosis is to have strong abdominal muscles and long, but not too strong, hip flexor muscles. The strong abdominal muscles pull the bottom of the pelvis upward and help keep the top of the pelvis tipped backward, eliminating excessive back curve (figure 16.2).

If the hip flexor muscles are too strong, or not long enough, they have the opposite effect of strong abdominal muscles; that is, they tip the top of the pelvis forward, causing excessive low back curve (lordosis). (See figure 16.3.) This is why it is important to have long, but not too strong, hip flexor muscles. As a general rule, flexibility exercises to lengthen the

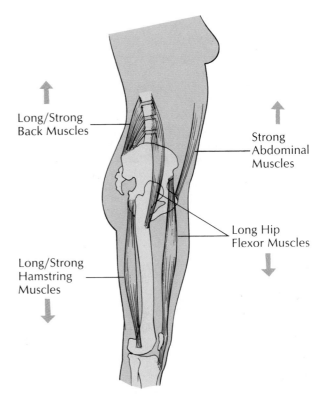

Figure 16.2
Balanced muscle strength and length permit good postural alignment

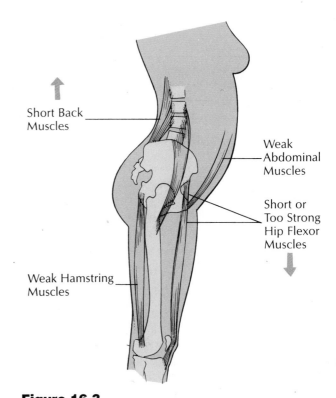

Figure 16.3
Unbalanced muscular development may cause poor posture or back problems.

Table 16.1
Backache Risk Factors: Activities or Characteristics That Predispose People to Suffer Back Pain

• Obesity	• Trunk muscle imbalance
	• Previous back problems
• Frequent bending over	• Participation in gymnastics, javelin throw, diving, weight lifting, skiing, football, rowing, and swimming butterfly
• Frequent lifting of heavy loads	
• Regular exposure to vibration	• Repetitive and large range hyperextensive lumbar movements or rapid acceleration or deceleration of spine
• Lack of lumbar flexibility	
• Lack of hamstring flexibility	• Increased age
• Weak trunk extensor muscles	
• Previous back surgery	• Osteoporosis

hip flexor muscles, as well as strength and endurance exercises for the abdominal muscles, are recommended. For obvious reasons, exercises to increase the strength of the hip flexor muscles are not recommended for those with back pain.

Abdominal ptosis can increase the risk of back pain.

If the abdomen sticks out too far over the belt line, problems with the back muscles can result. The extra weight of the protruding abdomen can cause lordosis by pulling the top of the pelvis forward. This can result in extra strain on the low back muscles and can precipitate muscle fatigue, soreness, or injury. Strengthening of the abdominal muscles and a loss of body fat, if you are overfat, are advised for this problem.

Poor posture, especially lordosis, can cause back strain and pain and can make the back more susceptible to injury.

The forward tilt of the pelvis may cause the sacral bone or one of the lumbar vertebrae to press on nerve roots with consequent low back pain and **sciatica.** To be on the safe side, some authorities advise those who have lordosis and weak abdominals to eliminate all exercises that hyperextend the spine. Incidence of lordosis is about the same for men as it is for women, except that women experience an added back strain during pregnancy.

Some people have a "flat back" (lumbar **kyphosis**) in the lower back region that can lead to backaches.

There is an increased interest among therapists in patients who lack a normal lordotic curve in the lumbar spine. Robin McKenzie's theories and exercises (1980, 1981, 1983) have become increasingly popular in the treatment of people who sit for long periods with the back flat and pelvis tilted backward or those who engage in prolonged bending, heavy lifting, and long standing with flat back postures.

These people may need to regain a normal lordotic curve and probably need to perform relaxed static stretches with the back in hyperextension, such as the press-up exercise. They may also benefit from the use of lumbar support (rolls or pillows) during sitting.

The Facts About Backaches and Neckaches

Backache has been called "a twentieth-century epidemic," "the nemesis of medicine," and "the albatross of industry" (Zamula 1989) because most people (60–80 percent of all Americans) will see a physician about a backache during their lifetimes.

Backache is second only to headaches as a common medical complaint. An estimated 30 to 70 percent of Americans have recurring back problems, and two million of those cannot hold jobs as a result. The nation's medical bill for backaches is $24 billion annually. It is the most frequent cause of inactivity in individuals under the age of forty-five. It most often affects people between the ages of twenty-five and sixty. Even teenagers have backaches. (One study indicated that 26 percent of teenagers have backaches.) Athletes also have backaches, but the condition is more common in people who are not highly fit.

The causes of backache are varied, but it is rarely a dramatic event such as trauma in a diving or an automobile accident.

Incorrect postures when standing, sitting, lying, or working are responsible for many back problems. Compounding this are weak muscles and muscular imbalance. Other causes of low back pain include improper exercises (concept 12); incorrect techniques in lifting and in sports; repetitive, forced hyperextension of the back; and other preventable causes. Some of these are reflected in the list of risk factors in table 16.1. (This list excludes known causes such as trauma, tumors, and congenital abnormalities.) What you may not know is that in 80 percent of the cases, physicians are unable to pinpoint the exact cause.

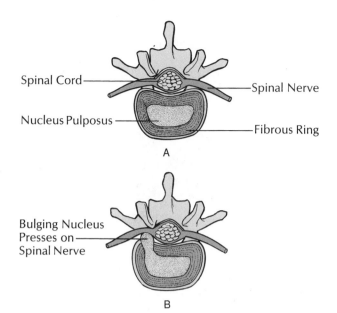

Figure 16.4
Normal disk (*A*) and herniated disk (*B*)

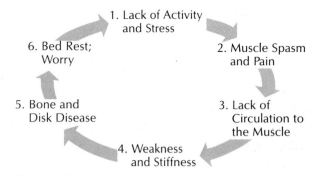

Figure 16.5
The vicious cycle of back pain

The overwhelming majority of backaches and neckaches are avoidable. A common cause of backache is muscular strain, frequently precipitated by poor body mechanics in daily activities or during exercise.

When lifting improperly, there is great pressure on the lumbar disks and severe stress on the lumbar muscles and ligaments. Many popular exercises place great strain on the back (see concept 12). Sleeping flat on the back or abdomen on a soft mattress can also cause lower back strain.

There is no such thing as a slipped disk.

Disk problems are frequently misunderstood. **Intervertebral disks** may herniate or rupture, but they do not slip (figure 16.4). Material from the pulpy center part of the disk (the nucleus pulposus) may bulge outward and press on spinal nerves, causing pain, and a protective reflex muscle spasm may occur to protect it. This causes a lack of circulation to the muscle and more pain, and more muscles tense up to prevent movement. Stiffness results and the muscles become weaker; chronic back pain may set in unless this vicious pain cycle can be stopped (see figure 16.5). If it persists, bones may develop spurs, disks may degenerate, the patient may go to bed and worry and tense up, and the cycle may go on indefinitely.

The disks in the lumbar area are subjected to greater compression and torque because they are at the bottom of the spine. They are, therefore, more apt to be damaged. Sudden twisting and flexion or extension movements, such as suddenly reaching for a ball in tennis or racquetball, may precipitate a **herniated disk.** It is more apt to happen when the disk is degenerated from overuse (figure 16.6). It is more

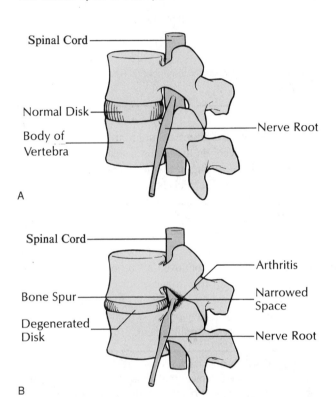

Figure 16.6
Normal disk (*A*) and degenerated disk with nerve impingement and arthritic changes (*B*)

common in men than women and in people who do heavy manual labor. Degenerated disks are normal with aging, but not uncommon in athletes. One study shows gymnasts' disks were comparable to the disks of sixty-five-year-old men. However, in spite of what popular literature and certain unethical "back doctors" may tell you, studies show that a herniated disk is *rarely* the cause of back pain—occurring in only 5 to 10 percent of the cases.

The neck is probably strained more frequently than the lower back.

The neck is constructed with the same curve and has the same mechanical problems as the lower back. The postural

Table 16.2
Some Risk Factors for Chronic Neck (and Shoulder) Pain

- Poor posture (especially cervical lordosis and kyphosis)
- In women, large breasts
- Weak neck muscles (especially flexors and rotators)
- Stress
- Job dissatisfaction
- Job monotony (repetitive motion or position)
- Degenerated disks
- Desk or chair too low or high
- Wearing bifocals (to read computer screen)
- Arthritis
- Previous neck injury
- Holding/carrying loads for long periods (e.g., purse, briefcase, baby)

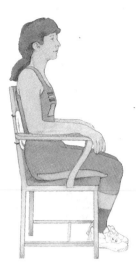

Figure 16.7
A proper chair and good posture can prevent back problems from prolonged sitting.

fault of **head forward** places a chronic strain on the posterior neck muscles. Tension in these muscles can lead to myofascial trigger points, causing headache or **referred pain** in the face, scalp, shoulder, arm, and chest.

> Kyphosis is a contributing factor in neck pain.

The more the upper back is flexed, the greater the compensating curve (**cervical lordosis**) in the neck. The sharpest angle is between the fourth and sixth cervical vertebrae, creating wear and tear (microtrauma) that accelerates disk degeneration and arthritic changes, which can ultimately result in nerve and artery impingement.

> The causes of chronic neck pain are many, and they have a complex interaction that varies with the individual and makes it difficult to diagnose and prevent or treat.

Some of the causes of chronic neck pain (and the often accompanying shoulder pain) include workplace design, poor posture, work habits, and physical fitness, and too much stress. The risk factors that predispose a person to suffering neck pain are listed in table 16.2.

Facts About Prevention and Intervention

> Practicing good body mechanics and posture can help prevent back problems.

Several practical suggestions for modifying everyday activities are listed here:

- To relieve back stress due to a swayback during prolonged standing, try to keep the lower back flat by propping one foot on a stool or rail; alternate feet occasionally. Dentists, hair dressers, barbers, and store clerks are particularly susceptible to back problems because they must stand while working.
- If your back arches excessively when sitting, use a hard chair with a straight back and armrests, placing the spine against it; keep one or both knees higher than the hips by crossing the legs (alternate sides) or by using a foot rest and keeping the knees bent. If your back flattens when you sit, use a lumbar roll behind your lower back. (See figure 16.7.)
- When driving a car, to avoid a swayback position place a hard seat and backrest combination over the seat of the automobile; pull the seat forward so the legs are bent when operating the pedals. If your back flattens when you drive, use a lumbar support pillow.
- When lying, keep the knees and hips bent; avoid lying on the abdomen. When lying on the back, a pillow or lift should be placed under the knees.
- Avoid improper lifting and carrying. Especially avoid bending over or straightening the spine while twisting. (This can be more damaging from a sitting position than from a standing position.)
- Do exercises to strengthen abdominal and hip extensors, and to stretch the hip flexors and lumbar muscles if they are tight.
- Avoid hazardous exercises (see concept 12).
- General exercises involving the entire body, such as walking, jogging, swimming, and bicycling are important in preventing weak or tight muscles.
- Warm up before engaging in strenuous activity.
- Get adequate rest and sleep. Avoid pushing yourself mentally or physically to the point of exhaustion.
- Vary the working position by changing from one task to another before feeling fatigued. When working at a desk, get up and stretch occasionally to relieve tension.

- Sleep on a firm mattress or place a three-fourths-inch-thick plywood board under the mattress.
- Avoid sudden, jerky back movements, especially twisting.
- The smaller the waistline, the lesser the strain on the lower back. Avoid obesity.

Practicing good body mechanics and posture can prevent or alleviate neck pain.

Some modifications of your daily activities are suggested here:

- Use appropriate back and seat supports when sitting for long periods.
- Use proper tools and equipment to reduce neck strain; for example, use a paint roller with an extension to reach overhead, thus reducing the need to hold the arms overhead and to hyperextend the neck.
- Maintain good posture when carrying heavy loads; don't lean forward, sideways, or backward.
- When sleeping use a good pillow that supports your head in a neutral position—not too high or too low.
- Adjust sports equipment to permit good posture; for example, adjust bicycle seat and handle bars to permit good body alignment.
- When you have a neckache,
  a. lie down;
  b. apply heat or ice;
  c. massage the neck and shoulders; and
  d. stretch the neck muscles.
- Avoid long periods of desk sitting or driving; take frequent breaks and adjust the seat and headrest for maximum support.
- To avoid injury, use safe sports equipment and techniques, e.g., proper helmet and cervical collar (if indicated); look before you dive in water.
- When shaving, don't tilt the head backward.
- Wash your hair in the shower rather than in the sink.
- Try to work at eye level; for example, when typing put the copy on a vertical typist's stand; when working above head level, get on a stool or ladder to avoid tipping the head back.
- Do not sit in front row theater seats so you don't have to tip your head back.

Organize work to save energy and avoid stooping or unnatural positions that cause strain.

- Sideward flexion of the trunk is more strenuous than forward trunk flexion.
- Avoid constant arm extension, whether forward or sideward.
- Whenever possible, sit while working but stand occasionally.

- The arms should move either together or in opposite directions. When the conditions allow, use both hands in opposite and symmetrical motions while working.
- Tools most often used should be the closest to reach.
- When working with the hands, the workbench or kitchen cabinet should be about 2 to 4 inches below the waist. The office desk should be about 29 to 30 inches high for the average man and about 27 to 29 inches high for the average woman.

The Facts About Dynamic Postures: Lifting and Carrying

The best method for lifting or carrying a given object depends upon its size, weight, shape, and position in space. However, here are some general principles that are applicable to lifting with both hands, including the weight lifting squats.

- *Stand close to the object and assume a wide base.* Stand in a forward-backward stride position with the object at the side of the body, or assume a side-stride position with the object between the knees. The purpose of the lifting from this position is to allow you to lift straight upward from a stable position, utilizing the most efficient leverage.
- *Keep the head up and the back fairly erect with the normal lordotic curve maintained, and bend at the hips and knees.* Squat, do not bend, regardless of how light the object may be. The back was never meant to be used as a lever for lifting. Avoid leaning forward to pick up objects without bending the knees because of the strain placed on the muscles and joints of the spine. This kind of back strain can occur when improperly making a bed or when lifting a child out of a crib.
- *Lower your body only as far as necessary, directly downward.* Squatting lower than is necessary is a waste of energy, but more importantly perhaps, deep knee bends can damage the structures of the knee joints.
- *Carry the object close to the body's center of gravity and no higher than waist level (except when carrying on the shoulder, head, or back).* When objects are carried in front of the body above the level of the waist, you must lean backward to balance the load, producing an undesirable arch in the lower back. Carrying loads at the midline of the body, such as in a knapsack or on the head or shoulders, is **effective** in reducing the stress on the skeletal system.
- *Grasp the object, tighten the lower back muscles, then lift with your leg muscles, keeping the object close to the body's **center of gravity*** (see figure 16.8). The leg

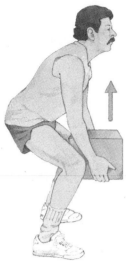

Figure 16.8
Maintain a normal curve in the back when lifting an object with both hands.

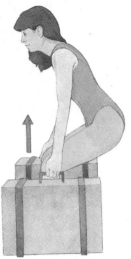

Figure 16.9
Divide a heavy load.

muscles are the strongest in the body. If the back is kept erect, use of the legs for lifting allows a maximal force to be applied to the load without wasting energy. Do not twist during the lift. If the object is heavy, hold your breath on the lift (this produces "trunk cavity pressurization," which helps to reduce the load on the spine). A lumbar belt may also help protect the spine.

- *Push or pull heavy objects, if this can be done efficiently, rather than lifting them.* Theoretically, it takes about thirty-four times more force to lift than to slide an object across the floor. The size, shape, and friction of the object determine whether or not it is feasible to push or pull it.

- *Divide the load if possible, carrying half in each hand/arm. If the load cannot be divided, alternate it from one side of the body to the other.* (See figure 16.9.) When walking with the weight carried on one side of the body, the force on the opposite hip is much greater than when the load is distributed on both sides. This is true even when the bilateral load is twice as great as the unilateral load. If the weight must be carried on only one side, the opposite arm should be raised to counterbalance the load and help keep the center of gravity over the base.

- *Avoid hyperextending the neck and the back when lifting and lowering an object from overhead. Any lift above waist level is inefficient.* Occasionally, you must reach overhead to lift an object from a high shelf. To avoid back and neck strain, climb a ladder or stand on a stool so you don't have to raise your arms over-

head. If this is not practical, reach for the object with your weight on the forward foot, and then step backward on the rear foot as the object is lowered.

- *Do not try to lift or carry loads too heavy for you.* The most economical load for the average adult is about thirty-five percent of the body weight. Obviously, with strength training, you can lift a greater load but heavy loads are a backache risk factor.

> One-handed lifts are executed with the same body mechanics as a two-handed lift, except for the use of one arm to support the trunk.

Some guidelines for one-handed lifting are included below (Boyce and Jackson 1991). (Remember to use the same squat technique as previously described for the two-handed lifts.)

A. *When lifting from the floor, follow these four steps:*
   1. Squat and support the weight of the trunk by putting the left hand on the floor while grasping the weight with the right.
   2. Remain in this position and lift the weight to the right thigh.
   3. Shift your upper body weight toward the right while the left hand moves from the floor to the left thigh.
   4. Push with the left hand on the thigh to help raise the trunk as the legs extend.

   Reverse these steps to return the weight to the floor.

B. *For one-arm upright rowing or for lifting loads from awkward, bent-over positions such as a car trunk or a baby's crib:*

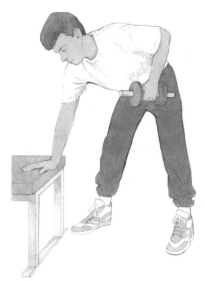

Figure 16.10
When lifting with one hand (as in upright rowing), support the trunk with the other hand.

Use a technique similar to the one-arm lift from the floor. Support the trunk with your free arm by leaning on something for support while lifting with the other arm. This saves the back muscles from having to do the work (see figure 16.10).

Facts About Exercises for Posture and Back/Neck Care

Exercise is one of the most frequently prescribed treatments for painful spines.

Treatments range from surgical removal of a disk or fusion, to more conservative measures such as injections, electrical stimulation, muscle relaxants, anti-inflammatory drugs, vapo-coolant spray, bracing, traction, bed rest, heat, cryotherapy, massage, and therapeutic exercise. Regardless of the treatment used, 70 to 85 percent of back patients recover spontaneously. Of those, 70 percent will have no symptoms by the end of three weeks and 90 percent will recover in two months (Tietz 1985). The various treatment modalities may simply make patients more comfortable or they may hasten the recovery.

Exercise has been found to be helpful in treating all kinds of chronic pain. (Resistance exercises and aerobic exercises have been particularly helpful in pain clinics.) Aerobic exercise is also known to help nourish the spinal disks.

Exercise can serve to prevent or correct some of the underlying causes of back and neck pain by strengthening weak muscles and stretching short ones. In the process of creating muscle balance, it improves postural alignment and body mechanics and relaxes muscle spasms.

Exercises for the correction of postural deviations are generally based on this assumption: if the problem is a functional deformity, regardless of the factors causing it, muscular imbalance will be present.

If the muscles on one side of a joint are stronger than the muscles on the opposite side of that joint, the body part is pulled in the direction of the stronger muscles. Corrective exercises are usually designed to strengthen the long, weak muscles and to stretch the short, strong ones in order to have equal pull in both directions. For example, those with lumbar lordosis may need to strengthen the abdominals and hamstrings, and stretch the lower back and hip flexor muscles (see figures 16.2 and 16.3).

Some people are unable to lift loads safely because tight and/or weak muscles may prevent them from using proper body mechanics.

Some people have backaches because they lift improperly. In many instances the poor technique is caused by muscle imbalance, such as hamstrings or gluteals too tight to permit the lower back to retain its normal curve during the squat and lift; or calf muscles too tight to allow the heels to remain on the floor during the squat; or abdominals too weak to support the back and quadriceps and gluteals too weak to lift the weight of the body and the load. Proper exercise could remediate these problems.

Specific exercises are sometimes needed to prevent or help rehabilitate posture, neck, and back problems.

Exercises included in previous concepts were presented with health-related fitness in mind. The exercises included in this concept are not really so different. They are either flexibility or strength exercises for specific muscle groups; however, each is selected specifically to help correct a postural problem or to remove the cause of neck and back pain. To that extent these exercises may be classified as "therapeutic." These same exercises may be called "preventative" because they can be used to prevent postural or spine problems. Whether therapeutic or preventative, the exercises will not be effective unless they are done faithfully and with the "FIT Formula" applied. Those who have back and neck pain should seek the advice of a physician to make certain that it is safe for them to perform the exercises.

Exercises for Good Posture and Care of the Neck and Back

The exercises suggested here should be performed as described until you are able to increase repetitions. Most people need to do all of these exercises regularly, but some may need to perform only selected exercises to meet their specific needs. Muscles depicted in color are those primarily involved in the exercise.

1. Isometric Neck Exercises

Purpose

To strengthen the neck muscles and prevent or correct forward head and cervical lordosis, as well as upper back and neck trigger points and pain.

Position

Sit; place one or both hands on the head as shown. Assume good head and neck posture by tucking the chin, flattening the neck, and pushing the crown of the head up (axial extension).

Movement

Apply resistance (a) sideward, (b) backward, and (c) forward. Contract the neck muscles to prevent the head and neck from moving. Hold six seconds; repeat each exercise up to six times.

Note

For neck muscles, it is probably best to use a little less than a maximal contraction, especially in the presence of arthritis, degenerated disks, or injury.

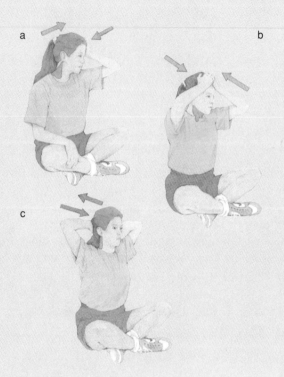

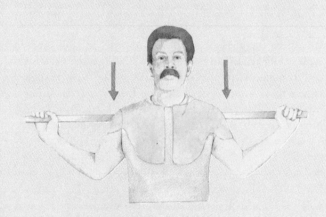

2. Wand Exercise

Purpose

To help prevent and correct round shoulders and kyphosis by stretching the muscles on the anterior side of the shoulder joint.

Position

Sit with wand grasped at ends. Raise wand overhead. Be certain that the head does not slide forward into a "poke neck" position. Keep the chin tucked and neck straight.

Movement

Bring wand down behind shoulder blades. Keep spine erect. Hold. Hands may be moved closer together to increase stretch on chest muscles.

Note

If this is an easy exercise for you, try straightening the elbows and bringing the wand to waist level in back of you.

3. Pectoral Stretch

Purpose

To stretch pectorals and prevent or correct kyphosis and round shoulders. (See exercise no. 5, p. 93.)

4. Side Bender

Purpose

To stretch trunk lateral flexors and help prevent and correct backaches by maintaining flexibility in the spine.

Position

Stand with feet shoulder width apart.

Movement

Stretch left arm overhead to right. Bend to right at waist reaching as far to right as possible with left arm; reach as far as possible to the left with right arm; hold. Do not let trunk rotate or lower back arch. Repeat on opposite side.

Note

This exercise is made more effective if a weight is held down at the side in the hand opposite the side being stretched. More stretch occurs also if the hip on the stretched side is dropped and most of the weight is borne by the opposite foot.

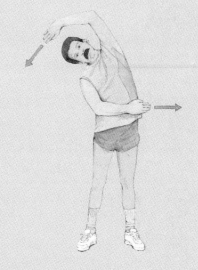

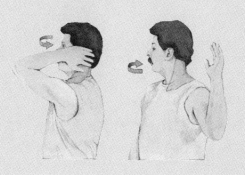

5. Neck Rotation Exercise

Purpose

This PNF exercise strengthens and stretches the neck rotators. It should always be done with the head and neck in axial extension (good alignment). It is particularly useful for relieving trigger point pain and stiffness.

Position

Place palm of left hand against left cheek; point fingers toward ear and point elbow forward.

Movement

Try to turn head and neck left while resisting with left hand. Hold six seconds. Relax and turn head to right as far as possible; hold ten seconds. Repeat four times; then repeat on opposite side.

6. Back-Saver Hamstring Stretch

Purpose

To stretch hamstrings and calf muscles, and help prevent or correct backache caused in part by short hamstrings.

Position

Sit on the floor with the feet against the wall or an immovable object. Bend left knee and bring foot close to buttocks. Clasp hands behind back.

Movement

Bend forward from hips, keeping lower back as straight as possible. Let bent knee rotate outward so trunk can move forward. Lean forward keeping back flat; hold and repeat on each leg.

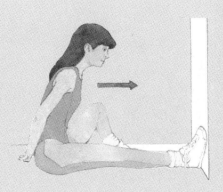

7. Hip and Thigh Stretcher

Purpose

To stretch hip flexor muscles, and help prevent or correct forward pelvic tilt, lumbar lordosis, and backache.

Position

Place right knee directly above right ankle and stretch left leg backward so knee touches floor. If necessary, place hands on floor for balance.

Movement

Press pelvis forward and downward; **hold.** Repeat on opposite side. *Caution: Do not bend front knee more than 90°.*

Note

Useful for those who have lordosis or lower back problems.

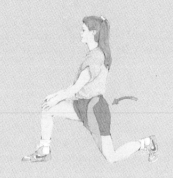

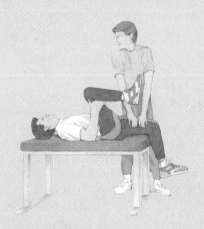

8. Low Back Stretcher

Purpose

To stretch hip flexors, gluteals, and lumbar muscles, and help prevent or correct lumbar lordosis and backache.

Position

Supine position.

Movement

Draw one knee up to the chest and pull thigh down tightly with the hands, then slowly return to the original position. Repeat with other knee. Do not grasp knee; grasp thigh. If a partner or a weight stabilizes the extended leg, the hip flexor muscles on that leg will be stretched.

9. Single Knee-to-Chest

Purpose

To stretch lower back, gluteals, and hamstring muscles and help prevent or correct lordosis and backache.

Position

Supine with knees bent.

Movement

Use hands on back of thigh to draw one knee to the chest, then extend the knee and point the foot toward the ceiling; hold. Return to the starting position by drawing the knee back to the chest before sliding the foot to the floor. Repeat with other leg.

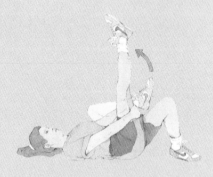

10. Double Knee-to-Chest

Purpose

To stretch lower back, gluteals, and hamstring muscles, and help prevent or correct lordosis and backache (advanced exercise).

Same as Single Knee-to-Chest, except use both legs simultaneously.

Note

If you are a back patient, this is more advanced than the preceding exercises and it should not be attempted until the others have been performed for three to four weeks.

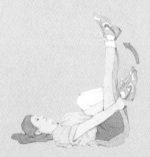

11. Calf Stretcher

Purpose

To stretch the calf muscles (gastrocnemius and soleus) to enable you to squat correctly when performing lifts.

Position

Face a wall with your feet two or three feet away. Step forward on left foot to allow both hands to touch the wall.

Movement

(1) Keep the heel of your right foot on the ground, toe turned in slightly, knee straight, and buttocks tucked in. Lean forward by bending your front knee and arms and allowing your head to move nearer the wall. Hold. (2) Bend right knee, keeping heel on floor. Hold. Repeat with the other leg.

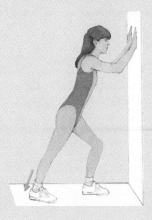

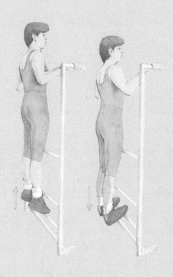

12. Lower Leg Stretcher

Purpose

Same as calf stretcher except it is a more advanced exercise. (See exercise no. 1, p. 91.)

13. Half-Squat with Weights

Purpose

To strengthen the muscles of the thighs and buttocks.

Position

Stand erect, feet turned out 45 degrees. Rest bar behind neck on shoulders. Spread hands in a comfortable position.

Movement

Squat slowly, keeping back straight, eyes ahead. Bend knees to 90 degrees; keep knees over feet. Pause, then stand. Repeat.

Note

Use spotters if barbell is used. A dumbbell may be held in each hand at side of body in place of barbell.

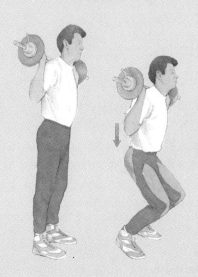

14. Pelvic Tilt

Purpose

To strengthen abdominals and help prevent or correct lumbar lordosis, abdominal ptosis, and backache.

Position

Supine with knees bent.

Movement

Tighten the abdominal muscles and tilt the pelvis backward; try to flatten the lower back against the floor. At the same time, tighten the hip and thigh muscles. Hold, then relax. Breathe normally during the contraction, do not hold the breath.

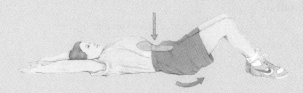

15. Reverse Curl

Purpose

To develop the lower abdominal muscles, correct abdominal ptosis, and prevent backache.

Position

Lie on the floor. Bend the knees, place the feet flat on the floor, and place arms at sides.

Movement

Lift the knees to the chest, raising the hips off the floor; do not let the knees go past the shoulders. Return to the starting position. Repeat.

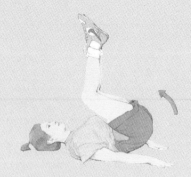

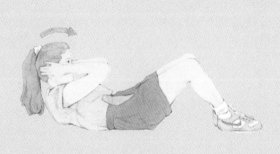

16. Crunch (Curl-Up)

Purpose

To develop the upper abdominal muscles, correct abdominal ptosis and lordosis; backache prevention.

Position

Assume a hook-lying position with arms extended or crossed with hands on shoulders or palms on ears. If desired, legs may rest on bench to increase difficulty. For less resistance, place hands at side of body (do *not* put hands behind neck). For more resistance, move hands higher.

Movement

Curl up until shoulder blades leave floor, then roll down to the starting position. Repeat.

17. Crunch with Twist (on Bench)

Purpose

To strengthen the oblique abdominals and help prevent or correct lumbar lordosis, abdominal ptosis, and backache.

Position

Lie supine with feet on bench, knees bent 90 degrees. Arms may be extended or on shoulders or hands on ears (the most difficult).

Movement

Same as crunch except twist the upper trunk so the right shoulder is higher than the left. Reach toward the right knee with the left elbow. Hold; return and repeat to the opposite side.

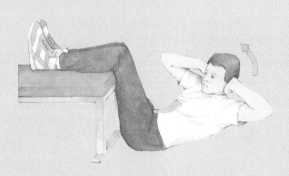

18. Sitting Tucks

Purpose

To strengthen the lower abdominals and increase their endurance; improve posture and prevent backache. (This is an advanced exercise.)

Position

Sit on floor with feet raised, arms extended for balance.

Movement

Alternately bend and extend legs without letting back or feet touch floor.

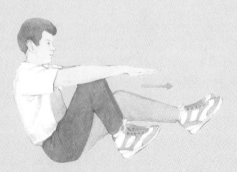

Exercises for Good Posture and Care of the Neck and Back *cont.*

19. Standing Crunch

Purpose

To strengthen abdominals, prevent or correct lordosis, abdominal ptosis, and backaches.

Position

Stand erect, holding ends of elastic resistance (tubes or bands) in each hand at shoulder level. Contract abdominals and tilt pelvis backward, flattening the lower back.

Movement

Pull on the elastic resistance by curling the chest toward the pubis, keeping the pelvis titled backward.

Note

A similar exercise may be performed on some resistance machines or with pulleys.

20. Arm Lift

Purpose

To strengthen scapular adductors and help prevent or correct round shoulders and kyphosis.

Position

a. Least difficult: lie prone with arms in reverse-T; forehead resting on floor.
b. More advanced—same as "a" except extend arms overhead and hold against the ears.

Movement

Maintain the arm position and contract the muscles between the shoulder blades, lifting the arms as high as possible without raising head and trunk. Hold; relax and repeat.

Note

If the arms are first pressed against the floor before lifting, this becomes a PNF exercise and range of motion may be greater.

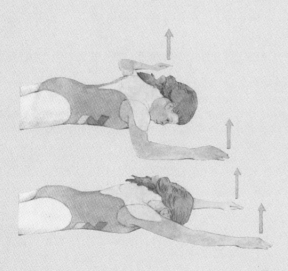

21. Seated Rowing

Purpose

To strengthen the scapular adductors (rhomboid and trapezius) and to prevent or correct kyphosis, round shoulders, head forward or cervical lordosis, and neck pain.

Position

Sit facing pulley, feet braced and knees slightly bent. Grasp bar, palms down with hands shoulder width apart.

Movement

Pull bar to chest, keeping elbows high, and return; repeat.

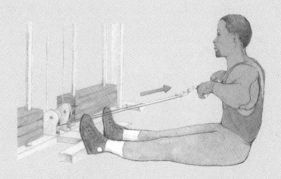

22. Upper Trunk Lift

Purpose

To develop upper back strength.

Position

Lie on a table or bench or a special purpose bench designed for trunk lifts with the upper half of the body hanging over the edge.

Movement

Have a partner stabilize the feet and legs while the trunk is raised parallel to the floor, then lower the trunk to the starting position. Place hands behind neck or on ears. Do not raise past the horizontal or arch the back.

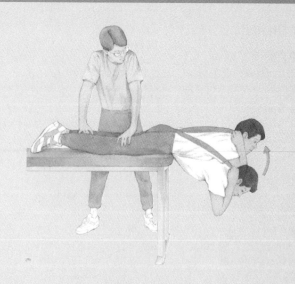

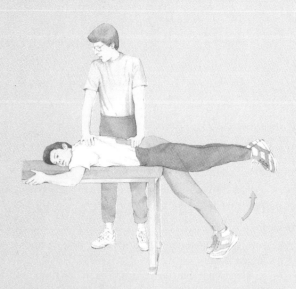

23. Lower Trunk Lift

Purpose

To develop low back and hip strength.

Position

Lie prone on bench or table with legs hanging over the edge.

Movement

Have a partner stabilize the upper back or grasp the edges of the table with hands. Raise the legs parallel to the floor and lower them. Do not raise past the horizontal or arch the back. Suggested progression: (1) Begin by alternating legs; when you can do 25 reps, (2) add ankle weights; when you can do 25 reps, (3) lift both legs simultaneously (no weights).

24. Press-Up (McKenzie Extension Exercise)

Purpose

To increase flexibility of lumbar spine, reduce tension on posterior disks and longitudinal ligaments, and restore normal lordotic curve, especially for those with a flat lumbar spine.

Position

Prone with hands under the face.

Movement

Slowly press up to a rest position on forearms; keep pelvis on floor. Relax and *hold* ten seconds. Repeat once; do several times a day. Progress to gradually straightening the elbows while keeping the pubic bone on the floor. *Caution:* Do *not* perform if you have lordosis or if it produces any pain or discomfort in the back or legs.

Note

A prone press-up will feel good as a stretch after doing abdominal strength or endurance exercises. This relaxed lordotic position can be performed while standing. Place the hands in the small of the back and gently arch the back and hold. This should feel good after sitting for a long period with the back flat.

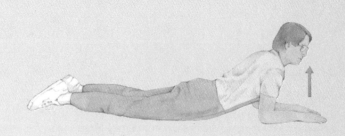

25. Bridging

Purpose

To strengthen hip extensors, especially gluteal muscles and help prevent and correct lordosis and forward pelvic tilt.

Position

Supine with knees bent and feet close to buttocks.

Movement

Contract gluteals, lifting buttocks and lower back off floor. Hold; relax; repeat. Do not allow the lower back to arch.

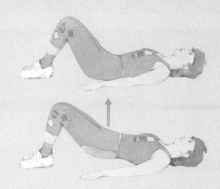

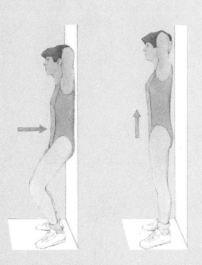

26. Wall Slide

Purpose

To help prevent or correct poor spinal alignment by teaching the feel of flattening the neck and back, and tilting the pelvis.

Position

Stand with heels 4 to 6 inches from wall, arms at sides.

Movement

Flatten neck and lumbar region to wall by flexing knees and sliding down wall until spine can be forced against it. Slide up wall, maintaining flat spine. Walk away from wall, keeping curves flat. Return to wall and check alignment. Repeat with hands behind neck and elbows touching wall. Repeat with arms at sides and sandbag on head. Repeated flexion and extension of the knees can develop strength in the quadriceps muscles on the front of the thigh.

27. Supine Trunk Twist

Purpose

To increase flexibility of spine and stretch rotator muscles.

Position

Lie supine, arms extended at shoulder level; left foot on right patella.

Movement

Twist the lower body by lowering left knee to touch floor on right. Turn head to left; try to keep shoulders and arms on floor.

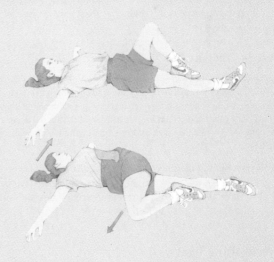

Suggested Readings

Back Owners Manual. Daly City, CA: Krames Communications. 1990.
   Neck Exercises for a Healthy Neck. San Bruno, CA: Krames Communications. 1990.

Boyce, R., and S. Jackson. "One-Arm Lifting for a Healthy Back." *Strategies* (Jan. 1991): 19–22.

Field, R. "How Humans Sit." *The American Way* (April 15, 1988): pp. 28–29.

Malvivaara, A. et al. "The Treatment of Acute Low Back Pain—Bed Rest, Exercise or Ordinary Activity." *New England Journal of Medicine,* Vol 332 No. 6. 1995, pp 351–335.

Teitz, C.C., and D. M. Cook, "Rehabilitation of Neck and Low Back Injuries." *Clinics in Sports Medicine: Rehabilitation of Injured Athletes* 4(1985):456.

Zamula, E. "Back Talk: Advice for Suffering Spines." *FDA Consumer* 23(1989):28.

Chart 16.1 Healthy Back Tests

These tests are among the ones used by physicians and therapists to make differential diagnoses of back problems. You and your partner can use them to determine if you have muscle tightness that may make you "at risk" for back problems. Discontinue any of these tests if they produce pain or numbness, or tingling sensations in the back, hips, or legs. Experiencing any of these sensations may be an indication that you have a low back problem that requires diagnosis by your physician. Partners should use *great caution* in applying force. Be gentle and listen to your partner's feedback.

Test 1—Back to Wall

Pass ☐ Fail ☐

Stand with your back against a wall, with head, heels, shoulders, and calves of legs touching the wall as shown in the diagram. Try to flatten your neck and the hollow of your back by pressing your buttocks down against the wall. Your partner should just be able to place a hand in the space between the wall and the small of your back.

- If this space is greater than the thickness of his/her hand, you probably have lordosis with shortened lumbar and hip flexor muscles.

Test 2—Straight-Leg Lift

Pass ☐ Fail ☐

Lie on your back with hands behind your neck. The partner on your left should stabilize your right leg by placing his/her right hand on the knee. With the left hand, your partner should grasp the left ankle and raise your left leg as near to a right angle as possible. In this position (as shown in the diagram), your lower back should be in contact with the floor. Your right leg should remain straight and on the floor throughout the test.

- If your left leg bends at the knee, short hamstring muscles are indicated. If your back arches and/or your right leg does not remain flat on the floor, short lumbar muscles or hip flexor muscles (or both) are indicated. Repeat the test on the opposite side. (Both sides must pass in order to pass the test.)

Test 3—Thomas Test

Pass ☐ Fail ☐

Lie on your back on a table or bench with your right leg extended beyond the edge of the table (approximately one-third of the thigh off the table). Bring your left knee to your chest and pull the thigh down tightly with your hands. Your lower back should remain flat against the table as shown in the diagram. Your right thigh should remain on the table.

- If your right thigh lifts off the table while the left knee is hugged to the chest, a tight hip flexor (iliopsoas) on that side is indicated. Repeat on the opposite side. (Both sides must pass in order to pass the test.)

Test 4—Ely's Test

Pass ☐ Fail ☐

Lie prone; flex right knee. Partner *gently* pushes right heel toward the buttocks. Stop when resistance is felt or when partner expresses discomfort.

- If pelvis leaves the floor or hip flexes or knee fails to bend freely (135 degrees) or heel fails to touch buttocks, there is tightness in the quadriceps muscles. Repeat with left leg. (Both sides must pass to pass the test.)

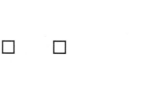
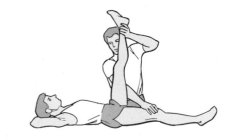
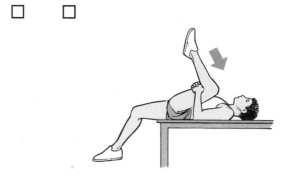
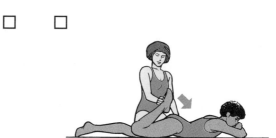

Chart 16.1 *Continued* 215

Test 5—Ober's Test

Pass ☐   Fail ☐

Lie on left side with left leg flexed 90 degrees at the hip and 90 degrees at the knee. Partner places right hip in neutral position (no flexion) and right knee in 90-degree flexion; partner then allows the weight of the leg to lower it toward the floor.

- If there is no tightness in the iliotibial band (fascia and muscles on lateral side of leg), the knee touches the floor without pain and the test is passed. Repeat on the other side. (Both sides must pass in order to pass the test.)

Test 6—Press-Up (Straight Arm)

Pass ☐   Fail ☐

Perform the press-up.

- If you can press to a straight-arm position, keeping your pubis in contact with the floor, and if your partner determines that the arch in your back is a continuous curve (not just a sharp angle at the lumbosacral joint), then there is adequate flexibility in spinal extension.

Test 7—Knee Roll

Pass ☐   Fail ☐

Lie supine with both knees and hips flexed 90 degrees, arms extended to the sides at shoulder level. Keep the knees and hips in that position and lower them to the floor on the right and then on the left.

- If you can accomplish this and still keep your shoulders in contact with the floor, then you have adequate rotation in the spine, especially at the lumbar and thoracic junction. (You must pass both sides in order to pass the test.)

Chart 16.2 Healthy Back Test Ratings

Classification	Number of Tests Passed
Excellent	7
Very good	6
Good	5
Fair	4
Poor	1–3

Chart 16.4 Posture *Rating Scale*

Classification	Total Score
Excellent	0–2
Very good	3–4
Good	5–7
Fair	8–11
Poor	12 or more

Chart 16.3 Posture Evaluation

Side View	Points	Back View	Points
Head forward	___	Tilted head	___
Sunken chest	___	Protruding scapulae	___
Round shoulders	___	Symptoms of scoliosis	
		Shoulders uneven	___
Kyphosis	___	Hips uneven	___
Lordosis	___	Lateral curvature of spine (Adam's position)	___
Abdominal ptosis	___	One side of back high (Adam's position)	___
Hyperextended knees	___		
Body lean	___	Total score ___	

CONCEPT ·17·

Planning for Physically Active Living

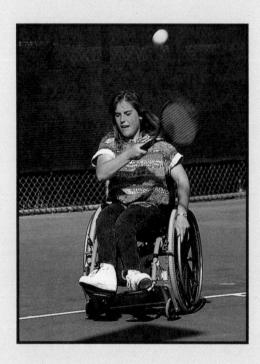

Concept 17

Planning for physically active living is essential to optimal physical fitness, health, and wellness.

Introduction

There is no single exercise program best suited for all people, nor is there one best lifestyle for health and wellness. When planning a program of exercise, it is important to consider your own unique needs and interests.

Health Goals for the Year 2000

- Increase the proportion of people who do daily exercise. (↑)
- Increase the proportion of people who engage in activity to promote cardiovascular fitness. (<>)
- Reduce the proportion of people who do no leisure-time physical activity. (<>)
- Increase the proportion of people who engage in activity to enhance muscular strength, muscular endurance, and flexibility. (<>)
- Increase the proportion of overfat people who use sound dietary practices and regular exercise to attain appropriate body weight. (<>)

Note: (↑) indicates progress toward goal, (↓) indicates regression from goal, and (<>) indicates either no change or lack of new data since 1990.

Terms

- **Behavioral Goal**   A statement of intent to perform a specific behavior (changing a lifestyle) for a specific period of time. An example would be, "I will walk for fifteen minutes each morning before work."
- **Fitness Goals**   A fitness goal is an outcome goal with a specific fitness score as the intended outcome.
- **Long-Term Goal**   A statement of intent to change behavior or achieve a specific outcome in a period of months or years.
- **Outcome Goal**   A statement of intent to achieve a specific test score (attainment of a specific standard) associated with good health or wellness. An example would be, "I will lower my body fat level by 3 percent."
- **Physical Activity Goals**   An exercise or physical activity goal is a behavioral goal with exercise as the intended behavior.
- **Short-Term Goal**   A statement of intent to change a behavior or outcome in a period of days or weeks.

Steps in Program Planning

There are several steps for planning an effective physical activity program

Step 1—Clarify your reasons for starting your physical activity program.

Clarifying your purposes for starting a physical activity program may help you to select activities that you will enjoy and continue for a lifetime. Different people have different reasons why they do or do not exercise regularly. At this time it would be useful to try to identify your reasons for starting a program.

Step 2—Identify your fitness needs.

If you have no medical problems, the second step in program planning is to test your physical fitness on each of the health-related components.

Step 3—Establish your short-term and long-term goals.

Having established both your reasons (step 1) and your needs (step 2), it is now possible to develop your **physical activity goals** and **fitness goals**. Some guidelines follow:

- **Be realistic.** The biggest problem with goal setting is that you may fail to meet your goals if they are too difficult to achieve. Failure to meet goals is discouraging. You should set goals that you have a realistic chance of achieving. This is especially true for short-term goals.

- **Focus on short-term goals first. Short-term goals** are easier to accomplish than long-term goals. Realistic short-term goals make you successful. One success leads to another. When you meet short-term goals, establish new ones.

- **Short-term goals should be physical activity or behavioral goals.** If you do physical activity regularly, fitness will improve. Beginners who establish short-term physical activity goals and stick with them will be successful. Because fitness goals take more time to reach, they make poor short-term goals. Physical activity is a behavior that anyone can do—it takes only effort. You can easily monitor a behavior to tell that you have met your goal. Outcomes such as fitness can be monitored, but when changes do not occur immediately you may get the feeling you have failed. **Outcome goals** or fitness goals are more appropriate **long-term goals.**

- **Long-term fitness goals should consider your heredity.** Your heredity limits your fitness. When establishing long-term fitness goals, be careful not to base them on what other people can do. You may be setting yourself up for failure. Be sure that the fitness outcomes you expect are based on health standards or scores slightly above what you can currently perform, rather than on performance scores of other people.

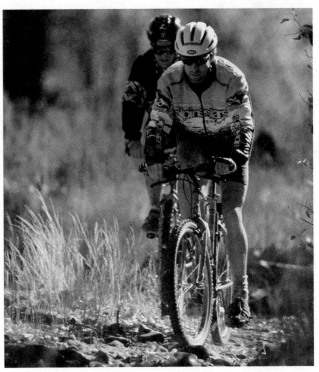

Select activities that you enjoy and that are good for meeting your own personal goals.

- **Consider maintenance goals as well as improvement goals.** There is a limit to the amount of fitness any person can achieve. You cannot improve forever. At some point it is reasonable to set "maintenance goals." Maintenance means staying active and fit when improvement goals have already been met.

- **Set goals that call for a lifestyle that you can maintain.** Physical activity and fitness for a lifetime mean maintaining your program forever. If you set exercise or fitness goals that are excessive, you may burn out and quit exercising entirely. Consider the long term in setting your goals.

- **Put your goals in writing.** It is easy to forget your goals if they are not in writing. Writing them helps establish a commitment to yourself and clearly establishes your goals. You can revise them if necessary. Written goals are not cast in concrete.

Step 4—Select activities that are best for meeting your goals.

In reading this text, you have learned about the benefits of different types of physical activities. Use this information to select activities to include in your program. The activities should adhere to the FIT (frequency, intensity, and time) formula for the various components of fitness. They should be safe and meet your personal needs and interests. Include activities you have enjoyed in the past, ones that you feel will meet your future goals, and those in which you are likely to persist for a lifetime.

Table 17.1
Weekly Physical Activity Program (Sample)

Chart 17.1 Weekly Physical Activity Program		

Daily Schedules
(List the activities and times of day for each activity.)

Monday	Tuesday	Wednesday

7:00 a.m. warm up, jog, cool-down
 	
7:30 a.m. flexibility exercises
 	
12:00 noon   warm-ups
      strength/me exercises
      1, 2, 3, 7 and other
      special exercises
      cool-down
	12:00 noon warm-up,
	      strength/me exercises
	      4, 5, 6 and 8
		7:00 a.m. warm up, jog, cool-down
		
		7:30 a.m. flexibility exercises
		
		12:00 noon same as Monday

Thursday	Friday	Saturday

12:00 noon   same as Tuesday
 	
1:00   warm-up
      slow pitch softball
      cool-down
	7:00 a.m. warm up, jog, cool-down
	
	7:30 a.m. flexibility exercises
	
	12:00 noon same as Monday
		9:30 mow the lawn
		
		12:00 noon same as Tuesday

Sunday	Flexibility Exercises			Strength and Muscular Endurance Exercises		
	Exercise	Time	Reps	Exercise	Sets	Reps
8:30 a.m. walk for one hour	1. lower leg stretches	15 sec.	3	1. biceps curls	3	8
	2. one-leg stretches	15 sec.	3	2. seated rowing	3	8
	3. lateral trunk stretches	15 sec.	3	3. push-ups	1	15
	4. wand exercise	15 sec.	3	4. leg press	3	8
				5. knee extension	3	8
				6. hamstring curl	3	8
				7. crunches	1	25
				8. upper back lift	1	8

Warm-Up and Cool-Down Activities	Other Special Exercises	
calf stretches back-saver toe stretch leg hug side stretch zipper one minute jog	1. isometric neck exercise 2. push up 3. double knee to chest	

Step 5—Write a weekly plan and do it!

You are more likely to perform your program if you put it in writing. To get you started, a sample **Weekly Physical Activity Program** is provided (see table 17.1). A blank weekly plan is provided in the Lab for you to write out your personal plan. Now do it! If you are going to adhere to this program, you must be able to manage your time. Time management is one of the keys to success. A hit-or-miss program may turn into no program at all. From the beginning, set aside a specific time and place for your activity. Place a high priority on your exercise time. Don't allow anything to interrupt your schedule. Build *physical activity* into your daily routine; make it as much a habit as taking a bath or eating regular meals. Some form of *physical activity* should be done at least three days per week and *is recommended for most days of the week.*

Step 6—Keep monthly records of physical activity and fitness.

Record keeping can help you stick with your physical activity program and can help you attain your fitness goals. Use a one-month calendar to keep track of your regular physical activity and of any fitness changes that occur. Steps in using the calendar are described in the Lab.

Step 7—Periodically reevaluate and modify your program.

The weekly program you write in step 5 may be an excellent one. However, as time goes by your needs, interests, and goals change. For this reason, you should periodically reevaluate and revise your personal program. If you become bored with certain activities, you may wish to drop them and add other new and interesting activities. Changes in the weather, the availability of facilities, and personal schedules may all require program changes. Each time you change your program, follow steps 1 through 6. It is not necessary to do the same program forever; the key is to have a program that meets your current needs, interests, and goals.

Suggested Readings

American College of Sports Medicine. *ACSM's Guidelines for Exercise Testing and Exercise Prescription.* 5th ed. Baltimore, MD: Williams and Wilkins, 1995.

American College of Sports Medicine. "The Recommended Quantity and Quality of Exercise for Developing and Maintaining Cardiorespiratory and Muscular Fitness in Healthy Adults." *Medicine and Science in Sports and Exercise* 22(1990):2.

Pate, R., et al. "Physical Activity and Public Health." *Journal of the American Medical Association* 273(1995):402.

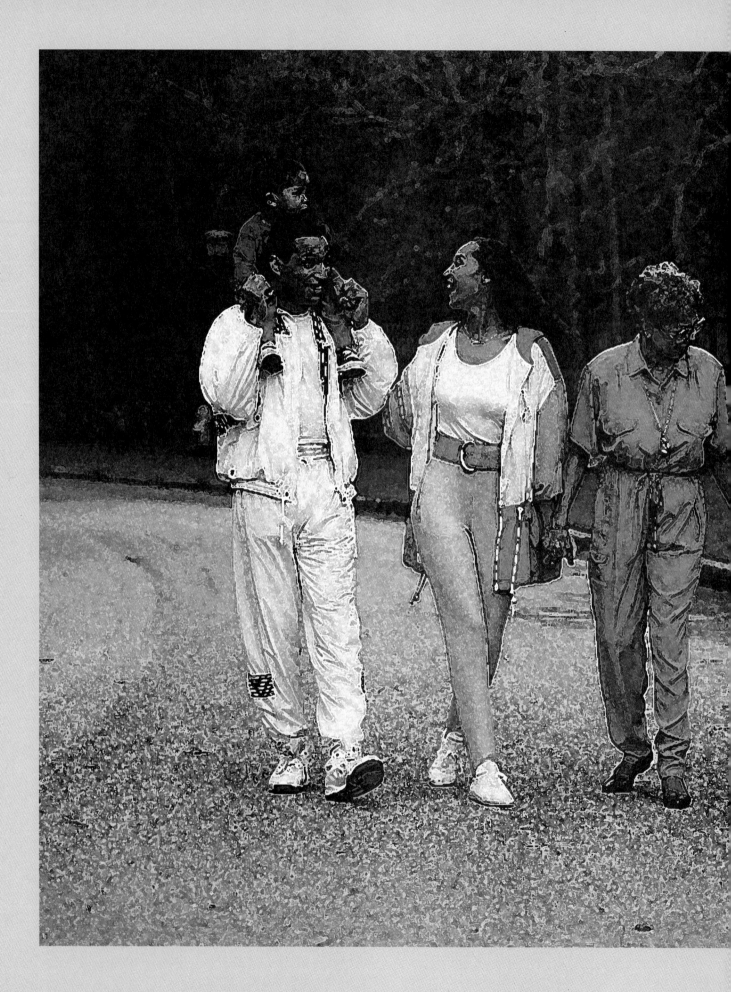

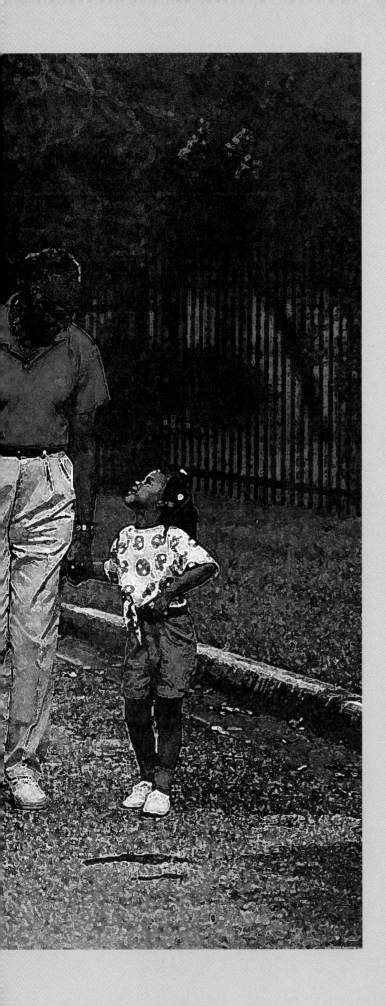

SECTION ·IV·

Healthy Lifestyles

CONCEPT ·18·

Wellness and Healthy Living

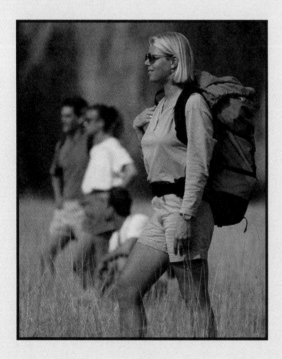

Concept 18

Wellness is the positive aspect of optimal health that can be enhanced by the adoption of healthy lifestyles.

Introduction

Goals for the nation's optimal health have been established in a comprehensive document entitled *Healthy People 2000*. The intent of the document was to establish reasonable goals that, with a conscientious effort, could be achieved by the year 2000. "The challenge of *Healthy People 2000* is to use the combined strength of scientific knowledge, professional skill, individual commitment, community support, and political will to enable people to achieve their potential to live full, active lives. It means preventing premature death and preventing disability, preserving a physical environment that supports human life, cultivating family and community support, enhancing each individual's inherent abilities to respond and to act, and assuring that all Americans achieve and maintain a maximum level of functioning." (Public Health Service 1991, p. 6) Clearly the goals for the nation emphasize all the components of optimal health, including **wellness,** as evidenced by a positive sense of well-being and quality living. A mid-decade review of *Healthy People 2000* objectives indicates that progress is being made in a majority of the priority health and wellness goals. Focusing on healthy lifestyles pays dividends.

Health Goals for the Year 2000

- Increase the span of life. (↑)
- Increase the span of optimally healthy life. (<>)

Note: (↑) indicates progress toward goal, (↓) indicates regression from goal, and (<>) indicates either no change or lack of new data since 1990.

Terms

- **Emotional Wellness**   A person's ability to cope with daily circumstances and to deal with personal feelings in a positive, optimistic, and constructive manner.
- **Health**   Health is optimal well-being that contributes to quality of life. It is more than freedom from disease and illness, though freedom from disease is important to good health. Optimal health includes high-level emotional, intellectual, physical, social, and spiritual wellness.
- **Intellectual Wellness**   A person's ability to learn and to use information to enhance the quality of daily living and optimal functioning.
- **Mental Wellness**   The goals for the nation's health refer to mental rather than emotional health and wellness. In this book mental wellness is considered to be the same as emotional wellness (see above).

- **Physical Wellness** A person's ability to function effectively in meeting the demands of the day's work and ability to use free time effectively. Physical wellness includes good physical fitness and the possession of useful motor skills.
- **Social Wellness** A person's ability to successfully interact with others and to establish meaningful relationships that enhance the quality of life for all people involved in the interaction (including self).
- **Spiritual Wellness** A person's ability to establish a values system and act on the system of beliefs as well as to establish and carry out meaningful and constructive lifetime goals. Spiritual wellness is often based on a belief in a force greater than the individual that helps one contribute to an improved quality of life of all people.
- **Wellness** Wellness is the integration of many dimensions, including emotional, intellectual, physical, spiritual, and social, that expands one's potential to live and work effectively and to make a significant contribution to society. Wellness is considered to be the positive component of good health. It reflects how one feels (a sense of well-being) about life as well as one's ability to function effectively.

The Facts About Wellness

> **Wellness** is the positive component of optimal **health.**

Death, disease, illness, and debilitating conditions are the negative components of health. Death is the ultimate opposite of optimal health. Disease, illness, and debilitating conditions obviously detract from optimal health. Wellness has been recognized as the positive component of optimal health as evidenced by a sense of well-being reflected in optimal functioning, a good quality of life, meaningful work, and a contribution to society (see figure 18.1).

> Wellness is the integration of all parts of health that expands one's potential to live and work effectively and to make a significant contribution to society.

Wellness is the integration of many dimensions, including **emotional (mental), intellectual, physical, social,** and **spiritual.** Each of the five sections of figure 18.1 is meant to illustrate the importance of each dimension to total wellness.

Throughout this book references will be made to the various wellness dimensions to help the reader understand the importance of each dimension to integrated total wellness. Wellness, however, is an integrated state of being that is better depicted as many threads that can be woven together to produce a larger, integrated fabric. Each specific dimension relates to each of the others and overlaps all others. The overlap is so frequent and so great that the specific contribution of each thread is almost indistinguishable when looking at the total (figure 18.2).

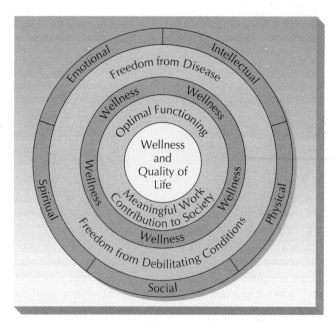

Figure 18.1
A model of optimal health and wellness

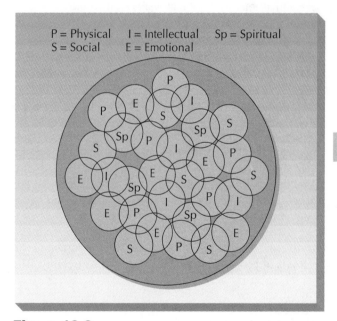

Figure 18.2
The integration of wellness dimensions

> Wellness reflects how one feels about life as well as one's ability to function effectively.

As noted in table 18.1, a positive total outlook on life is essential to wellness. A total positive outlook is impacted by each of the wellness dimensions. A well person is one who is satisfied in his/her work, who is spiritually fulfilled, enjoys leisure time, is physically fit, is socially involved, and has a positive emotional-mental outlook. This person is happy and fulfilled. Many experts believe that a positive total outlook is a key to wellness.

The way one perceives each of the dimensions of wellness affects total outlook. Researchers have used the term "self-perceptions" to describe the feelings people have about their competence in each area of wellness. Many believe that self-perceptions are more important than actual performance when it comes to various wellness dimensions. For example, a person who has an important job may find less meaning and job satisfaction than another person with a much less important job.

Apparently one of the important factors for a person who has achieved high-level wellness and a positive life's outlook is the ability to reward himself/herself. A good self-reward system allows a person to feel good about self. Some people seem unable to give themselves credit for their life's experiences. The development of a system that allows a person to positively perceive the self is important. Of course, the adoption of positive lifestyles that encourage improved self-perceptions is also important. The questionnaire in the Lab Resources Materials of this concept will help you assess your self-perceptions of the various wellness dimensions. For optimal wellness it would be important to find positive feelings about each dimension.

Feelings of wellness are important for people with disease and disability.

All people can benefit from enhanced wellness. Wellness, an improved quality of life, is possible for everyone, regardless of disabilities or disease states. Evidence is accumulating to indicate that people with a positive outlook are better able to resist the progress of disease and illness. Thinking positive thoughts has been associated with enhanced results from various medical treatments and better results from surgical procedures.

Because self-perceptions are important to wellness, positive perceptions of self are especially important to the wellness of people with disease, illness, and disability. The

Table 18.1
The Dimensions of Wellness

–	Wellness Dimensions	+
Depressed	Emotional-Mental	Happy
Ignorant	Intellectual	Informed
Unfit	Physical	Fit
Lonely	Social	Involved
Unfulfilled	Spiritual	Fulfilled
Negative	Total Outlook	Positive

concepts of wellness and optimal health must be considered in light of one's heredity and personal disabilities and disease states.

Wellness is a useful term that may be used by quacks as well as experts.

Healthy People 2000 recognizes that optimal health comes from an improved quality of life and " . . . is best measured by citizens' sense of well-being" (Public Health Service 1991, p. 6). Experts support the importance of wellness to optimal health.

Unfortunately, some individuals and groups have tried to identify wellness with products and services that promise benefits that cannot be documented. Because "well-being" is a subjective feeling that is hard to document, it is easy for quacks to make claims of improved wellness for their product or service without facts to back them up.

"Holistic health" is a term that is similarly abused. Optimal health includes many areas (see figure 18.2), thus the term holistic (total) is appropriate. In fact the word "health" originates from a root word meaning *wholeness*. Nevertheless, care should be used when considering services and products that make claims of wellness and/or holistic health to be sure that they are legitimate.

The Facts About Healthy Lifestyles

Three strategies are commonly employed in efforts designed to achieve optimal health for all people.

Disease and illness treatment, disease and illness prevention, and health and wellness promotion are three different strategies used to achieve optimal health. Disease and illness treatment includes efforts to treat and cure common diseases and illnesses that threaten society and are likely to result in pain, suffering, hospitalization and/or premature death. Much of the burden for this strategy falls to those in the medical and health professions.

Disease and illness prevention includes efforts to prevent rather than treat health problems. Though medical and public health agencies have a considerable responsibility in this area, much of the burden for implementing this strategy rests with communities and individuals within these communities.

Health and wellness promotion includes efforts to alter personal lifestyles to enhance the quality of life that " . . . enables people to achieve their potential to live full, active lives" (Public Health Service 1991, p. 6). Whereas the treatment and prevention strategies focus on death, disease, and illness, promotion strategies focus on wellness.

Table 18.2
Healthy Lifestyles

- Exercising regularly
- Eating properly
- Managing stress
- Avoiding destructive habits
- Practicing safe sex
- Adopting good safety habits
- Learning first aid
- Adopting good personal health behaviors
- Seeking and complying with medical advice
- Being an informed consumer
- Protecting the environment
- Managing time effectively

The principal path to wellness is health promotion associated with altering lifestyles.

Just as physical fitness is a state of being that is altered by regular physical activity, wellness is a state of being (see figures 18.1 and 18.2) that is altered by one's behaviors. Lifestyles are behaviors that are partially or totally in your own control. Some of the healthy lifestyles considered to be very important to optimal wellness are presented in table 18.2.

Participating in Physical Activity Regularly

As noted throughout this book, regular physical activity is associated with the reduced risk of many diseases. Regular physical activity is a positive addiction. It is habit-forming, but the result of the habit is positive, not negative. Regular exercise can be fun and can improve the quality of life. It is interesting to note that people who exercise regularly are likely to adopt other healthy lifestyles. For example, regular exercisers are more likely than sedentary individuals to visit a physician for preventive examinations, practice preventive dentistry, and wear seat belts.

Eating Properly (Good Nutrition)

Good eating habits can help you feel and look your best. Failure to eat properly can result in many health problems. It has been shown that six of the ten leading causes of death in North America are linked to improper nutrition. Millions of teenagers and adults regularly modify their diet in an attempt to assume control of the way they look and of their health. Unfortunately, many of these dietary modifications have a negative rather than positive impact on health. Making *appropriate* changes in eating patterns is the key. Eating properly is a goal that is achievable.

Managing Stress

Nearly 30 million professionals and executives who rank among the highest in annual earnings indicate that they would like to find a way to get away from their steady diet of stress and tension. Reducing stress in your life and learning to cope with stress are associated with feelings of well-being and an improved quality of life. Stress reduction is possible for most people with alterations in lifestyle. (See concept 20 for ways to reduce stress.)

Avoiding Destructive Habits

Among the most destructive habits are the use of tobacco and alcohol, and the abuse of drugs (See table 18.3.) These are lifestyle or health behaviors over which you have personal control, but once they are adopted they are exceptionally difficult to eliminate.

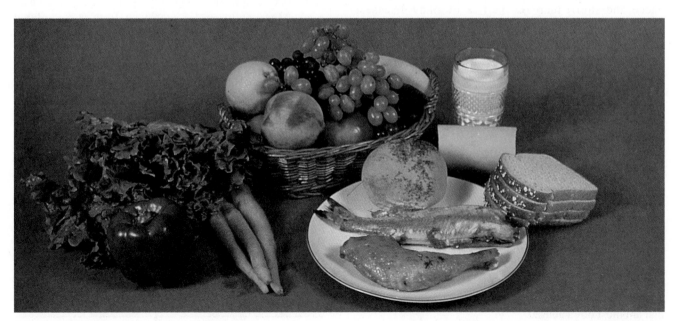

A healthy lifestyle includes eating healthy foods.

Table 18.3
Facts About Destructive Habits

Effects of the Tobacco Habit

- Smokers have five times the risk of heart attack as nonsmokers.
- Smoking tobacco is directly related to cancer (lung, oral, throat), emphysema, and other respiratory diseases.
- Use of smokeless tobacco is associated with heart disease and cancer.
- Pregnant women who smoke increase the risk of health problems for their unborn babies.
- Secondhand smoke (smoke created by smokers) can cause health problems for people who breathe it.

Facts About the Abuse of Alcohol

- Alcohol abuse is a known cause of traffic accidents, violent crimes, allergic reactions, and child and spouse abuse.
- Alcohol abuse is associated with diseases of the liver, cardiovascular system, digestive system, and nervous system, to name but a few.
- Alcohol use by pregnant women can result in medical problems for the unborn child.

Facts About the Abuse of Drugs

- Illegal or illicit drug use is associated with violent crimes, traffic accidents, the increased risk of diseases such as AIDS, suicide, absenteeism, and decreased work production, among other problems.
- Legal drugs taken in improper amounts, too frequently, or in combination with other drugs are associated with many of the same health problems as illegal drugs and alcohol.
- Anabolic steroid use has health risks and has been shown to be related to use of other illegal or illicit drugs.

Smoking cigarettes, cigars, and pipes as well as the use of smokeless tobacco products, such as chewing tobacco and snuff, increase the risk of many diseases. Though it is best not to start using these products, stopping the use of tobacco after years of use is beneficial to health. Unfortunately, it is very difficult to stop smoking.

Addiction to alcohol is another disease that is difficult to conquer. Seventy percent of all American adults consume alcohol. Alcohol is a depressant to the central nervous system and can have other negative effects on the body, mind, and society.

Abuse of drugs is a destructive health habit that can result from abuse of legal or illegal drugs. Among the legal drugs most often abused are caffeine and various over-the-counter drugs. Caffeine is a stimulant found in many drinks including coffee, tea, and soft drinks. In 1980 it was classified as an addicting drug. Many adults also abuse over-the-counter drugs and prescription drugs with the intent of reducing health problems. Tranquilizers and sedatives (depressants), analgesics (pain relievers), antidepressants, and amphetamines (stimulants) are among the legal drugs that are most often abused.

Illicit drugs such as cocaine (coke and crack), marijuana, the opiates (heroin, morphine, codeine, and others), the psychedelics (LSD, mescaline, designer drugs), the deliriants (PCP and others), and inhalants are illegal addicting drugs abused by a large number of Americans. As many as 40 percent of young adults try drugs, and] many become addicted. One in ten of those who do not use illicit drugs are affected each day by people who do abuse these drugs.

Good health and wellness would dictate avoidance of illegal drugs, responsible use of medication, and limited use of legal drugs such as over-the-counter drugs and those found in foods or drinks.

Practicing Safe Sex

Though sexually transmitted diseases (STD) are not currently among the leading killers, they are the source of much pain and suffering. The human immunodeficiency virus (HIV) that causes acquired immunodeficiency syndrome (AIDS) is now a major health problem. HIV/AIDS is a worldwide health problem that has reached epidemic proportion. Many STDs can be cured but others, such as HIV/AIDS, have no cure. Healthy lifestyles are the key to prevention of the most common STDs, including chlamydia, genital herpes and warts, gonorrhea, hepatitis B, HIV/AIDS, and syphilis (see table 18.4).

Adopting Good Safety Habits

Accidents are a major cause of death in North America, accounting for more than 6 percent of all deaths in the United States. In addition, they result in many disabilities and problems that can detract from good health and wellness. All accidents cannot be prevented, but it is possible to adopt habits that greatly reduce the risk of accidents. Deaths from automobile accidents can be greatly reduced by regular use of seat belts. The proper maintenance of play and work equipment can greatly reduce injury and death rates. Many children die each year from water-related accidents that can be prevented by proper supervision, the

Table 18.4
Factors Associated with Reduced Risk of STDs

- Abstaining from sexual activity.
- Limiting sexual activity to a noninfected partner. A lifetime partner who never has sex with other people or never uses illegal injection drugs is the only "safe" partner.
- Avoiding sexual activity or other activity that puts you in contact with semen, vaginal fluids, or blood.
- Using a new condom (latex) every time you have sex, especially with a partner who is not known to be "safe."
- Using a water-based lubricant with condoms (petroleum-based lubricants increase risk of condom failure).
- Never sharing a needle or drug paraphernalia.

use of proper safety devices such as life jackets, and knowledge of cardiopulmonary resuscitation. Proper storage of guns, use of smoke alarms, proper use of ladders, and proper maintenance of cars, motorcycles, and bicycles can also reduce accident risk.

Learning First Aid

Many deaths could be prevented if persons at the site of emergencies were able to administer first aid. Because they can prevent death, all people should be familiar with cardiopulmonary resuscitation (CPR) and the Heimlich maneuver for assisting a person who is choking. Many agencies give extensive classes in first aid taught by qualified experts. It is best to learn these procedures in such a class. First aid for minor injuries and poisoning and for control of bleeding are other important procedures.

Adopting Good Personal Health Behaviors

Many of the healthy lifestyles already discussed are good personal health habits. There are other simple personal health behaviors that are important to optimal health. These behaviors may be considered elementary because they are often taught in school and at home at a very young age. Still, are many adults who fail to adopt these behaviors on a regular basis. Examples include regular brushing and flossing of the teeth; care of ears, eyes, and skin; proper sleep habits; proper innoculations for disease prevention and good posture. Health behaviors that prevent sexually transmitted diseases are also important.

Seeking and Complying with Medical Advice

Some people purposely avoid seeking the advice of a physician because they fear that something may be wrong. This occurs in spite of the evidence that delay in treatment greatly increases the risk of death for many diseases that can be cured or controlled. In addition to medical readiness exams for unhealthy people beginning exercise, regular preventive medical exams are important. After age forty, a yearly preventive exam is recommended for all people. Young adults probably need a regular medical examination less often, but a regular examination is important for all people to help in the early diagnosis of problems. Regular self-examination for breast cancer is recommended, as are periodic mammograms and Pap tests for women (especially after age forty). For men, regular testicular exams and a prostate test are recommended. Other important behaviors that should be considered are listed below:

- Be familiar with the symptoms of the most common medical problems in our culture.
- If symptoms are present, seek medical help. Many deaths could be prevented if the early warning signs of medical problems were heeded.

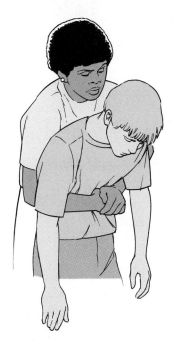

Learn first aid such as the Heimlick Manevuer.

- If medical advice is given, comply. It is not uncommon for people to stop taking medicine when symptoms stop rather than taking the full amount of medicine prescribed.
- If you doubt the advice given, seek a second opinion.

Being An Informed Consumer

Each year too many people purchase health services and products that are ineffective and often dangerous. Extensive advertising of quack health products, often by celebrities, bombards all of us. It is important to investigate so-called health products and services of all kinds (see concept 22).

Protecting the Environment

A recent national poll indicated that 70 percent of the adult population felt that the public was not concerned enough about the environment. If fact, more than half felt that there was an immediate need to take drastic action to protect the environment. Concern for the environment has increased in recent years as indicated by the fact that more than eight of ten households now indicate that they voluntarily recycle newspapers, glass, or aluminum. We have not been as actively involved in other lifestyle changes that would help protect the environment (see table 18.5).

Unlike lifestyle behaviors such as regular exercise or managing stress, behaviors that help protect the environment may not have immediate wellness benefits. Experts are quick to point out, however, that protecting the environment may be one of the most important things that we can do over time to guarantee quality of living for our children and the generations to come.

Table 18.5
Adult Involvement in Behaviors to Protect the Environment

Lifestyle Behavior	Percent of Involvement
• Recycle paper, glass, aluminum, oil, etc.	86%
• Cut energy use.	73%
• Avoid buying or using aerosol sprays.	68%
• Cut water use.	68%
• Replace inefficient automobile.	67%
• Contribute to environmental or conservation group.	51%
• Avoid nonrecyclable goods.	49%
• Car pool or use public transportation.	46%
• Boycott company's unsafe products.	28%
• Use cloth rather than disposable diapers.	25%
• Do environmental or conservation volunteer work.	18%

Source: Data from the Gallup Poll, 1991.

Managing Time Effectively

Central to the concept of wellness are working efficiently and making a significant contribution to society. Working effectively requires a commitment of time. A social contribution requires time for special causes, and social wellness requires a commitment of time to family and friends. Similarly, each of the other dimensions of wellness requires a time commitment. A healthy lifestyle is one that allocates time efficiently to insure that appropriate time is allocated to behaviors that contribute to each wellness dimension, and ultimately to total wellness.

More Facts About Wellness and Healthy Lifestyles

> Moderation is a good rule for lifestyle modification and wellness promotion.

In many ways, the things that enrich your life and lead to quality living can also be the source of problems. Some stress (eustress) makes life interesting; too much stress is considered distressful. Regular exercise contributes to good health and wellness. Too little or too much could be detrimental. This is true of almost any lifestyle. A moderate lifestyle can make life interesting and enjoyable without creating the risk of health problems.

> A balanced lifestyle is important for promoting wellness.

"All work and no play makes Jack a dull boy" is a saying that illustrates the problem with an unbalanced lifestyle. If work is the only focus of your life, it detracts from good health and wellness. A balanced lifestyle includes interesting work and enjoyable leisure as well as balance on the other dimensions of wellness.

> Personal control is critical to altering lifestyles for wellness promotion.

Many health problems are associated with health behaviors that can be modified through lifestyle changes. To make positive lifestyle changes, you must believe that changing your lifestyle can help you prevent illness and achieve wellness. If you believe that optimal health is outside of your personal control, you will probably not make lifestyle changes.

> Healthy lifestyles learned early in life are most likely to be maintained throughout life.

Research suggests that behaviors that are learned at a very young age and that become a habit are more likely to be maintained throughout life. For this reason, education concerning healthy lifestyles should be started in the formative years. Simple health behaviors such as brushing the teeth, when begun early in life, are often maintained throughout life.

> It is never too late to adopt positive lifestyles to promote optimal health.

The negative impact of unhealthy living may have effects that are irreversible. Severe malnutrition, for example, could result in stunted growth and other problems that are permanent. Nevertheless, many problems associated with unhealthy lifestyles can be improved or eliminated by changing personal living habits. For example, recent research indicates that stopping smoking, even among people who smoked for years, reduces the risk of heart disease and cancer. Proper exercise and techniques for stress reduction can help reduce back pain and improve the quality of life for people with back problems, even those who have had chronic problems.

Suggested Readings

Bruess, C., and G. Richardson, *Decisions for Health,* 4th ed. Dubuque, IA: Brown & Benchmark Publishers, 1995.

Cancer Facts and Figures—1995. Atlanta: American Cancer Society, 1995.

Health Letters Associates. *Wellness Made Easy: 101 Tips for Better Health.* Berkeley: University of California, Berkeley, Wellness Letter, 1990.

1995 Heart Facts Reference Sheet. Dallas: American Heart Association, 1995.

McGinnis, M., and P. Lee. "Healthy People 2000 at Mid Decade." *Journal of the American Medical Association* 273(1995):1123.

Public Health Service. *Healthy People 2000: National Health Promotion and Disease Prevention Objectives.* Washington, DC: U.S. Government Printing Office, 1991. (DHHS Pub. No. PHS 91–50212.)

Siegel, B. S. *Love, Medicine, and Miracles.* New York: Harper and Row, 1986.

LAB RESOURCE MATERIALS

Scoring the Wellness Perceptions Questionnaire

1. Score four points for an X marked in the first box of each row. Score a three for the second box, a two for the third box, and a one for the fourth box in each row.

2. Each question represents one of the wellness dimensions in figure 18.1. The following questions represent these wellness dimensions: 1 = emotional, 2 = intellectual, 3 = physical, 4 = social, 5 = spiritual, and 6 = general.

3. To determine a total wellness score, sum the numbers for the six questions.

4. Use chart 18.1 to determine your wellness ratings.

Chart 18.1 Wellness *Rating Scale*

	Individual Wellness Dimensions	Total Wellness
Excellent	4	21–24
Good	3	18–20
Marginal	2	12–17
Low	1	11 or less

Chart 18.2 Self-Perceptions of Wellness Questionnaire

Directions: There are four possible responses for each question. Place an X in *one* of the four boxes for *each* question.

Sample Question: A person who likes ice cream a lot would mark the box as indicated below.

Some people like ice cream very much.	**but**	Other people do not like ice cream at all.

Especially true for me	True for me		Not true for me	Especially not true for me
⊠	☐		☐	☐

1. Some people are happy most of the time. **but** Other people feel depressed much of the time.

Especially true for me	True for me		Not true for me	Especially not true for me
☐	☐		☐	☐

2. Some people are well informed about health and wellness. **but** Other people are ignorant of the facts concerning their health and well-being.

Especially true for me	True for me		Not true for me	Especially not true for me
☐	☐		☐	☐

3. Some people are physically fit. **but** Other people are not so fit physically.

Especially true for me	True for me		Not true for me	Especially not true for me
☐	☐		☐	☐

4. Some people have a lot of friends and are very involved socially. **but** Other people do not have many friends and are often lonely.

Especially true for me	True for me		Not true for me	Especially not true for me
☐	☐		☐	☐

5. Some people feel fulfilled spiritually. **but** Other people are not so fulfilled spiritually.

Especially true for me	True for me		Not true for me	Especially not true for me
☐	☐		☐	☐

6. Some people have a very positive outlook on life— they are optimistic. **but** Other people have a more negative outlook on life— they are pessimistic.

Especially true for me	True for me		Not true for me	Especially not true for me
☐	☐		☐	☐

Scoring and Interpreting the Healthy Lifestyle Questionnaire (Chart 18.3)

Score the questionnaire using the following method.

1. For questions 1, 3, 4, 6, 10, 11, 15, 16, 17, 18, 19, 21, 22, 23, and 24 assign the following point values to answers: never = 1, sometimes = 2, often = 3, and regularly = 4.

2. For questions 2, 9, 12, 13, and 14 assign the following point values to answers: no = 1 and yes = 4.

3. For questions 5, 7, 8, and 20 assign the following point values to answers: never = 4, sometimes = 3, often = 2, and regularly = 1.

4. Calculate a total Healthy Lifestyle Score by adding the number of points for all 24 questions.

5. Subscores for each of the nine different lifestyle areas can be calculated by summing the scores of the two questions in each area. Interpret the questionnaire using the following information. In general, a total score of 72 or higher on the Healthy Lifestyle Questionnaire would indicate a healthy lifestyle as it would suggest that you choose the healthy alternative "often." This, however, can be deceiving. You might have a score of 72 or higher and eat high-fat meals regularly or smoke regularly. In other words, scores on individual subscores are also important. For most scales, a score of six or higher merits a "good" rating, though a score of 8 is preferred.

Chart 18.3 The Healthy Lifestyle Questionnaire

Using the Healthy Lifestyle Questionnaire

The purpose of this questionnaire is to help you analyze your lifestyle and to help you in making decisions concerning good health and wellness for the future. Information on this Healthy Lifestyle Questionnaire is of a very personal nature. For this reason, this questionnaire is not one that is designed to be handed in to your instructor. It is for your information only. Answer each question as honestly as possible and use the scoring information to help you assess your lifestyle.

Directions: Place an "x" in one box for each question based on your own personal behaviors.

Exercise and Fitness	Never	Sometimes	Often	Regularly
1. I do moderate to vigorous exercise at least three times a week for 15 to 30 minutes.	☐	☐	☐	☐

	No			Yes
2. I rate in the good fitness zone on the five components of health-related physical fitness.	☐			☐

Nutrition	Never	Sometimes	Often	Regularly
3. I eat three regular meals daily that contain the recommended servings from the food pyramid.	☐	☐	☐	☐
4. I limit the amount of saturated fat (solid at room temperature), salt, and simple sugar in my diet.	☐	☐	☐	☐

Stress	Never	Sometimes	Often	Regularly
5. My normal daily activities expose me to stressful situations.	☐	☐	☐	☐
6. I do exercises or other relaxation techniques that help me reduce my stress levels.	☐	☐	☐	☐

Destructive Habits	Never	Sometimes	Often	Regularly
7. I smoke or use other tobacco products.	☐	☐	☐	☐
8. I abuse alcohol or drugs (legal or illegal).	☐	☐	☐	☐

Safe Sex Habits	No			Yes
9. I abstain from sex or limit sexual activity to a safe partner.	☐			☐

	Never	Sometimes	Often	Regularly
10. I practice other safe procedures for avoiding STDs.	☐	☐	☐	☐

Safety Habits	Never	Sometimes	Often	Regularly
11. I use seat belts and adhere to the speed limit when I drive in an automobile.	☐	☐	☐	☐

	No			Yes
12. I have a smoke detector in my home and check it regularly to see that it is working effectively.	☐			☐

First Aid	No			Yes
13. I can perform CPR effectively if called on in an emergency.	☐			☐
14. I can perform the Heimlich maneuver effectively if called on in an emergency.	☐			☐

Personal Health Habits	Never	Sometimes	Often	Regularly
15. I brush my teeth at least two times a day and floss at least once a day.	☐	☐	☐	☐
16. I get an adequate amount of sleep each night.	☐	☐	☐	☐

Seeking and Complying with Medical Advice	Never	Sometimes	Often	Regularly
17. I have medical check-ups and seek medical advice when symptoms are present.	☐	☐	☐	☐
18. When I receive advice and/or medication from a physician including medication, I follow the advice and take the medication as prescribed.	☐	☐	☐	☐

Being an Informed Consumer	Never	Sometimes	Often	Regularly
19. I read product labels and investigate the effectiveness of products before I buy them.	☐	☐	☐	☐
20. I buy and use food supplements and other so-called "health" foods without advice from an M.D. or R.D.	☐	☐	☐	☐

Protecting the Environment	Never	Sometimes	Often	Regularly
21. I recycle paper, glass, or aluminum.	☐	☐	☐	☐
22. I practice other environmental protection such as car pooling and conserving energy.	☐	☐	☐	☐

Managing Time Effectively	Never	Sometimes	Often	Regularly
23. I find time for family and friends.	☐	☐	☐	☐
24. I make time for leisure and recreation.	☐	☐	☐	☐

CONCEPT
19
Nutrition

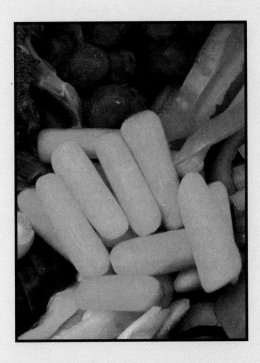

Concept 19

The amount and kinds of food you eat affect your health and wellness.

Introduction

In spite of the fact that nutrition is an advanced science, many myths and misconceptions prevail. These are propagated by commercial interests. Product sales are advanced by the public's (and even physicians' and educators') superstitions and ignorance of the facts.

In this concept some basic nutrition guidelines are presented to inform the reader and dispel various nutrition myths. Since superstition seems to thrive particularly among athletes, coaches, and those interested in high-level performance, a special section is presented on nutrition and physical performance.

Because nutrition affects us all, it is important that we are knowledgeable about the subject. It is far too complicated to cover even the fundamentals in these pages; therefore, the reader is encouraged to enroll in a nutrition course taught by a registered dietitian or to study reliable books, journals, or government documents such as *The Surgeon General's Report on Nutrition and Health* and *Nutrition and Your Health: Dietary Guidelines for Americans* (4th ed.). (See suggested readings.)

Health Goals for the Year 2000

- Reduce dietary fat, especially saturated fat intake. (↑)
- Increase the complex carbohydrates in the diet. (<>)
- Increase the calcium intake in the diet. (<>)
- Decrease the salt and sodium in the diet. (<>)
- Reduce the incidence of iron deficiency. (<>)
- Increase the proportion of people who use food labels. (↑)

Note: (↑) indicates progress toward goal, (↓) indicates regression from goal, and (<>) indicates either no change or lack of new data since 1990.

Terms

- **Amino Acids**   Twenty-two basic building blocks of the body that make up proteins.
- **Antioxidants**   Vitamins (C, E, and plant forms of A or beta carotene) which are thought to inactivate "activated oxygen molecules" sometimes called "free radicals". Free radicals are naturally created by human cells but are also caused by environmental factors such as smoke and radiation. Free radicals may cause cell damage which leads to disease. If antioxidant vitamins work, they would inactivate the free radicals before they do their damage.
- **Basal Metabolic Rate (BMR)**   Metabolic rate at rest.
- **Carbohydrate Loading**   Extra consumption of complex carbohydrates in the days prior to a long, sustained performance.
- **Cellulose**   Indigestible fiber (bulk) in foods.

- **Ergogenic Aid** In this concept, this term will refer to a nutritional supplement claimed by its promoters to improve performance.
- **Essential Amino Acids** Eight basic amino acids that the human body cannot produce and that must be obtained from food sources.
- **Fiber** Indigestible bulk in foods.
- **Glycogen** A source of energy stored in the muscles and liver that is necessary for sustained physical activity.
- **Metabolic Rate (MR)** The rate at which the body produces heat that is measured in calories; an indication of the body's activities, including exercise and normal body functions.
- **Recommended Daily Allowance (RDA)** The minimum amount of a specific nutrient that should be included in the daily diet to meet current health needs.
- **Saturated Fat** Dietary fat that is usually solid at room temperature and comes primarily from animal sources.
- **Trans Fatty Acids** Fats that result when liquid oil has hydrogen added to it to make it more solid. "Hydrogenation" transforms unsaturated fats so that they take on characteristics of saturated fats, as is the case for margarine and shortening.
- **Unsaturated Fat** Monounsaturated or polyunsaturated fat that is usually liquid at room temperature and comes primarily from vegetable sources.
- **Vegan** A strict vegetarian who not only excludes all forms of meat from the diet, but also excludes dairy products and eggs.

The Facts About Basic Nutrition

> The amount and kinds of food you eat affect your health and well-being.

There are about forty-five to fifty nutrients in food that are believed to be essential for the body's growth, maintenance, and repair. These are classified into six categories: carbohydrates (and fiber), fats, proteins, vitamins, minerals, and water. The first three provide energy, which is measured in calories. Specific dietary recommendations for each of the six nutrients are presented later in this concept.

The Food and Nutrition Board of the National Academy of Sciences—National Research Council has established **recommended daily allowances (RDA)** for each nutrient. To help assure that you select foods containing the essential elements, the board has classified foods into groups, each of which should be included in the daily diet. The quantity of nutrients recommended varies with age and other considerations; for example, a young, growing child needs more calcium than an adult, and pregnant women or postmenopausal women need more calcium than other women.

Some foods contain some of all six classes of nutrients (e.g., whole wheat bread) whereas others (e.g., sugar) contain only one. No food is a "complete" food because none contains all of the specific essential nutrients.

> Eating the recommended servings of food from the Food Guide Pyramid will provide key nutrients and enable a person to meet the dietary recommendations outlined in this concept.

The Food Guide Pyramid (see figure 19.1) was designed to guide people in the selection of nutritious food. Selecting the appropriate number of servings from each portion of the pyramid will assure inclusion of necessary nutrients in the diet. A greater number of servings is recommended from the foods near the base of the pyramid (complex carbohydrates) with fewer servings from the upper levels. Foods from the lower level of the pyramid are "nutritionally dense," meaning that they have more nutrients per calorie than low-density foods. For example, a 200-calorie piece of Boston cream pie (from tip of pyramid) has very few vitamins and minerals and is high in fat and refined carbohydrates, whereas 200 calories of tuna has very little fat, 100 percent of the RDA for protein, niacin, vitamin B_{12}, and substantial B_6 and phosphorus. Eating nutritionally dense food is particularly important for someone on a low-calorie diet. For example, it is difficult to get all the essential nutrients in a 1000- to 1200-calorie diet unless foods are chosen carefully.

> Counting food servings is important to assuring that adequate choices are made from the pyramid.

Figure 19.2 provides you with an idea of what constitutes a serving for each food group. Use this information to help you see if you have made the appropriate number of choices from the pyramid. *Healthy People 2000* goals for nutrition specifically target fruits and vegetables as important to the diet of all Americans. The goal is to consume 5 servings per day of these foods. Recent studies indicate that only 32 percent of American adults meet this goal. Of the vegetables Americans eat, 11 percent are consumed as french fries. Clearly many adults need to focus more on getting adequate fruit and vegetable servings each day.

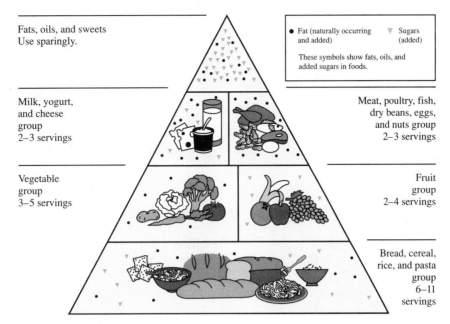

Figure 19.1
The Food Guide Pyramid
Source: Data from the U.S. Department of Agriculture

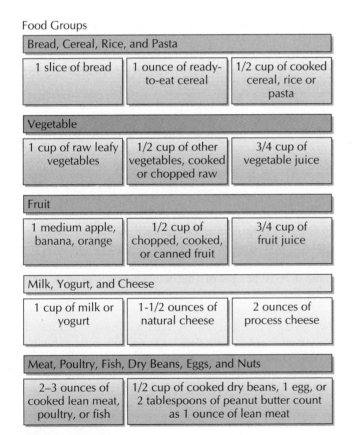

Food Groups

Bread, Cereal, Rice, and Pasta		
1 slice of bread	1 ounce of ready-to-eat cereal	1/2 cup of cooked cereal, rice or pasta

Vegetable		
1 cup of raw leafy vegetables	1/2 cup of other vegetables, cooked or chopped raw	3/4 cup of vegetable juice

Fruit		
1 medium apple, banana, orange	1/2 cup of chopped, cooked, or canned fruit	3/4 cup of fruit juice

Milk, Yogurt, and Cheese		
1 cup of milk or yogurt	1-1/2 ounces of natural cheese	2 ounces of process cheese

Meat, Poultry, Fish, Dry Beans, Eggs, and Nuts	
2–3 ounces of cooked lean meat, poultry, or fish	1/2 cup of cooked dry beans, 1 egg, or 2 tablespoons of peanut butter count as 1 ounce of lean meat

Figure 19.2
What counts as a serving?
Source: Data from the U.S. Department of Agriculture

New dietary guidelines are available to help you plan for sound nutrition.

Federal law requires the publication of national dietary guidelines every five years. The most recent guidelines are illustrated in figure 19.3. These guidelines are intended to supplement previous guidelines and the food guide pyramid in helping Americans select a nutritious diet. Among the major differences in these guidelines from previous ones are: an emphasis on selecting a variety of foods in the diet; an emphasis on foods from the base of the pyramid; an emphasis on physical activity as part of balancing calories; a recognition that vegetarian diets can be sound when properly selected; and a change in weight standards (age-neutral standards) so as not to allow weight gain as people grow older (see concept 13).

The Facts About Nutrition and Good Health

The number of calories needed per day depends upon the body's metabolic rate (MR), which, in turn, depends upon such factors as age, sex, size, muscle mass, glandular function, emotional state, climate, and exercise.

Your **basal metabolic rate (BMR)** is the basis for your caloric needs. The higher the BMR, the more calories you

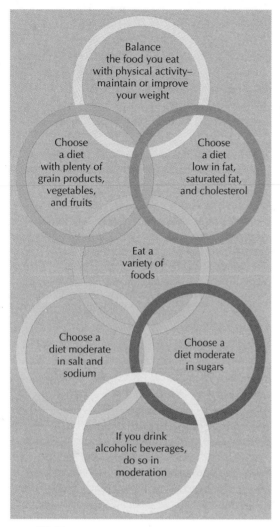

Figure 19.3
Dietary Guidelines for Americans

Source: Data from *Home and Garden Bulletin No. 232,* 4th edition, December 1995. U.S. Department of Agriculture, U.S. Department of Health and Human Services, Washington, DC.

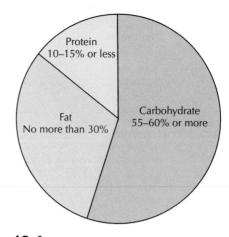

Figure 19.4
Recommended dietary intake

Excess fat in the diet, particularly saturated fat, is associated with an increased risk of disease and is inversely related to optimal health.

burn at rest. Your **metabolic rate (MR)** is a combination of your BMR and calories expended in normal daily activities. The MR is usually higher in males, young people, large people, lean and muscular people, and in nervous people; in cold and hot weather; and during exercise.

A moderately active college-age woman needs about 2000 calories per day, whereas a moderately active man of the same age needs about 2800 calories. A female athlete in training might burn 2600 to 4500 calories; a male athlete in training might expend 3500 to 6000. If your weight remains at the optimum, the caloric content of your diet is correct. If weight varies from optimal, the caloric content of the diet may need to be altered.

The three sources of calories in the diet are fat, protein, and carbohydrates. The typical adult consumes too much fat and too little carbohydrate, especially complex carbohydrates. A goal is to reduce the amount of dietary fat and increase the amount of complex carbohydrate in the diet of the average adult (see figure 19.4).

Humans need some fat in their diet because fats are carriers of vitamins A, D, E, and K. They are a source of essential linoleic acid, make food taste better, and provide a concentrated form of calories, which serve as an important source of energy during moderate to vigorous exercise. Fats have twice the calories per gram as carbohydrates.

There is evidence that excessive total fat in the diet is associated with atherosclerotic cardiovascular disease and breast, prostate, and colon cancer as well as obesity. **Saturated fats** come primarily from animal sources such as red meat, dairy products, and eggs, but they are also found in some vegetable sources such as coconut and palm oils. They are considered most likely to contribute to the health problems mentioned above. In addition, excess saturated fat in the diet contributes to increased cholesterol, and increased LDL (low-density lipoprotein) cholesterol in the blood. It is for this reason that it is recommended that no more than 10 percent of your total calories consist of saturated fats.

Unsaturated fats, also a part of a normal diet, are of two basic types: polyunsaturated and monounsaturated. Polyunsaturated fats are derived principally from vegetable sources such as safflower, cottonseed, soybean, sunflower, and corn oils (Omega-6 fats), and cold water fish sources such as salmon and mackerel (Omega-3 fats). Monounsaturated fats are derived primarily from vegetable sources including olive, peanut, and canola oil.

Unsaturated fats are generally considered to be less likely to contribute to cardiovascular disease, cancer, and obesity than saturated fats. When polyunsaturated fats (Omega-6) are substituted for saturated fats, there is a reduction in total cholesterol and LDL cholesterol in the blood, but there may be a decrease in HDL (high-density lipoprotein) cholesterol as well. However, when monounsaturated fats are substituted for saturated fats, total cholesterol and LDL cholesterol are thought to decrease without an accompanying decrease in the desirable HDL. There is very limited evidence that Omega-3 unsaturated fats may inhibit cancers, but Omega-6 fats may not have the same effect. Fish oils have been shown to reduce triglycerides, but there is no conclusive evidence that they are especially successful in reducing blood cholesterol.

Humans produce their own cholesterol even when dietary cholesterol is limited. Still, there is evidence that high dietary cholesterol can increase the risk of atherosclerosis and coronary heart disease. Principal sources of dietary cholesterol are organ meats, some shellfish, and egg yolks.

Recent evidence indicates that foods such as margarine and shortening containing hydrogenated fats or **trans fatty acids** can result in greater total blood cholesterol levels and higher LDL levels. This suggests that food containing trans fatty acids should be limited in the diet. Also, experts have recommended that future food labels stipulate the amounts of trans fatty acids included in processed foods.

It is interesting that the new dietary guidelines have changed the wording concerning fat in the diet (see figure 19.4). Formerly, it was recommended that "30 percent or less" of the diet should consist of fat. The new wording states that "no more than 30 percent" of the diet should be from fat. This change was made to downplay the notion that "the lower the fat the better". While the experts want to encourage lower fat in the diet, they also want to emphasize that some fat is necessary in a healthy diet.

The discussion of fat in the diet would not be complete without a discussion of "Olestra," a product sometimes referred to as "fake fat" which was recently approved by the FDA for use in foods. Olestra is a synthetic fat substitute which passes through the gastrointestinal system without being digested. Thus foods cooked with Olestra have fewer calories. For example, a chocolate chip cookie cooked in a normal way would have 138 calories while an Olestra cookie would have 63. One ounce of normal potato chips contains 160 calories while the same amount prepared using Olestra has 70. Many consumer groups opposed the approval of Olestra because it has possible side effects. A warning label must be included on this product noting these possible effects. The label reads: *"This product contains Olestra. Olestra may cause abdominal cramping and loose stools. Olestra inhibits the absorption of some vitamins and other nutrients. Vitamins A, D, E, and K have been added."* Consumer groups are concerned that consumers may not eat less fat even when they eat foods with Olestra, but rather will feel that they can eat more of foods not especially dense in nutrients. One thing is certain—Olestra does not add significantly to the nutritional value of food. Its only value would be to reduce calories and fat in the diet. If it does not do this, as many experts expect it won't, it will not enhance your diet and could have negative consequences (see warning label).

Dietary Recommendations: Fat

- Total fat in the diet should consist of no more than 30 percent of the total calories consumed.
- Saturated fat in the diet should be no more than 10 percent of total calories consumed.
- Polyunsaturated and monounsaturated fats should be substituted for saturated fat in the diet.
- Dietary cholesterol should be limited to 300 milligrams per day.

Dietary Implementation: Fat

- Substitute lean meat, fish, poultry, nonfat milk, and other low-fat dairy products for high-fat foods.
- Reduce intake of fried foods, especially those cooked in saturated fats (often true of fast-food restaurants), desserts with high levels of fat (many cookies and cakes), and dressings with high-fat levels.
- Limit dietary intake of foods high in cholesterol such as egg yolks, organ meats, and shellfish.
- Use monounsaturated or polyunsaturated fats for cooking.
- Limit the amount of trans fatty acids in the diet and in cooking.
- Though two or three servings of fish per week may be prudent because of its content of Omega-3 polyunsaturated oils, there is not sufficient evidence to endorse a fish-oil dietary supplement.
- Be careful of the total elimination of a single food source from the diet. For example, the elimination of meat and dairy products could result in iron or calcium deficiencies, especially among women and children.

> For optimal health, carbohydrates, especially complex carbohydrates, should be the principal source of calories in the diet.

Complex carbohydrates are known as starches and include fruits, vegetables, whole-grain breads, and cereals. These foods are nutritionally dense and also contain **cellulose** (popularly known as **fiber**). Cellulose does not provide nutrition and is not digested, but is considered essential for the bulk it provides for efficient digestion.

Research evidence shows that diets high in complex carbohydrates such as whole-grain cereals, legumes, vegetables, and fruits are associated with a low incidence of lung, colon, esophagus, and stomach cancer as well as coronary heart disease. Some of this benefit may be due to the fact that complex carbohydrate diets are likely to be low in saturated fat. Water-soluble fiber, such as pectin and oat bran, has recently been shown to produce small reductions in total blood cholesterol independent of the effects of reduced dietary fat. Long-term studies indicate that high-fiber diets may also be associated with a lower risk of diabetes mellitus, diverticulosis, hypertension, and gallstone formation. It is not known whether these health benefits are directly attributable to high dietary fiber or other effects associated with the ingestion of vegetables, fruits, and cereals in the diet. Complex carbohydrates may also be beneficial to health because they provide rich sources of vitamins and minerals. The possible benefits of consuming a diet high in complex carbohydrates and certain vitamins are discussed in the section on vitamins. For the reasons mentioned above, the new dietary guidelines for Americans place a special emphasis on complex carbohydrates (see figure 19.3).

Simple carbohydrates are sugars such as sucrose, lactose, maltose, glucose, and fructose. They are nutritionally low in density and are commonly found in foods considered to possess "empty calories" such as candy and soft drinks. The national dietary guidelines note that "the body cannot tell the difference between naturally occurring and added sugars because they are identical chemically." This statement was added to counter the public perception that some types of sugars are better than others. Food high in simple carbohydrates do not, however, have the same benefits to health as do the complex carbohydrates. Foods high in simple carbohydrates are often high in fat as well. Simple carbohydrates, especially sucrose, a sugar often found in candy and soft drinks, have also been shown to increase the incidence of dental caries. Research has not shown that sugar consumption, among those who have an adequate diet, is a risk factor for diseases such as cancer and heart disease. It should be noted that athletes and other active people who need supplemental calorie intake to maintain body weight may need to consume more carbohydrates, including simple carbohydrates, than those who are sedentary. Increasing carbohydrates in the diet is more desirable than supplementing proteins or consuming higher amounts of fat.

Dietary Recommendations: Carbohydrates

- Total carbohydrate in the diet should account for 55 percent or more of total calories consumed.
- Simple carbohydrates should be limited to 15 percent or less of total calories consumed, except for very active people.
- High-fiber foods should be included in the daily diet.

Dietary Implementation: Carbohydrates

- Consume at least five servings of vegetables and/or fruits each day. Servings of green and yellow vegetables as well as citrus fruits are recommended. A serving of vegetables equals approximately one-half cup. A serving of fruit equals one medium-size piece.
- Consume at least six servings of complex carbohydrates such as breads, cereals, and/or legumes. A serving of legumes or cereal equals approximately one-half cup. A serving of bread is one slice, or one roll or muffin.

- Limit intake of desserts, baked goods, and other foods high in simple sugars or empty calories.
- Dietary fiber supplements other than in the form of food (such as oat bran) are not recommended unless prescribed for medical reasons.

Protein is the basic building block for the body, but dietary protein constitutes a relatively small amount of daily calorie intake.

It is said that proteins are the building blocks of your body because all body cells are made of protein. Proteins are formed from twenty-two different **amino acids.** More than 100 proteins are made up of these amino acids. Fourteen of these amino acids are made in your own body, but eight **essential amino acids** are not. You must consume foods that contain these eight essential amino acids if your body is to function properly. Certain foods, called "complete proteins," contain all eight essential amino acids. Examples of complete proteins are meat, dairy products, and fish. Incomplete proteins contain some, but not all, of the essential amino acids. Examples of incomplete proteins are beans, nuts, and rice.

Experts agree that there are no known benefits and some possible risks to consuming diets exceptionally high in animal protein. Certain cancers and coronary heart disease risk have been associated with high dietary intake of animal protein. Researchers are not certain whether the increased risk of contracting these diseases due to a high intake of animal protein is because of the protein itself or the fact that diets high in animal protein are also high in fat. There is evidence that excessive protein intake can lead to urinary calcium loss, which can be dangerous, especially for women.

Some scientists are concerned that restriction of animal protein might result in lower than necessary dietary intake of essential nutrients such as iron, especially for women and children. If the recommendations suggested in this section are followed, this should not be a problem. It is not our intent to suggest that animal protein should not be part of the normal diet, but rather consumption of animal protein be restricted somewhat, especially when the fat content is high. In fact, the most recent dietary guidelines for Americans for the first time include a statement indicating that "vegetarian diets are consistent with the Dietary Guidelines for Americans and can meet Recommended Dietary Allowances for nutrients. You can get enough protein as long as the variety and amounts of foods consumed are adequate." It is noted that **vegans** must supplement the diet with vitamin B_{12} because the only source is from animal foods. The Guidelines also emphasize the need for vegans to take care that, especially for children, adequate vitamin D and calcium are contained in the diet because most people get these nutrients from milk products.

People who eat a variety of foods including meat, dairy products, eggs, and plants rich in protein virtually always eat more protein than the body needs. Eating a variety of foods assures that all essential amino acids are consumed. Because of problems associated with excessive protein intake and health problems encountered by those who have used protein supplements; the latter are not recommended. In fact, many of the more serious health problems resulting from the consumption of dietary supplements are associated with excessive protein intake.

Dietary Recommendations: Protein

- Protein in the diet should account for 15 percent or less of the total calories consumed.
- Protein in the diet should exceed the RDA of .8 grams per kilogram (2.2 pounds) of a person's desirable weight. This is about 36 grams for a 100-pound person.
- Protein in the diet should *not* exceed twice the RDA (1.6 grams per kilogram of a person's desirable weight).
- Vegetarians or those who severely limit the intake of animal products must be especially careful to eat combinations of foods that assure adequate intake of essential amino acids and vegans should supplement their diets with vitamin B$_{12}$.

Dietary Implementation: Protein

- Consume at least two servings of lean meat, fish, poultry, and dairy products (especially those low in fat content) or adequate combinations of foods such as beans, nuts, and rice in the diet.
- Dietary supplements of protein such as tablets and powders are *not* recommended.

Adequate vitamin intake is necessary to good health and wellness, but excessive vitamin intake is *not* necessary and can be harmful.

Consuming foods containing the minimum RDA of each of the vitamins is essential to the prevention of disease and maintenance of good health. Consuming foods high in carotinoid and retinoid is recommended because these foods are associated with the reduced risk of some forms of cancer. Carotinoid- and retinoid-rich foods such as green and yellow vegetables, carrots, and sweet potatoes contain high amounts of vitamin A. Diets high in vitamin C (citrus fruits and vegetables) and vitamin E (green leafy vegetables) are also associated with reduced risk of cancer. One recent study indicated that diets high in vitamin E are associated with reduced risk of heart disease. It has been hypothesized that vitamins C, E, and carotinoid-rich foods act as **antioxidants** which help prevent cancer and other forms of disease. Most experts point out that selecting more servings from the second level of the food pyramid is wise strategy, but they recommend caution concerning the use of vitamin supplements.

Nevertheless, a number of respected health and wellness publications and popular books have advocated antioxidant supplements including beta carotine (a plant product that is converted to vitamin A in the body) and vitamins

C and E. Those making the recommendation to take relatively high amounts of these vitamins do so based on the theory that the antioxidant vitamins protect the body from cell damaging "free radicals" resulting from environmental pollution. They also assumed that supplements of these vitamins had the same health effect as good food high in vitamin content. Several very recent large scale studies have shown either no benefit from beta carotene supplements or have shown that the supplements may have negative effects. One study was discontinued early because of higher heart disease and lung cancer among the supplement group. While some advocates of antioxidants still recommend supplements of vitamins C and E, most have backed off recommendations for beta carotine based on the results of the studies cited above.

Just as some have advocated antioxidant supplements, others have not. For example, the National Council Against Health Fraud (1994) says "the fact is that the value of antioxidants has been more an illusion created by the vitamin hucksters than scientific reality." Also, the committee that developed the dietary guidelines for Americans chose to emphasize good food rather than food supplements. Most experts agree. Some foods that are especially rich in vitamins and minerals are considered nutrition "allstars" and make good dietary choices (see table 19.1).

While one type of supplement for all people is not deemed wise, there is little doubt that certain segments of the population do not eat a balanced diet and as a matter of national policy many foods have been fortified. National policy dictates that milk be fortified with vitamin D, low-fat milk with vitamins A and D, and margarine with vitamin A. These foods were selected because they are common food sources for growing children. Recently the FDA announced that breads, flours, rice, grits and other grain products would be fortified with Folic acid because of the evidence that such fortification would help reduce birth defects. Less than half of young women get sufficient Folic acid (a B vitamin) and such deficiencies are related to birth defects. Also, there is some evidence that this vitamin can help reduce risk of heart disease. The public policy of food fortification continues to emphasize consuming a variety of healthy foods (in this case fortified foods) rather than the use of supplements.

Sometimes supplements are needed to meet specific nutrient requirements for specific groups. For example, older people and others may need a vitamin D supplement if they get little exposure to sunlight, and iron supplements are often recommended for pregnant women. Daily vitamin supplements at or below the RDA are considered safe, but are rarely needed by people who eat a variety of foods as recommended by the food guide pyramid. However, excess doses of vitamins have been shown to cause health problems. For example, excessively high amounts of vitamin C are dangerous for 10 percent of the population who inherit a special gene related to health problems. Excessively high amounts of vitamin D are toxic and mothers who take too much vitamin A risk birth defects to unborn children.

Table 19.1
The Top Ten Antioxidant All-Stars

	C (mg)	Beta caro-tene (mg)	E (mg)	Folacin (mg)
Broccoli (½ cup cooked)	49	0.7	0.9	53
Cantaloupe (1 cup cubed)	68	3.1	0.3	27
Carrot (1 medium)	7	12.2	0.3	10
Kale (½ cup cooked)	27	2.9	3.7	9
Mango (1 medium)	57	4.8	2.3	31
Pumpkin (½ cup canned)	5	10.5	1.1	15
Red bell pepper (½ cup raw)	95	1.7	0.3	8
Spinach (½ cup cooked)	9	4.4	2.0	131
Strawberries (1 cup)	86	—	0.3	26
Sweet potato (1 medium, cooked)	28	14.9	5.5	26
Adult RDA or suggested intake	60	5–6	8–10	180–200

Runners-up: Brussels sprouts, all citrus fruits, tomatoes, potatoes, other berries, other leafy greens (dandelion, turnip, and mustard greens, swiss chard, arugula), cauliflower, green pepper, asparagus, peas, beets, and winter squash.

Source: Reprinted with permission from the *University of California at Berkeley Wellness Letter,* © Health Letter Associates, 1994.

Dietary Recommendation: Vitamins

- Vitamins in the amounts equal to the RDAs should be included in the diet each day.

Dietary Implementation: Vitamins

- A diet containing the food servings recommended for carbohydrates, proteins, and fats will more than meet the RDA standards.
- Extra servings of green and yellow vegetables, citrus and other fruits, and other nonanimal food sources high in fiber, vitamins, and minerals are wise (especially foods from the nutrition all-stars).
- Those who eat a sound diet as described in this concept do not need a vitamin supplement. Those who insist on taking a daily vitamin supplement are advised not to take daily amounts larger than the RDA and only after following the guidelines for dietary supplements suggested later in this concept.
- Those with special needs should seek medical advice before selecting supplements and should inform medical personnel as to amounts and content of all supplements (vitamin or other).

Adequate mineral intake is necessary for good health and wellness, but excessive mineral intake is *not* necessary and can be harmful.

Like vitamins, minerals have no calories and provide no energy for the body. They are important in regulating various bodily functions. Two particularly important minerals are calcium and iron. Calcium is important to bone, muscle, nerve, blood development and function, and has been associated with reduced risk of heart disease. Iron is necessary for the blood to carry adequate oxygen. Other important minerals are phosphorus, which builds teeth and bones; sodium, which regulates water in the body; zinc, which aids in the healing process; and potassium, which is necessary for proper muscle function.

RDAs for minerals are established to determine the amounts of each necessary for healthy day-to-day functioning. A sound diet provides all of the RDA for minerals. Evidence indicating that some segments of the population may be mineral deficient have led to the establishment of health goals identifying a need to increase mineral intake.

A recent National Institutes of Health consensus statement indicates that a large percentage of Americans fail to get enough calcium in their diet and emphasizes the need for increased calcium—particularly for women who are pregnant, postmenopausal women, and people over 65 who need 1500 mg/day, which is higher than previous RDA amounts. The NIH also indicated that a total intake of 2000 mg/day of calcium is safe and that adequate vitamin D in the diet is necessary for optimal calcium absorption to take place. Though getting these amounts in a calcium-rich diet is best, calcium supplementation for those not eating properly seems wise. Check with your physician or a dietitian before you consider a supplement because individual needs vary. Several of the suggested readings at the end of this concept provide information on the topic.

Another concern is iron deficiency among very young children and women of childbearing age. These groups need to ensure adequate iron in the diet. Also, a decrease in salt and sodium intake is a health goal established for people of all ages because of the association of dietary salt and sodium with elevated blood pressure. Eating the appropriate number of servings from the food pyramid provides all the minerals necessary for meeting the RDA for minerals. Nutrition goals for the nation emphasize the importance of adequate servings of foods rich in calcium, such as green leafy vegetables and milk products; adequate servings of foods rich in iron, such as beans, peas, spinach, or meat; and reduced salt in the diet.

Dietary Recommendations: Minerals

- Minerals in amounts equal to the RDAs should be taken in the diet each day.
- In general, a dietary supplement of calcium is not recommended for the general population; however, supplements may be appropriate for adults who do not eat well (up to 1000 mg/day). For postmenopausal women, a calcium supplement is recommended (up to 1500 mg/day for those who do not eat well). A supplement may also be appropriate for those who restrict calories. Consult with a registered dietitian or a physician regarding amounts and types of supplements.
- Salt should be limited in the diet to no more than 4–6 grams per day, and even less would be desirable (3 grams). Three grams equals one teaspoon of table salt.

Dietary Implementation: Minerals

- A diet containing the food servings recommended for carbohydrates, proteins, and fats will more than meet the RDA standards.
- Extra servings of green and yellow vegetables, citrus and other fruits, and other non-animal sources of foods high in fiber, vitamins, and minerals are recommended as a substitute for high-fat foods.
- In general, people who eat a sound diet as described in this concept do *not* need a mineral supplement. Those who insist on taking a daily mineral supplement are advised not to take daily amounts larger than the RDA (except as specified for calcium, above) and only after following the guidelines for dietary supplements suggested later in this concept.

Water is a critical component in the healthy diet.

Though water is not in the food pyramid because it contains no calories, provides no energy, and provides no key nutrients, it is very important to health and survival. Water is a major component of most of the foods you eat, and more than half of all body tissues are comprised of it. Regular water intake maintains water balance and is critical to many important bodily functions.

Dietary Recommendations and Implementation: Water

- In addition to foods containing water, the average adult needs about two quarts of water every day. Water intake must be increased even more for active people and those in hot environments.

Beverages other than water are a part of many diets. Some beverages can have an adverse effect on good health.

Coffee, tea, soft drinks, and alcoholic beverages are often substituted for water in the diet. Too much caffeine consumption has been shown to cause symptoms such as irregular heartbeat in some people. Tea has not been shown to have similar effects, though this may be because tea drinkers typically consume less volume than coffee drinkers and tea has less caffeine per cup than coffee. Both beverages contain caffeine, as do many soft drinks, though drip coffee typically contains two to three times the caffeine of a typical cola drink.

Excessive consumption of alcoholic beverages can have negative health implications because the alcohol often replaces nutrients. Excessive alcohol consumption is associated with the increased risk of heart disease, high blood pressure, stroke, and osteoporosis. Long-term, excessive alcoholic beverage consumption leads to cirrhosis of the liver, and the increased risk of hepatitis and cancer. Alcohol consumption during pregnancy can result in low birth weight, fetal alcoholism, and other damage to the fetus. The National Dietary Guidelines indicate that alcohol used in moderation can "enhance the enjoyment of meals" and is associated with a lower risk of coronary heart disease for some individuals.

Dietary Recommendations and Implementation: Beverages

- Servings of coffee, tea, and soft drinks should not be substituted for water and/or other beverages or foods such as low-fat milk, fruit juices, or foods rich in calcium, which provide sources of key nutrients.
- Daily servings of beverages containing caffeine should be limited to no more than three.
- If you are an adult and you choose to drink alcohol, do so in moderation. The latest dietary guidelines for Americans indicate that moderation includes no more than one drink per day for women and no more than two drinks per day for men (one drink equals 12 ounces of regular beer, 5 ounces of wine—small glass, or one average-size cocktail—1.5 ounces of 80 proof alcohol).

Facts About Sound Eating Practices

Healthy snacks can be an important part of good nutrition.

Snacking is not necessarily bad. For those interested in losing or maintaining their current weight, small snacks of appropriate foods can help fool the appetite. For those interested in gaining weight, snacks can provide additional calories. The key is proper selection of the foods for snacking. For those trying to maintain or lose weight, the calories consumed in snacks will probably necessitate limiting the calories consumed at meals.

As with your total diet, the best snacks are those that are nutritionally dense. Too often, snacks are high in calories, fats, simple sugar, and salt. Check the content of snacks. Even foods sold as "healthy snacks," such as granola bars, are often high in fat and simple sugar. Some common snacks such as chips, pretzels, and even popcorn are high in salt and may be cooked in fat.

Some suggestions for healthy snacks include ice milk instead of ice cream, fresh fruits, vegetable sticks, popcorn not cooked in fat and with little or no salt, crackers, and nuts with little or no salt.

Consistency (with variety) is a good general rule of nutrition.

Eating regular meals every day, including a good breakfast, is wise. Many studies have shown breakfast to be an important meal. One-fourth of the day's calories should be consumed at breakfast. Skipping breakfast impairs performance because blood sugar levels drop in the long period between dinner the night before and lunch the following day. Eating every four to six hours is wise.

Moderation is a good general rule of nutrition.

Just as too little food can cause problems, excessive intake of various nutrients can cause problems. More is not always better. Moderation (neither too much nor too little) in choices of foods is advised.

It is not necessary to permanently eliminate foods that you really enjoy, but some of your favorite foods may not be among the best of choices. Enjoying special foods on occasion is part of moderation. The key is to limit choices that are not consistent with the recommendations made in this concept.

Careful selection of food choices is important for those who rely on fast foods as a significant part of their diet.

More and more Americans rely on fast foods as part of their normal diet. Unfortunately, many fast foods are poor nutritional choices. Many hamburgers are high in fat. French fries are high in fat because they are usually cooked in saturated fat. Even choices deemed to be more nutritious, such as chicken or fish sandwiches, are often high in fat and calories because they are cooked in fat and covered with special high-fat/high-calorie sauces.

Dietary Recommendations: Fast Foods

- Become informed about the content of fast foods before you make your selection.

The Facts About Nutrition and Physical Performance

In general, the nutrition rules described in the previous pages apply to all people, whether active or sedentary, but there are some additional nutrition facts that are important for exercisers and athletes. This information is outlined in table 19.2.

Carbohydrate loading and carbohydrate replacement during exercise can enhance sustained aerobic performances exceeding one hour in length.

Athletes and vigorously active people must maintain a high level of readily available fuel, especially in the muscles. Adequate complex carbohydrate consumption is the best way to assure this.

Prior to an activity that will require extended duration of physical performance (more than one hour in length, such as a marathon), **carbohydrate loading** can be useful. Carbohydrate loading is accomplished by resting one or two days before the event and eating a higher than normal amount of complex carbohydrates. This procedure helps prevent the depletion of muscle **glycogen,** which is necessary for sustained performance. However, this procedure could cause problems for those with diabetes, hypertriglycemia, and kidney disorders.

Ingesting carbohydrate solutions during long, sustained exercise can also aid in performance by preventing or forestalling muscle glycogen depletion. Taking in fluids with less than 5 percent sugar helps prevent dehydration and replenishes energy stores. These solutions should be taken regularly in long, sustained performances. After long, sustained performances, the consumption of carbohydrates within fifteen to thirty minutes can aid in rapid replenishment of muscle glycogen, which may be important to future performances. Carbohydrate drinks are *not* helpful for short (less than an hour) endurance activity.

The timing may be more important than the makeup of the pre-event meal.

It is probably best to eat about three hours before competition or heavy exercise to allow time for digestion. Generally, the athlete can make his or her food selection on the

Table 19.2
Dietary Recommendations for Athletes and Active People

Fat	Active people, like everyone else, should restrict fat, especially saturated fat.
Protein	The American Dietetics Association (ADA) recommends 1.0 grams per kg of body weight for active people such as athletes. This is higher than the .8 per kg recommended for normal adults. A normal healthy diet easily meets this need so protein above 15 percent of the diet is not recommended, nor are protein supplements (including amino acids).
Carbohydrates	Because active people often expend calories in amounts considerably above normal, extra calories are necessary in the diet. Carbohydrates are the best source. To avoid excess fat and protein intake, carbohydrates (especially complex carbohydrates) may constitute as much as 70 percent of total calorie intake.
Vitamins and Minerals	Those in activities for which caloric restriction may be encouraged, such as wrestling, must be especially careful in the food choices they make. Also, female athletes should consider a calcium supplement after consultation with an expert. This is especially true for those who are amenorrheic and/or are involved in extensive training.

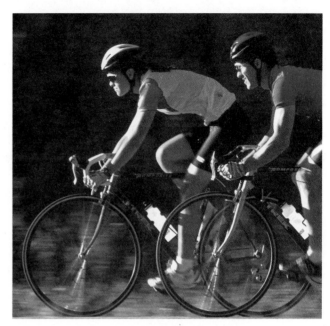

Good nutrition is essential for active people.

basis of past experience. Tension, anxiety, and excitement are more likely to cause gastric distress than is food selection. It is generally accepted that fat intake should be minimal because it digests more slowly; "gas formers" should probably be avoided: and proteins and high-cellulose foods should be kept to a moderate amount prior to prolonged events to avoid urinary and bowel excretion. Two or three cups of liquid should be taken to ensure adequate hydration.

Ingestion of simple carbohydrates (sugar, candy) within an hour or two prior to an event is *not* recommended because it may cause an insulin response that results in weakness and fatigue. Sometimes they cause stomach distress, cramps, or nausea.

It should be noted that the excitement associated with competition is probably the main reason for having a special diet before participation. Because many people who exercise regularly usually are not competing, there is little reason to alter normal diet before regular exercise. Likewise, there is no need to delay exercise for long periods after the meal if exercise is moderate and noncompetitive.

The Facts: Nutrition Quackery

The Food and Drug Administration has labeled the "health food" racket as the most widespread quackery in the United States.

Whether athletic or sedentary, the individual on a well-balanced diet does *not* benefit from special organic foods, phosphate, alkaline salts, choline, lecithin, wheat germ, honey, gelatin, aspartates, brewer's yeast, or royal jelly unless prescribed for medical purposes by a physician. Because these products do not produce the special benefits claimed for them, their use and/or sale can be considered nutritional quackery.

Claims for foods in advertisements may *not* provide accurate information about the nutritional value of the foods.

Until recently, food labels have failed to provide useful information concerning the nutritional values of foods. Recently Congress enacted laws to make food labels more uniform and to protect consumers. Now products sold in stores must meet specified standards to be able to use words such as "fat free" on the label. For example, a food

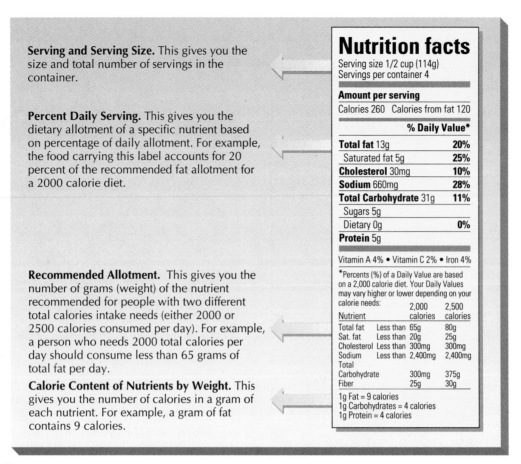

Serving and Serving Size. This gives you the size and total number of servings in the container.

Percent Daily Serving. This gives you the dietary allotment of a specific nutrient based on percentage of daily allotment. For example, the food carrying this label accounts for 20 percent of the recommended fat allotment for a 2000 calorie diet.

Recommended Allotment. This gives you the number of grams (weight) of the nutrient recommended for people with two different total calories intake needs (either 2000 or 2500 calories consumed per day). For example, a person who needs 2000 total calories per day should consume less than 65 grams of total fat per day.

Calorie Content of Nutrients by Weight. This gives you the number of calories in a gram of each nutrient. For example, a gram of fat contains 9 calories.

Nutrition facts

Serving size 1/2 cup (114g)
Servings per container 4

Amount per serving

Calories 260   Calories from fat 120

	% Daily Value*
Total fat 13g	20%
Saturated fat 5g	25%
Cholesterol 30mg	10%
Sodium 660mg	28%
Total Carbohydrate 31g	11%
Sugars 5g	
Dietary 0g	0%
Protein 5g	

Vitamin A 4% • Vitamin C 2% • Iron 4%

*Percents (%) of a Daily Value are based on a 2,000 calorie diet. Your Daily Values may vary higher or lower depending on your calorie needs:

Nutrient		2,000 calories	2,500 calories
Total fat	Less than	65g	80g
Sat. fat	Less than	20g	25g
Cholesterol	Less than	300mg	300mg
Sodium	Less than	2,400mg	2,400mg
Total Carbohydrate		300mg	375g
Fiber		25g	30g

1g Fat = 9 calories
1g Carbohydrates = 4 calories
1g Protein = 4 calories

Figure 19.5
Using food labels
Source: Data from the U.S. Food and Drug Administration.

must have less than one-half of a gram of fat per serving (50 grams) to be labeled "fat free," and it must have less than 3 grams per serving to be labeled "low fat." To be labeled "low in saturated fat," a food must have less than 15 percent of its calories from saturated fat.

The labels required on foods sold in stores (see figure 19.5) provide information based on diets of 2000 calories per day. As noted earlier in this concept, the number of calories you consume depends on your age, body size, gender, metabolic rate, and activity level. The 2000-calorie value is better suited for children and women than for men, who typically consume more calories in a day. Values must be adjusted for those whose daily calorie intake is above 2000 calories.

In spite of recent improvements in food labeling, consumers must continue to be wary of deceptive advertising. While the use of words such as "light" or "low fat" has been regulated to some extent, consumers should be sure that products live up to claims made for them.

Even with recent efforts to regulate dietary supplements, many fall outside the current regulations and use false or deceptive advertising. It is wise to read food labels, to ask for information about food content in restaurants, and to be wary of claims about supplements advertised for health or fitness improvement.

For most people, dietary supplements, when taken in excess of amounts known to be beneficial to good health, can be considered as nutritional quackery.

The most common forms of nutritional quackery involve nutritional supplements containing protein, vitamins, and minerals. Before taking any of these supplements, consider the following guidelines:

• *Analyze the content of your diet before making decisions about its quality.* If you assume your current diet is not adequate, on what do you base the assumption? It is recommended that you do a dietary analysis to determine the quality of your diet. This is best done by logging your food intake for several days and determining the content of the foods eaten. Expert assistance may be useful in conducting a dietary analysis.

• *Have a medical exam to see if you have any symptoms of nutritional deficiencies.*

• *Consult an expert (physician or dietitian) about your nutritional needs.* Most experts will recommend changes in your diet if they decide that you are not getting proper nutrition. Only in special cases will

Table 19.3
Some Commonly Misrepresented Dietary Supplements Alleged to Enhance Performance

Product	Claim	The Facts
Plant steroids	• Alleged to promote muscle development similar to animal steroids.	• Plant steroids do not promote muscle mass gains in humans.
Trace elements (ex: chromium picolinate)	• Alleged to promote muscle development.	• No evidence of effectiveness. It could lead to anemia if taken in excess. One recent study indicates possible link to cancer and chromosome damage.
Amino acids (ex: arginine, lysine)	• Alleged to promote increases in human growth hormone that lead to increased muscle mass.	• Some evidence that increased HGH results from intake of amino acids, but little evidence of resulting muscle mass increases. There is risk in taking the high doses recommended by sellers. Banned in Canada.
Protein supplements	• Alleged muscle mass gains.	• No evidence of effectiveness, some are not digestible. Not superior to dietary protein as some claim, and far more costly. Overuse can lead to excess loss of body water, diarrhea, abdominal cramps, and altered kidney function.
Caffeine	• Alleged to enhance endurance performance.	• Inconsistent results. Banned by Olympic rules. Some negative health consequences.
Vitamin supplements (ex: B complex, B_{15})	• Alleged stress reduction and performance enhancement.	• No evidence of benefits to those who are not vitamin deficient. B_{15} (pangamic acid) is not a vitamin and can be harmful. No evidence of stress-reducing effects.
Minerals (ex: iron)	• Alleged that athletes and active people need more than other people.	• Some evidence that active people have increased need, but the consensus is that a sound diet provides for those needs.
Hormones (ex. melatonin)	• Claims to enhance sex life, combat aging, and reduce disease risk.	• Effects not known, especially long term. All sales banned in some European countries: a prescription is required in Canada. Hormones are powerful substances that can produce unexpected results. Actual content of product is not regulated so there is no certainty of content. Users are considered to be "human guinea pigs" by some experts.

Note: FDA standards have not been set for many advertised products. For this reason the consumer cannot be assured of the exact content of products, and product safety cannot be assured. This is illustrated by the recall of products containing the amino acid L-tryptophan after the deaths of 32 people were linked to its use.

supplements be recommended. Be aware that the term "nutritionist" is one that virtually anyone can use, and the qualifications of such a person should be checked thoroughly before considering him or her an expert. Registered dietitians with a degree (RD) in nutrition are considered qualified and recognized as experts.

• *Beware of people selling products who imply that the Food and Drug Administration (FDA) is conspiring to keep you from getting products.* As one FDA official indicates, "the goal is simple: We want people to have access to products that are safe, and we want to assure consumers that claims made about the health and nutritional benefits are truthful (Farley, 1995, p. 3)." Those who discredit the FDA are often trying to sell something that does not work and may be guilty of fraud and/or quackery. Between 1990 and 1993 FDA took action against 188 products considered to be dietary supplements on the grounds that they made unsubstantiated claims about serious medical conditions.

> People who are interested in enhancing physical performance are especially subject to nutrition quackery.

A food or nutrition product thought to enhance performance is considered to be an **ergogenic aid.** Many of the products that are alleged to be ergogenic aids can be classified as quack products because they do not enhance performance as promised and are often exceptionally expensive. In some cases so-called "performance-enhancing supplements" are dangerous to health and wellness. Examples of products that are misrepresented in terms of potential performance-enhancing benefits are dietary supplements such as vitamins, minerals, proteins and amino acids, and plant steroids. Among the most often misrepresented products are protein and amino acid supplements, sometimes referred to as "steroid alternatives." Table 19.3 lists some of these.

> Claims for products alleged to promote weight loss are especially likely to be fraudulent.

Recently the Federal Trade Commission (FTC) studied weight-loss programs, including some of the most famous dietary supplement programs. The FTC forced many of the companies to abandon false claims they used in their advertising. Before making a choice consumers are urged to ask questions about the health risks of a program; the data supporting program effectiveness; costs of the program; long-term program effectiveness; and expert supervision of the program.

> Recent legislation should help regulate the content and claims of food supplements but will not totally protect the consumer.

The Dietary Supplements Health and Education Act that was passed in 1994 is considered by many experts to be a compromise between some health food manufacturers who want no regulation of dietary supplements (such as vitamins, minerals, proteins, and herbs) and those who want strict control of these substances. This Act stipulates that labeling must be truthful and non-misleading. Claims concerning disease prevention, treatment, or diagnosis must be substantiated or they can not appear on the product. Labeling of supplements similar to food labels will be implemented to help the consumer know the exact content of products. Consumers are cautioned that "third party literature" can still be used in health stores. This is literature that can be distributed separate from the product, thus allowing stores to make claims for products that may not be substantiated. Many experts fear that this will result in false promises and quackery. Consumers should also know that the new legislation does not allow the FDA to regulate dietary supplements as food additives.

Suggested Readings

"The Antioxidant Scare," *National Council Against Health Fraud Newsletter* 17(May–June 1994):1.

"Beta Carotine Pills: Should You Take Them?" *University of California at Berkeley Wellness Letter.* 12(April 1996):1.

"Calcium: Vital for Women and Men." *Consumer Reports on Health* 6(1994):13.

Clark, N. "Water: The Ultimate Nutrient." *Physician and Sportsmedicine* 23(1995):21.

Farley, D. "Making Sure Hype Doesn't Overwhelm Science." *FDA Consumer,* 56(1996), 1.

Lemonick, M. D. "Is America Ready for Fat-Free Fat?" *Time.*147, (1996): 53.

National Institute of Health. "Optimal Calcium Intake." *Consensus Development Conference Statement, June 1994.* Available from NIH Office of Medical Applications Research.

Public Health Service. *The Surgeon General's Report on Nutrition and Health.* Washington, DC: Department of Health and Human Services, 1988, Pub. No. 88–50210.

"The Supplement Story: Can Vitamins Help?" *Consumer Reports.* 57(1992):12.

U.S. Department of Agriculture and U.S. Department of Health and Human Services. *Nutrition and Your Health: Dietary Guidelines for Americans (4th ed.).* Washington, DC: U.S. Department of Agriculture and U.S. Department of Health and Human Services, 1995.

U.S. Department of Agriculture and U.S. Department of Health and Human Services. *Report of the Dietary Guidelines Advisory Committee.* Washington, DC: U.S. Department of Agriculture and U.S. Department of Health and Human Services, 1995.

LAB RESOURCE MATERIALS

Chart 19.1 Dietary Habits Questionnaire

Yes	No	
☐	☐	1. Do you eat regular meals?
☐	☐	2. Do you eat a good breakfast daily?
☐	☐	3. Do yo eat lunch regularly?
☐	☐	4. Does your diet contain about 55%–60% carbohydrates with a high concentration of fiber?
☐	☐	5. Are less than one-fourth of the carbohydrates you eat simple carbohydrates?
☐	☐	6. Does your diet contain 10%–15% protein?
☐	☐	7. Does you diet contain less than 30% fat?
☐	☐	8. Do you limit the amount of saturated fat in your diet?
☐	☐	9. Do you limit salt intake to acceptable amounts?
☐	☐	10. Do you get adequate amounts of vitamins in your diet without a supplement?
☐	☐	11. Do you eat regularly from all food groups?
☐	☐	12. Do you drink adequate amounts of water?
☐	☐	13. Do you get adequate minerals in your diet without a supplement?
☐	☐	14. Do you limit your caffeine and alcohol consumption to acceptable levels?
☐	☐	15. Is your average calorie consumption for the two-day period reasonable for your body size and for the amount of calories you normally expend?

_____ Total number of "Yes" answers

Chart 19.2 Dietary Habits *Rating Scale*

Score	Rating
14–15	Very Good
12–13	Good
10–11	Marginal
9 or less	Poor

CONCEPT 20

Stress Management and Relaxation

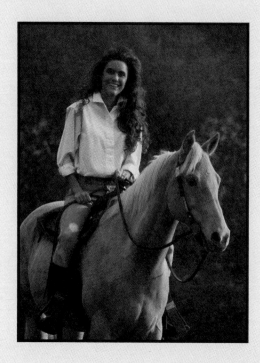

Concept 20

Mental and physical health are affected by an individual's ability to avoid or adapt to stress.

Introduction

Stress can trigger an emotional response that, in turn, evokes the autonomic nervous system to a "fight or flight" response. This adaptive and protective mechanism stimulates the ductless glands to hypo- or hyperactivity in preparation for what is perceived as a threat or assault on the whole organism. In some instances, this alarm reaction of the body may be essential to survival, but when evoked inappropriately or excessively, it may be more harmful than the effects of the original stressor. For example, a fight-or-flight response may cause a coronary spasm that could lead to a heart attack.

Health Goals for the Year 2000

- Fewer people reporting stress-related problems. (↑)
- Help those with stress to reduce or control it. (<>)

Note: (↑) indicates progress toward goal, (↓) indicates regression from goal, and (<>) indicates either no change or lack of new data since 1990.

Terms

- **Adaptation**   The body's efforts to restore normalcy.
- **Anxiety**   A state of apprehension with a compulsion to do something; excessive anxiety is a tension disorder with physiological characteristics.
- **Chronic Fatigue**   Constant state of entire body fatigue.
- **Distress**   Negative stress, or stress that contributes to health problems.
- **Eustress**   Positive stress, or stress that is mentally or physically stimulating.
- **Neuromuscular Hypertension**   Unnecessary or exaggerated muscle contractions; excess tension beyond that needed to perform a given task; also called hypertonus.
- **Physiological Fatigue**   A deterioration in the capacity of the neuromuscular system as the result of physical overwork and strain; also referred to as "true" fatigue.
- **Psychological Fatigue**   A feeling of fatigue usually caused by such things as lack of exercise, boredom, or mental stress that results in a lack of energy and depression; also referred to as "subjective" or "false" fatigue.
- **Relaxation**   The release or reduction of tension in the neuromuscular system.
- **Stress**   The nonspecific response (generalized adaptation) of the body to any demand made upon it in order to maintain physiological equilibrium.
- **Stressor**   Anything that produces stress or increases the rate of wear and tear on the body.

The Facts About Stress and Tension

All living creatures are in a continual state of **stress** (some more, some less).

There are many kinds of **stressors.** Environmental stressors include heat, noise, overcrowding, climate, and terrain. Physiological stressors may be such things as drugs, caffeine, tobacco, injury, infection or disease, and physical effort.

Emotional stressors are the most frequent and important stressors affecting humans. Some people refer to these as "psychosocial" stressors. These include life-changing events, such as a change in work hours or line of work, family illnesses, problems with superiors, deaths of relatives or friends, and increased responsibilities. In school, pressures such as grades, term papers, and oral presentations may induce stress. Approximately ⅔ of adults indicate that they feel "great stress" at least one day a week.

Too little stress (**hypostress**) is undesirable and distressful.

Stress is not always harmful. In fact, too little stress, sometimes called "rust out," is not good for optimal health. Moderate stress may enhance behavioral adaptation and is necessary for maturation and health. It stimulates psychological growth. It has been said that "freedom from stress is death" and "stress is the spice of life."

Individuals tend to adapt best to moderate stress.

You would expect mild stress to produce mild **adaptations,** and strong stress to produce strong adaptive responses, but this is not so. High levels of threat tend to evoke ineffective, disorganized behavior. Figure 20.1 shows this relationship between stress and adaptive responses.

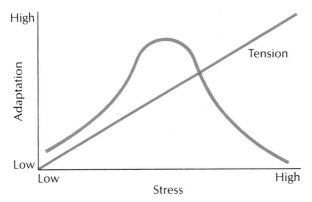

Figure 20.1
Stress and adaptive responses

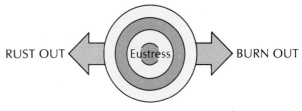

Too Little — Distress   Too Much — Distress

Figure 20.2
Stress target zone

The amount of stress that you can adapt to comfortably is what Hans Selye (1978) calls **eustress** (see figure 20.2) and would, in a sense, be our target zone for stress. Selye is generally regarded as "the father of the modern stress concept."

Excessive stress reduces the effectiveness of the immune system.

Between 50 and 70 percent of all illnesses are linked to the stress response. Too much stress—**distress**—can result in various health disorders. Some mental and physical conditions that can be psychosomatic (or stress caused) include high blood pressure and heart disease; psychiatric disorders, such as depression and schizophrenia; indigestion; colitis; ulcers; headaches; insomnia; diarrhea; constipation; increased blood clotting time; increased cholesterol concentration; diuresis; edema; and low back pain. Other serious diseases, such as cancer, can be influenced by a person's state of mind.

In some cases, there is considerable time between a major stressor and the onset of a disease, so we do not always associate the two. With too much stress, rather than "rust out" we "burn out" (see figure 20.2).

Individuals react and adapt differently to different stressors.

What one person finds stressful may not be stressful to another person, and stress affects people differently. It mobilizes some to greater efficiency, while it confuses and disorganizes others. For example, skydiving or riding a roller coaster would be thrilling for some people, but for others it would be a very stressful and unpleasant experience.

An individual's response to stress depends upon the intensity of the threat, the type of situation in which it occurs, and such personal variables as cultural background, tolerance levels, past experience, and personality. You can't make a racehorse out of a turtle and vice versa. Some people react to stress by biting their nails; others eat too much, chain smoke, or drink excessively.

An individual's capacity to adapt is not a static function, but fluctuates with energy, drive, and courage. The better your fitness, the better you can withstand the rigors of tension without becoming susceptible to illness or other disorders.

Stress can be self-induced and pleasurable, or unpleasurable.

Some people may deliberately place themselves in stressful situations; for example, athletes place themselves under maximum strain; lawyers and surgeons may be challenged by difficulties; and pregnant women accept the psychological and physiological stress of bearing children. Self-induced stress may also be an unpleasant but necessary interlude that cannot be avoided. For example, there is a risk of falling that is necessary in learning to ride a bicycle.

Occupations are common sources of stress, and some are more stressful than others.

One study showed that the twelve most stressful jobs were: laborer, secretary, inspector, clinical lab technician, office manager, foreman, manager/administrator, waiter/waitress, machine operator, farm owner, miner, and painter. Air traffic controllers also have a very stressful job. Business and industry often hire psychologists to counsel employees about occupational stress to help reduce absenteeism, boredom, and the number of accidents and resignations.

Fatigue and **neuromuscular hypertension** are closely related.

High levels of tension are a source of fatigue. Fatigue from lack of rest or sleep, emotional strain, pain, disease, and muscular work may produce too much muscle tension. **Fatigue** may be either **psychological** or **physiological** in origin, but both can result in a state of exhaustion or **chronic fatigue** with neuromuscular hypertension.

Neuromuscular hypertension may be both a cause and an effect of stress.

Anxiety is an emotional response caused by stressors, and it is manifested in muscular tension. Tension is a primary index of stress. One form of this tension is seen in the unnecessary "bracing" or "splinting" action of muscles—the clinched jaw, hunched shoulders, and white knuckles, or muscles contracting where they are not needed. They may stay contracted for long periods, often without your being aware of it. Muscular tension may also be physical in origin, resulting from overuse of a muscle group. This tension can cause muscle spasms and pain that, in turn, become additional stressors. Trigger points and the myofascial pain syndrome that lead to backache and headache are good examples of excess muscular tension. (See concept 16 on back and neck aches.)

Some tension is normally present in muscles and contributes to the adjustment of the individual to the environment.

Some tension is needed to remain awake, alert, and ready to respond. In fact, a certain degree of tension aids some types of mental activity. It appears that each individual has an optimum level of tension to facilitate the thought process. However, too much tension can inhibit some types of mental activity and physical skills (such as those requiring accuracy and steadiness in postures that must be held for long periods).

The Facts About Stress Management

The first step in managing stress is to recognize the causes and to be aware of the symptoms.

You need to recognize the situations in your life that are the stressors. Try to identify the things that make you feel "stressed-out." Everything from minor irritations, such as traffic jams, to major life changes such as births, deaths, or job loss can be stressors. Or a stress overload of just too many demands on your time can make you feel that you are no longer in control. You may feel so overwhelmed that you become depressed.

Make yourself aware of how your body feels when you are under stress. Are the muscles beginning to tighten? Are you gritting your teeth, gripping the steering wheel tightly, drumming your fingers, patting your foot, or hunching your shoulders? Can you feel your heart beating faster, your breathing rate becoming faster and more shallow? Are you perspiring, shaking, or getting a headache?

The second step is to use some type of **relaxation** technique for relief of symptoms.

When you are aware of what stress does to your body, you can do something to relieve those symptoms immediately as well as on a regular and more long-term basis. You can slow your heart and respiration. You can relax tense muscles. You can clear your mind, and relax mentally and emotionally. Several techniques for relaxing are described later in this concept.

The third step is to seek solutions for avoiding some of the stressors and for controlling your lifestyle.

The following are a few suggestions for managing stress:

- Take one thing at a time. You can't do it all at once. Decide which things you can do and which things can be postponed.
- Take action instead of worrying about it. Make a decision about how to solve the problem, then do it.

- If there is no acceptable solution, then accept what cannot be changed. Try to change your feelings about it. Make the best of it and get on with life.
- Think positively. Talk to yourself and visualize yourself succeeding. Think that you *will* pass the exam. You *will* make the free throw. You *will* be cool, calm, and collected as you make your oral presentation. Thinking negative thoughts is distressing in itself and sets you up for failure; it can become a self-fulfilling prophecy.
- Change the way you perceive a stressor. Look at it as a challenge or as a way to learn. Try to see humor in the situation. Look at the bright side.
- Don't try to escape a problem by pretending it doesn't exist. Dulling your senses with alcohol, drugs, or other excesses doesn't make it go away.
- Don't let the little things bother you. Benjamin Franklin reminded us that "little strokes fell great oaks." Small hassles may not be worth the stress you let them create for you. One cardiologist said: "Rule 1 is don't sweat the small stuff; and rule 2 is, it's all small stuff and if you can't fight it and you can't flee—go with the flow" (American Heart Association 1984).
- Be willing to make adjustments. The old saying, "A branch that is able to bend will not break," is applicable to dealing with stress. Try to be flexible in what you want and when you want it.
- Rank the demands on your time in order of priority, and manage your time effectively so the more important things get done. If you are trying to do too much, you may need to get rid of some responsibilities or delegate them to someone else. You must also learn to say "No" to new responsibilities.
- Balance work with rest and play. "Moderation in all things" is still a good adage. Give some priority to proper rest, recreational activities, and diversion in order to prevent "burnout." Diversion can be a temporary change from one activity to another (e.g., change from studying to mowing the lawn) or a change of scenery. You may even need a change of job or a vacation.
- Find and use a support system. Everyone needs someone to turn to for support when he/she is feeling overwhelmed. Support can come from friends, family members, clergy, a teacher, a coach, or a professional counselor. One study of athletic injuries has shown that those who were the most stressed were injured more often, and those who had the poorest support system were the most likely to be injured (Andersen and Williams 1988).

A fourth step you can take in managing stress is to be as fit and healthy as possible.

The more fit and healthy you are, the better able you are to cope with stress. Selye (1977) believes physical fitness serves as a sort of "inoculation against stress"; others have called it a "buffer."

Some methods of relieving tension are less desirable or are not recommended.

There is no magic cure for stress or tension, but there are a variety of therapeutic approaches. Some treatments are less desirable than others because they act only as "crutches" or "fire extinguishers" and do not get at the root of the problem. Hypnosis may lead to fantasy and dependency. Alcoholic beverages, tranquilizers, and painkillers may give temporary relief and may be prescribed by a physician as part of the treatment, but they do not resolve the problem and may even mask symptoms or cause further problems such as addiction. Drugs do not provide a long-term solution to chronic tension. Contrary to vitamin and mineral advertisements, there are no proven benefits to supplementing the diet with such products as vitamin C or special "stress" formulations.

Exercise is one of the best ways to relieve stress and aid muscle tension release.

Exercise is especially useful to relieve white-collar job stress. Studies show that regular exercise decreases the likelihood of stress disorders and reduces the intensity of the stress response. It also shortens the time of recovery from an emotional trauma. Its effect tends to be short term, so one must continue to exercise regularly for it to have a continuing effect. Exercise is not like a measles vaccine where one inoculation is good for life.

Aerobic exercise is believed to be especially effective in reducing anxiety and relieving stress (though a wide variety of other activities are also good). It reduces the levels of epinephrine and norepinephrine, the catecholamines that prepare a person for fight or flight, and thus reduces the end result of stress. Exercise can also act as a diversion and as a cathartic, or a release for frustration and anger, and can enhance one's self-esteem. Whatever your choice of exercise, it is likely to be more effective as an antidote to stress if it is something you find enjoyable. (See table 2.3 in concept 2, for some other psychological benefits of exercise.)

The Facts About Methods of Relaxation

Stretching exercises and rhythmical exercises especially aid in relaxation.

People who work long hours at a desk can release tension by getting up frequently and stretching, by taking a brisk walk down the hall, or by performing "office exercises" (see Lindsey and Gorrie 1989).

Exercising to music or to a rhythmic beat has been found to be relaxing and even "hypnotic." Some exercises are designed specifically for relaxation. Examples can be found on pages 251–252.

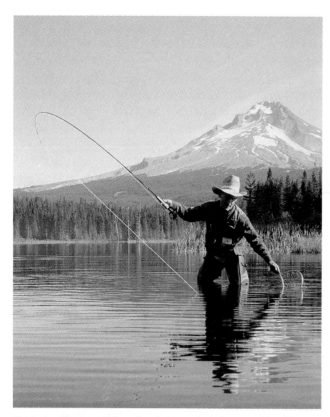

Taking a "time out" to relax is important for good health.

Massage, heat, and deep breathing aid relaxation of tense muscles.

Gentle effleurage, a type of massage; heat in the form of a hot bath (or shower or sauna); and deep breathing with prolonged exhalation when combined with conscious relaxation techniques described in this concept are effective means for relaxing tense muscles for most people.

There are several satisfactory methods of releasing tension through techniques of conscious relaxation.

In some way not fully understood, certain involuntary bodily functions can be controlled by an act of will (voluntarily). Relaxation of the muscles is a skill that can be learned through practice just as other muscle skills are learned, and it works! It is no gimmick.

Conscious relaxation techniques usually employ the "three Rs" of relaxation: (1) reduce mental activity, (2) recognize tension, and (3) reduce respiration.

Five examples of these systems are described here:

- *"The Quick Fix"*—To get relief from a stressful situation during the day, take a "time out" for five or ten minutes; find a quiet place away from the situation with as few distractions as possible. Sit, loosen your clothes, take off your shoes, and close your eyes. Then follow these steps: (1) Inhale deeply for about four seconds; then exhale, letting the air out slowly for about eight seconds (twice as long as the inhalation). Do this several times. (2) Mentally visualize a pleasant image, such as a peaceful lake or stream; continue to relax and breathe deeply. (3) When your time is up, breathe deeply and stretch luxuriously; go back to your work refreshed and with a changed attitude. You may need to do this several times a day.

- *Jacobson's Progressive Relaxation Method*—You must be able to recognize how a tense muscle feels before you can voluntarily release the tension. In this technique, contract the muscles strongly, then relax. Each of the large muscles is relaxed first, and later the small ones. The contractions are gradually reduced in intensity until no movement is visible. Always, the emphasis is placed on detecting the feeling of tension as the first step in "letting go," or "going negative." Jacobson (1978), a pioneer in muscle relaxation research, emphasized the importance of relaxing eye and speech muscles, because he believed these muscles trigger reactions of the total organism more than other muscles. A sample contract-relax exercise routine for relaxation is presented on page 252.

- *Autogenic (Self-generated) Relaxation Training*—Several times daily, sit or lie in a quiet room with eyes closed. Block out distracting thoughts by passively concentrating on pre-selected words or phrases. This technique has been used to focus on heaviness of limbs, warmth of limbs, heart rate regulation, respiratory rate and depth regulation, and coolness in the forehead. It evokes changes opposite to those produced by stress. Research has shown that people who are skilled in this technique can decrease oxygen consumption, change the electrical activity of the brain, slow the metabolism, decrease blood lactate, lower body temperature, and slow the heart rate.

- *Biofeedback-Autogenic Relaxation Training*—Biofeedback training utilizes machines that monitor certain physiological processes of the body and provide visual or auditory evidence of what is happening to normally unconscious bodily functions. When combined with autogenic training, subjects have learned to relax and reduce the electrical activity in their muscles, lower blood pressure, decrease heart rate, change their brain waves, and decrease headaches, asthma attacks, and stomach acid secretion. It has also been helpful in treating phobias, stage fright, drug abuse, sexual dysfunction, stuttering, and other psychological problems (Greenberg 1990).

- *Imagery*—Thinking autogenic phrases, you can visualize such feelings as "sinking into a mattress or pillow," or you can think of being a "limp, loose-jointed puppet with no one to hold the strings." You can imagine being a "half-filled sack of flour resting on an uneven surface" or pretend to be "a sack of granulated salt left out in the rain, melting away." Some people seem to respond better to the concept of "floating" than to feeling "heavy." It also

includes visualizing pleasant, relaxing scenes as mentioned in the description of "The Quick Fix." You attempt to place yourself in the scene and experience all of the sounds, colors, and scents. Whatever the image you wish to conjure, imagery can help take your mind off anxieties and distractions and, at the same time, release unwanted tension in the muscles using the principle of "mind over matter."

RELAXATION EXERCISES

1. **Neck Stretch** Roll the head slowly in a half circle from 9:00 to 8:00 to 7, 6, 5, 4, and 3, then reverse from 3 to 9. Close your eyes and feel the stretch. Do *not* make a full circle by tipping the head back. Repeat several times.

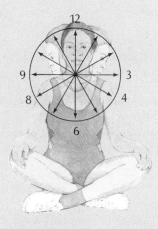

3. **Trunk Stretch and Drop** Stand and reach as high as possible; tiptoe and stretch every muscle, then collapse completely, letting knees flex and trunk, head, and arms dangle. Repeat two or three times. Inhale on the stretch and exhale on the collapse.

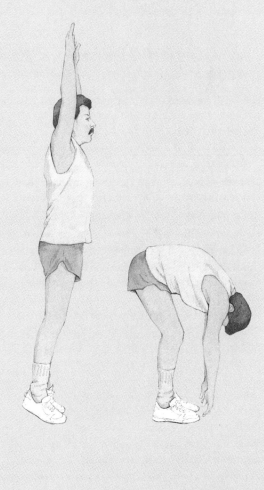

2. **Shoulder Lift** Hunch the shoulders as high as possible (contract) and then let them drop (relax). Repeat several times. Inhale on the lift; exhale on the drop.

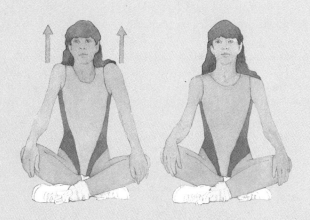

RELAXATION EXERCISES *cont.*

4. Trunk Swings Following the "trunk stretch and drop" (preceding illustration), remain in the "drop" position and with a minimum of muscular effort, set the trunk swinging from side to side by shifting the weight from one foot to the other, letting the heels come off the floor alternately. Keep the entire body (especially the neck) limp.

5. Tension Contrast With arms extended overhead, lie on your side. Tense the body as stiff as a board, then let go, and relax, letting the body fall either forward or backward in whatever direction it loses balance. Continue letting go for a few seconds after falling and allow yourself to feel like you are still sinking. Repeat on the other side.

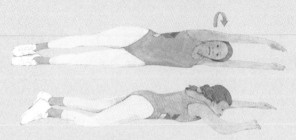

CONTRACT-RELAX EXERCISE ROUTINE FOR RELAXATION*

1. Hand and forearm—Contract your right hand, making a fist; hold 3 counts; relax and keep letting go 6–10 counts. Repeat, then do left fist, then both fists.

2. Biceps—Flex both elbows and contract your biceps; hold 3 counts; relax and continue relaxing 6–10 counts. Repeat.

3. Triceps—Same as biceps except extend both elbows, contract the triceps on the back of the arm. Repeat.

4. Relax both hands, forearms, and upper arms.

5. Forehead—Raise your eyebrows and wrinkle your forehead; hold 3 counts; relax and continue relaxing 6–10 counts.

6. Cheeks and nose—Make a face; wrinkle your nose and squint; hold 3 counts; relax and continue relaxing 6–10 counts.

7. Jaws—Clench your teeth 3 counts; relax 6–10 counts.

8. Lips and tongue—With teeth apart, press lips together and press tongue to roof of mouth; hold 3 counts; relax 6–10 counts.

9. Neck and throat—Push head backward while tucking chin, pushing against floor or pillow if lying; if sitting, push against high chair-back; hold 3 counts; relax for 6–10 counts.

10. Relax forehead, cheeks, nose, jaws, lips, tongue, neck, and throat. Relax hands, forearms, and upper arms.

11. Shoulder and upper back—Hunch shoulders to ears; hold 3 counts; relax 6–10 counts.

12. Relax lips, tongue, neck, throat, shoulders, and upper back.

13. Abdomen—Suck in abdomen; hold 3 counts; relax 6–10 counts.

14. Lower back—Contract and arch the back; hold 3 counts; relax 6–10 counts.

15. Thighs and buttocks—Squeeze your buttocks together and push your heels into the floor (if lying) or against a chair rung (if sitting); hold 3 counts; relax 6–10 counts.

16. Relax shoulders and upper back, abdomen, lower back, thighs, and buttocks.

17. Calves—Pull instep and toes toward shins; hold 3 counts; relax 6–10 counts.

18. Toes—Curl toes; hold 3 counts; relax 6–10 counts.

19. Relax every muscle in your body.

Note: Eventually, you should progress to a combination of muscle groups and gradually eliminate the "contract" phase of the program. Refer to Jacobson's relaxation method p. 251 for more instruction or read Jacobson's (1978) or Greenberg's (1996) books.

Suggested Readings

Coleman, D., and J. Gurin. Eds. *Mind/Body Medicine.* Fairfield, OH: Consumer Reports Books, 1993.

Greenberg, J. S. *Comprehensive Stress Management.* 5th ed. Dubuque, IA: Brown & Benchmark Publishers, 1996.

Greenberg, J. S. *Coping with Stress: A Practical Guide.* 3rd ed. Dubuque, IA: Wm. C. Brown Publishers, 1990.

Jacobson, E. *You Must Relax.* New York: McGraw-Hill, 1978.

Lindsey, R., and D. D. Gorrie. *Survival Kit for Those Who Sit.* Laguna Beach, CA: Publitec Editions, 1989.

Selye, H. *The Stress of Life.* 2nd ed. New York: McGraw-Hill, 1978.

Seward, B. L. *Managing Stress.* Boston: Jones & Bartlett Publishers, 1994.

LAB RESOURCE MATERIALS

THE LIFE EXPERIENCE SURVEY*

Listed below are a number of events that sometimes bring about change in the lives of those who experience them and necessitate social readjustment. Please check those events that you have experienced in the past year and indicate the time period during which you experienced each event. Be sure that all check marks are directly across from the items to which they correspond.

Also, for each item checked indicate the extent to which you viewed the event as having either a positive or negative impact on your life at the time the event occurred. That is, indicate the type and extent of impact that the event had. A rating of −3 would indicate an extremely negative impact. A rating of 0 suggests neither a positive nor a negative impact. A rating of + 3 would indicate an extremely positive impact.

Section I of the test is for everyone. It provides three extra blanks (numbers 45, 46, and 47) for you to list any recent experiences that have had an impact on your life but that were not mentioned in the preceding items.

Section II of the test is designed for students only. If there are school-related experiences that have had a noticeable impact on your life but are not listed, you may list them in one or more of the three blanks in Section I.

Note: Some items apply only to males and some apply only to females; these are indicated in the survey.

*From Irwin G. Sarason, James H. Johnson, and Judith M. Siegel. "Assessing the Impact of Life Changes: Development of the Life Experiences Survey" in *Journal of Consulting and Clinical Psychology*, 46(5):932–46. Copyright 1978 by the American Psychological Association. Adapted by permission.

THE LIFE EXPERIENCE SURVEY cont.

Section I	0–6 mos.	7–12 mos.	Extremely Negative	Moderately Negative	Somewhat Negative	No Impact	Slightly Positive	Moderately Positive	Extremely Positive
1. Marriage	___	___	−3	−2	−1	0	+1	+2	+3
2. Detention in jail or comparable institution	___	___	−3	−2	−1	0	+1	+2	+3
3. Death of spouse	___	___	−3	−2	−1	0	+1	+2	+3
4. Major change in sleeping habits (much more or less sleep)	___	___	−3	−2	−1	0	+1	+2	+3
5. Death of close family member:									
a. mother	___	___	−3	−2	−1	0	+1	+2	+3
b. father	___	___	−3	−2	−1	0	+1	+2	+3
c. brother	___	___	−3	−2	−1	0	+1	+2	+3
d. sister	___	___	−3	−2	−1	0	+1	+2	+3
e. child	___	___	−3	−2	−1	0	+1	+2	+3
f. grandmother	___	___	−3	−2	−1	0	+1	+2	+3
g. grandfather	___	___	−3	−2	−1	0	+1	+2	+3
h. other (specify) ___	___	___	−3	−2	−1	0	+1	+2	+3
6. Major change in eating habits (much more or much less food intake)	___	___	−3	−2	−1	0	+1	+2	+3
7. Foreclosure on mortgage or loan	___	___	−3	−2	−1	0	+1	+2	+3
8. Death of a close friend	___	___	−3	−2	−1	0	+1	+2	+3
9. Outstanding personal achievement	___	___	−3	−2	−1	0	+1	+2	+3
10. Minor law violations (traffic ticket, disturbing the peace, etc.)	___	___	−3	−2	−1	0	+1	+2	+3
11. *Male:* Wife's/girlfriend's pregnancy *Female:* Pregnancy	___	___	−3	−2	−1	0	+1	+2	+3
12. Changed work situation (different working conditions, working hours, etc.)	___	___	−3	−2	−1	0	+1	+2	+3

THE LIFE EXPERIENCE SURVEY cont.

Section I	0–6 mos.	7–12 mos.	Extremely Negative	Moderately Negative	Somewhat Negative	No Impact	Slightly Positive	Moderately Positive	Extremely Positive
13. New job	___	___	−3	−2	−1	0	+1	+2	+3
14. Serious illness or injury of close family member									
a. father	___	___	−3	−2	−1	0	+1	+2	+3
b. mother	___	___	−3	−2	−1	0	+1	+2	+3
c. sister	___	___	−3	−2	−1	0	+1	+2	+3
d. brother	___	___	−3	−2	−1	0	+1	+2	+3
e. grandfather	___	___	−3	−2	−1	0	+1	+2	+3
f. grandmother	___	___	−3	−2	−1	0	+1	+2	+3
g. spouse	___	___	−3	−2	−1	0	+1	+2	+3
h. child	___	___	−3	−2	−1	0	+1	+2	+3
i. other (specify) ___	___	___	−3	−2	−1	0	+1	+2	+3
15. Sexual difficulties	___	___	−3	−2	−1	0	+1	+2	+3
16. Trouble with employer (in danger of losing job, being suspended, demoted, etc.)	___	___	−3	−2	−1	0	+1	+2	+3
17. Trouble with in-laws	___	___	−3	−2	−1	0	+1	+2	+3
18. Major change in financial status (a lot better off or a lot worse off)	___	___	−3	−2	−1	0	+1	+2	+3
19. Major change in closeness of family members (deceased or increased closeness)	___	___	−3	−2	−1	0	+1	+2	+3
20. Gaining a new family member (through birth, adoption, family member moving in, etc.)	___	___	−3	−2	−1	0	+1	+2	+3
21. Change of residence	___	___	−3	−2	−1	0	+1	+2	+3
22. Marital separation from mate (due to conflict)	___	___	−3	−2	−1	0	+1	+2	+3
23. Major change in church activities (increased or decreased attendance)	___	___	−3	−2	−1	0	+1	+2	+3
24. Marital reconciliation with mate	___	___	−3	−2	−1	0	+1	+2	+3
25. Major change in number of arguments with spouse (a lot more or a lot less arguments)	___	___	−3	−2	−1	0	+1	+2	+3
26. *Married Male:* Change in wife's work outside the home (beginning work, ceasing work, changing to a new job) *Married Female:* Change in husband's work (loss of job, beginning new job, retirement, etc.)	___	___	−3	−2	−1	0	+1	+2	+3
27. Major change in usual type and/or amount of recreation	___	___	−3	−2	−1	0	+1	+2	+3
28. Borrowing more than $10,000 (buying a home, business, etc.)	___	___	−3	−2	−1	0	+1	+2	+3
29. Borrowing less than $10,000 (buying car, TV, getting school loan, etc.)	___	___	−3	−2	−1	0	+1	+2	+3
30. Being fired from job	___	___	−3	−2	−1	0	+1	+2	+3
31. *Male:* Wife/girlfriend having abortion *Female:* Having abortion	___	___	−3	−2	−1	0	+1	+2	+3
32. Major personal illness or injury	___	___	−3	−2	−1	0	+1	+2	+3
33. Major change in social activities; e.g., parties, movies, visiting (increased, or decreased participation)	___	___	−3	−2	−1	0	+1	+2	+3
34. Major change in living conditions of family (building new home, remodeling, deterioration of home, neighborhood, etc.)	___	___	−3	−2	−1	0	+1	+2	+3
35. Divorce	___	___	−3	−2	−1	0	+1	+2	+3
36. Serious injury or illness of close friend	___	___	−3	−2	−1	0	+1	+2	+3

Section I	0–6 mos.	7–12 mos.	Extremely Negative	Moderately Negative	Somewhat Negative	No Impact	Slightly Positive	Moderately Positive	Extremely Positive
37. Retirement from work	___	___	–3	–2	–1	0	+1	+2	+3
38. Son or daughter leaving home (due to marriage, college, etc.)	___	___	–3	–2	–1	0	+1	+2	+3
39. Ending of formal schooling	___	___	–3	–2	–1	0	+1	+2	+3
40. Separation from spouse (due to work, travel, etc.)	___	___	–3	–2	–1	0	+1	+2	+3
41. Engagement	___	___	–3	–2	–1	0	+1	+2	+3
42. Breaking up with boyfriend/girlfriend	___	___	–3	–2	–1	0	+1	+2	+3
43. Leaving home for the first time	___	___	–3	–2	–1	0	+1	+2	+3
44. Reconciliation with boyfriend/girlfriend	___	___	–3	–2	–1	0	+1	+2	+3
Other recent experiences that have had an impact on your life. List and rate.	___	___	–3	–2	–1	0	+1	+2	+3
45. _____	___	___	–3	–2	–1	0	+1	+2	+3
46. _____	___	___	–3	–2	–1	0	+1	+2	+3
47. _____	___	___	–3	–2	–1	0	+1	+2	+3

Section II: For Students Only	0–6 mos.	7–12 mos.	Extremely Negative	Moderately Negative	Somewhat Negative	No Impact	Slightly Positive	Moderately Positive	Extremely Positive
48. Beginning new school experience at a higher academic level (college, graduate school, professional school, etc.)	___	___	–3	–2	–1	0	+1	+2	+3
49. Changing to a new school at same academic level (undergraduate, graduate, etc.)	___	___	–3	–2	–1	0	+1	+2	+3
50. Academic probation	___	___	–3	–2	–1	0	+1	+2	+3
51. Being dismissed from dormitory or other residence	___	___	–3	–2	–1	0	+1	+2	+3
52. Failing an important exam	___	___	–3	–2	–1	0	+1	+2	+3
53. Changing a major	___	___	–3	–2	–1	0	+1	+2	+3
54. Failing a course	___	___	–3	–2	–1	0	+1	+2	+3
55. Dropping a course	___	___	–3	–2	–1	0	+1	+2	+3
56. Joining a fraternity/sorority	___	___	–3	–2	–1	0	+1	+2	+3

Scoring the Life Experience Survey

1. Add all of the negative scores to arrive at your own distress score (negative stress).
2. Add all of the positive scores to arrive at a eustress score (positive stress).
3. It is possible to calculate scores for the last six months, or for the last year. The more recent the incident, the more likely it will be distressful.

Chart 20.1 *Rating Scale* for Life Experiences and Stress

	Sum of Negative Scores (Distress)	Sum of Positive Scores (Eustress)
May need counseling	14+	
Above average stress	9–13	
Average	6–9	9–10
Below average stress	<6	

CONCEPT ·21·

Adhering to Physical Activity and Other Healthy Lifestyles

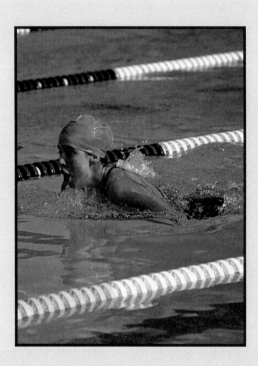

Concept 21

No matter how good your physical activity or lifestyle plan, if you do not carry it out you will not reap its benefits.

Introduction

You have read about the benefits of physical activity and the amount necessary for developing each of the physical components of fitness. Now the challenge is to make physical activity a permanent part of your lifestyle. Physical activity adherence or exercise adherence are terms used in this concept to describe staying with a plan for a lifetime. Many of the factors that help you to adhere to active lifestyles also help you adhere to other healthy behaviors. Once you have identified the factors that help you stay with or adhere to a physical activity program you can develop some self-management skills. Learning self-management skills can aid in adherence to other healthy lifestyles as well.

Health Goal for the Year 2000

▬ Increase the proportion of people who do regular physical activity. (↑)

Note: (↑) indicates progress toward goal, (↓) indicates regression from goal, and (<>) indicates either no change or lack of new data since 1990.

Terms

▬ **Adherence** Adopting a healthy behavior such as regular physical activity or sound nutrition as part of your lifestyle.

▬ **Enabling Factor** Anything that helps you to carry out your healthy lifestyle plan.

▬ **Mental Practice** Imagining yourself going through the performance of a skill without actually physically performing it.

▬ **Overlearning** To practice a skill repeatedly in an attempt to make the skill a habit.

▬ **Paralysis by Analysis** Overanalysis of skill behavior. This occurs when more information is supplied than the performer can really use or when concentration on too many details of skill results in interference with performance.

▬ **Positive Addiction** Exceptional adherence; the formation of a habit that is exceptionally difficult to break but that has positive rather than negative consequences.

▬ **Predisposing Factor** Anything that makes you more likely to decide that you should make a healthy lifestyle such as regular physical activity a part of your normal routine.

▬ **Reinforcing Factor** Anything that provides encouragement to maintain healthy lifestyles such as physical activity for a lifetime.

- **Self-confidence** The belief that you can be successful at something; for example, the belief that you can be successful in sports and physical activities, and can improve your physical fitness.
- **Self-criticism** Punishing yourself or getting angry with yourself because you did not perform as well as you think you should; negative "self-talk."
- **Self-management Skills** Skills that you can learn to help you adhere to healthy lifestyles such as regular physical activity. Examples include goal setting, time management, and program planning skills.
- **Skill Analysis** Breaking the performance of a skill into component parts and critically evaluating each phase of the performance.

Facts About Changing to Healthy Lifestyles

> People do not make lifestyle changes overnight. Rather, people progress forward and backward through several stages of change.

The goal for all people should be to get to practice healthy behaviors for a lifetime. A person who has accomplished this would have achieved the level of maintenance (see figure 21.1). People at the maintenance stage are true adherers, they have the "good health and wellness habit." At the other extreme are people who virtually never practice healthy behaviors such as regular physical activity. These people are at the precontemplation stage. Not only do they *not* practice specific healthy lifestyles such as regular physical activity, they are not even considering doing it.

Rather than trying to get people to move from the precontemplation stage directly to the maintenance stage, it is probably more effective to help them move through several more gradual stages. First, it is important to get people to contemplate a change, to start thinking about it. Helping people with **predisposing factors** discussed later in this concept will help in this change. Next, it is useful to help people who are contemplating change to begin planning. Putting your plans in writing is an important step toward taking action. Planning to improve **enabling factors** will help move you to the action stage.

People at the action stage have begun to change their behavior, but it is sporadic. Both enabling and **reinforcing factors** are important at this stage. These factors can help you meet the goal of moving on to the maintenance stage.

Two examples will help you better understand the stages that you go through in making changes in healthy lifestyles. Example 1: A smoker who is in the stage of precontemplation would say, "I don't want to stop smoking, leave me alone." At the contemplation stage the smoker might say, "I am thinking about cutting down." At the preparing stage the smoker may have purchased a nicotine

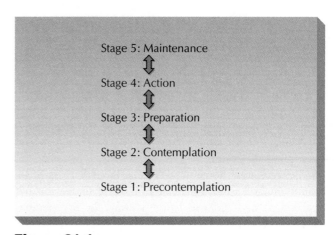

Figure 21.1
The stages of change for lifestyle behavior adherence
Source: Data from B. H. Marcus et al., 1992.

patch but may not have taken any direct action. At the action stage the smoker will have tried to stop or cut back on smoking. At the maintenance stage the smoker will have stopped smoking for an extended period of time. The factors that will help a smoker adopt the healthy lifestyle of nonsmoking will vary depending on the stage. Example 2: The same general stages would occur for physical activity. A totally sedentary person who is not thinking about doing any exercise is a precontemplator. When the person starts to consider the possibility of some activity, a shift to contemplation has been made. Preparation might be joining a health club or buying special exercise clothes. At the action stage a person would be doing some activity but may not have maintained it for a period of time. A person at the maintenance stage will have been doing activity for a relatively long period of time.

Learning about predisposing, enabling, and reinforcing factors can help you move through the stages of change. While many of the examples relate to the regular physical activity as a healthy lifestyle you will see that the stages of change and the factors that promote adherence and maintenance apply to many healthy lifestyles such as sound nutrition, stress management, personal health practices, consumer behavior, and avoiding destructive habits.

The Facts About Predisposing Factors

> Knowledge predisposes you to adherence.

Many people have misconceptions about healthy lifestyles. For example, dispelling misconceptions about physical activity and acquiring knowledge can help you know the value of exercise, how to perform it without injury, and how to get the most from your efforts. By itself, knowledge does not guarantee that you will start a lifelong program. However, a sound fitness and exercise education is one **predisposing factor** to lifetime physical activity.

Holding the beliefs that physical activity and fitness are important predisposes you to adherence.

A belief is something that you think is true. It may or may not be based on fact. If you believe that physical activity is important, you are more likely to be a regular exerciser than if you do not believe it is important. For example, if you believe that exercise helps you sleep better, you may do it regularly even if there is little scientific evidence that the belief is true. Some experts think that believing in the importance of a healthy lifestyle is more important than real knowledge about it. Unfortunately, the reverse may also be true. For example, if you believe physical activity is of no value, even though it is, you may be less likely to do it. Sound beliefs based on knowledge are likely to lead to **physical activity** or **exercise adherence,** as well as adherence to other healthy lifestyles.

Enjoyment predisposes you to adherence.

Enjoyment is a subjective feeling. It is hard to explain why some people enjoy physical activity and others do not. What is clear is that many people who enjoy exercise would probably choose to do it even if it did not contribute to optimal health and well-being. In fact, some people would probably do it even if it had negative consequences. This is evidenced by the fact that some people participate in sports when they are injured or ill. Some experts believe that knowledge and beliefs can improve one's attitude or positive feelings about physical activity. It may also be true that people who enjoy exercise are motivated to learn more about it and are more likely to believe that it is good for them. Since all people do not enjoy the same activities, it is important that you identify the form of physical activity that you most enjoy if you are to adhere to it.

Feeling comfortable about the way you look predisposes you to physical activity adherence.

If you are self-conscious about the way you look you may avoid physical activity because you feel that people might make fun of you. The feeling of self-consciousness is probably more important than actual appearance. Some people who are very fit and attractive feel uncomfortable in exercise clothes and in formal exercise classes or facilities. Being too fat, quite lean, or unfit does not always lead to feelings of self-consciousness. Some things you can do to reduce self-consciousness include: wearing exercise clothes that cover your body, avoiding exercise in highly visible places, exercising with supportive friends, listening to music, or finding other ways to keep you from thinking about what other people think about you. In reality, they may be admiring your dedication!

Self-confidence predisposes you to adherence.

If you have **self-confidence** you are more likely to engage in healthy lifestyles than those who lack self-confidence. Lack of confidence can result from lack of experience, pressure from others, comparisons to other people or unrealistic standards, lack of skill, and many other factors. Perhaps the most important reason for low self-confidence is **self-criticism.** If an activity makes you angry with yourself, it undermines your confidence. Improving your skills may reduce self-criticism. Selecting an activity that requires less skill may also help. Jogging/running, walking, cycling, swimming, and home calisthenics are quite popular because they do not produce self-criticism. Also, since self-criticism is often based on comparisons to other people, it is important to remember that most people are far more critical of themselves than of other people. The most competent people do not always have the most confidence. Some people with good skills lack confidence, and some with lesser skills exhibit high confidence.

Self-motivation predisposes you to adherence.

If you are self-motivated you do things for personal or internal reasons. You do not rely on external incentives such as money, awards, or even recognition as a source of motivation. The reasons why some people have self-motivation is not entirely clear. However, we do know that people who start exercise early in life and who have not depended on external rewards to enjoy their exercise are most likely to have self-motivation. Reliance on external rewards such as trophies, money, and other material rewards has been shown to undermine self-motivation. This is evidenced by the fact that some athletes perceive performance in their sport as work rather than play. Self-motivation is highest when you are not threatened by failure and when the activity is one that you typically enjoy.

People with a previous history of involvement in physical activity are more likely to adhere to it than those who have not participated regularly.

You **can** teach an old dog new tricks! It is possible to get a habitual non-exerciser to become active. However, the people most likely to become active in the future are those who have been active in the past. Of course, if you have a history of participating in activity you are also likely to enjoy it, to be self-confident, and to be self-motivated. If you do not have a history of regular exercise, there is nothing you can do about it. However, there are things you can do to change your knowledge, beliefs, attitudes, self-confidence, and self-motivation.

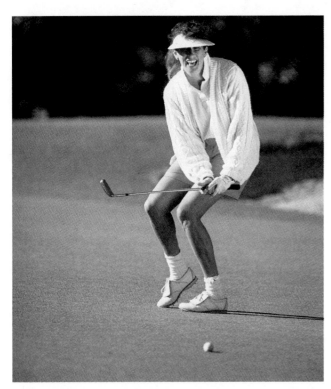
Skills enable you to be active.

The Facts About Enabling Factors

Possessing skill enables you to adhere to healthy lifestyles.

Having sports and other physical skills enables you to adhere to the healthy lifestyle of being physically active. But you do not have to be a great performer to enjoy sports and physical activity. The key is to have enough skill to feel competent. It is advisable to practice and perhaps seek instruction to enhance enjoyment of a lifetime activity, especially if you are unskilled. People with greater skill are more likely to get involved because they are more likely to be successful. However, there is another way to increase satisfaction from sports participation. Research suggests that you must be 65 to 75 percent as good as your partner if either of you is to enjoy the activity. For this reason, it is not only advisable to improve your skills, but you should find a playing partner or group of similar ability. Sports skills are just one example of skills that enable you to practice healthy lifestyles. Another example is stress management skills which enable you to relax and reduce the anxieties of daily living.

There are certain guidelines that can be followed to enable you to become skilled in physical activities.

- *When learning a new activity, concentrate on the general idea of the skill first; worry about details later.* For example, a diver who concentrates on pointing the toes and keeping the legs straight at the end of a flip may land flat on his/her back. To make it all the way over, the diver should concentrate on merely doing the flip. When the general idea is *mastered,* then concentrate on details.
- *The beginner should be careful not to emphasize too many details at one time.* After the general idea of the skill is acquired, the learner can begin to focus on the details, one or two at a time. Concentration on too many details at one time may result in **paralysis by analysis.** For example, a golfer who is told to keep the head down, the left arm straight, and the knees bent, cannot possibly concentrate on all of these details at once. As a result, neither the details nor the general idea of the golf swing are performed properly.
- *Once the general idea of a skill is learned, a **skill analysis** of the performance may be helpful.* Be careful not to overanalyze; it may be helpful to have a knowledgeable person help you locate strengths and weaknesses. Movies and videotapes of performances have been known to be of help to learners.
- *In the early stages of learning a lifetime sport or physical activity, it is not wise to engage in competition.* Beginners who compete are likely to concentrate on beating their opponent rather than on learning a skill properly. For example, in bowling, the beginner may abandon the newly learned hook ball in favor of the "sure thing" straight ball. This may make the person more successful immediately, but is not likely to improve the person's bowling skills for the future.
- *To be performed well, lifetime sports skills must be **overlearned.*** Oftentimes, when you learn a new activity, you begin to play the game immediately. The best way to learn a skill is to overlearn it, or practice it until it becomes habit. Frequently, games do not allow you to overlearn skills. For example, during a game is not a good time to learn the tennis serve because there may be only a few opportunities to serve. For the beginner, it would be much more productive to hit many services (overlearn) with a friend until the general idea of the serve is well learned. Further, the beginner *should not* sacrifice speed to concentrate on serving for accuracy. Accuracy will come with practice of a properly performed skill.

- *When unlearning an old (incorrect) skill and learning a new (correct) skill, a person's performance may get worse before it gets better.* For example, a golfer with a baseball swing may want to learn the correct golf swing. It is important for the learner to understand that the score may worsen during the relearning stage. As the new skill is overlearned, skill will improve as will the golf score.
- *Mental practice may aid skill learning.* Mental practice may benefit performance of motor skills, especially if the performer has had previous experience in performing the skill. Mental practice can be especially useful in sports when the performer cannot participate regularly because of weather, business, or lack of time.
- *For beginners, practicing in front of other people may be detrimental to learning a skill.* Research indicates that an audience may inhibit the beginner's learning of a new sports skill. This is especially true if the learner feels that his or her performance is being evaluated by someone in the audience.

> Possessing good physical fitness enables you to adhere to physical activity.

You may feel that you are unable to do certain physical activities because you might get injured. Possessing health-related fitness can reduce the risk of injury and fatigue. Both injury and fatigue are sources of inactivity. Skill-related fitness also aids in the performance of physical activities, though it is not a requirement for enjoying them. Perhaps you do not exercise because you lack fitness, and this leads to further lack of fitness. The best solution to breaking the inactivity cycle is to begin your program with a modest amount of exercise in an activity that you enjoy. Gradually take advantage of more rigorous activities when your fitness improves. There is evidence that people who begin exercise to improve fitness are likely to adopt other healthy lifestyles as well.

> Accessibility to facilities and equipment enables you to adhere to physical activity.

Repeatedly, people indicate that they are unable to do regular physical activity because the facilities are too far from home, the weather is bad, or the cost of using facilities is too great. These reasons may be merely excuses for not doing regular exercise. On the other hand, the easier it is to adhere, the more likely you are to do it. It is important that you find a place to exercise near or in the home, that you find a place to exercise when the weather is bad, and that you find a way to exercise that is within your budget. There are many forms of exercise that can be done at home at little or no cost. If you do not enjoy these,

you should investigate public recreation opportunities. You may need to be creative. Some people who walk regularly go to nearby covered shopping malls to walk when the weather is bad. Others use old bicycle inner tubes as a substitute for resistance machines or plastic bottles as a substitute for weights.

Accessibility is important to other lifestyles as well. For example, if good food is accessible people are more likely to consume it. Poor people, for example, often have poorer diets than those of greater financial means. Accessibility of appropriate personal health supplies such as tooth brushes, floss, and soap all enable one to practice healthy behaviors. Without accessibility, you may be unable to adhere to good health practices.

> Selecting a type of physical activity that is not too difficult enables you to adhere.

Corporate fitness programs have higher dropout rates when the physical activity provided is exceptionally vigorous. Beginners are especially likely to adhere to programs that are moderate. More vigorous exercise may lead to injury and is more likely to be perceived as too difficult. Beginners should start gradually. Also, they might want to make ratings of perceived exertion to learn to modify exercise that seems too difficult.

The Facts About Reinforcing Factors

> Family and spouse support reinforces adherence.

When family members support your behavior, you are likely to continue it. Family and spouse support is considered a **reinforcing factor** to most healthy lifestyles including regular physical activity. However, physical activity may take time away from family activities. If family members, especially one's spouse, feel that exercise is interfering with family obligations, activity may diminish. It is important to involve family members and friends in planning for physical activity and other healthy lifestyles.

> Support from friends and peers reinforces adherence.

People who live in communities where regular physical activity is typical are reinforced to persist in activity. Exercising with friends helps one adhere. Finding friends with similar interests and abilities is also important. An exercise leader who is encouraging and supportive can also reinforce exercise adherence. If you especially enjoy the social aspects of physical activity you should consider joining a sports or exercise group and/or choose sports and activities

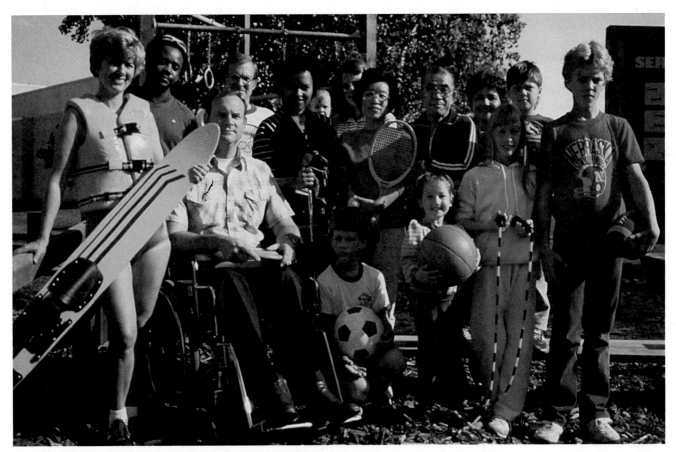
Support from friends and family reinforces exercise adherence.

with a social component. Peer support is very important in all lifestyle changes, particularly smoking and other destructive behaviors. A primary reason for starting smoking is the influence of peers.

Being successful reinforces adherence (success breeds success).

Some people avoid doing certain things because they see them as sources of failure. If done properly, anyone can succeed in physical activity. Some other suggestions are listed here.

- *Do not equate success with winning.* Sports psychologists agree that one problem experienced by many adults is that they cannot enjoy competitive activities unless they win. Though most people enjoy winning, it must be realized that only 50 percent of the participants in most activities can win. Playing well and enjoying the sport also makes you a "winner."

- *Avoid comparing yourself and your accomplishments to those of other people.*
- *Consider gradual improvement over the long-term improvement as a successful accomplishment.*
- *Try using a handicap system when competing with those of unequal skill.* Such systems as those used in golf and bowling can be adapted for other activities to help "even up" the competition.
- *Sports competition may or may not make exercise fun.* Some people especially enjoy competition. Others, however, avoid competitive activities because they have not had success in competitive games. Whatever the benefits of regular physical activity, none should be exaggerated to the point of detracting from a fuller life. Overemphasis on sports can cause anxiety and even neurosis. In fact, some people create stress for themselves by being excessively competitive, increasing their chances of getting stress-related diseases.

A physician's advice is the reason most often mentioned for
doing regular physical activity. It is also a leading reason
why people decide to stop smoking. Too often, the doctor's
advice is given after a health problem already exists. When
medical doctors, insurance companies, and employers place
an emphasis on healthy lifestyles and preventing health
problems, it sends a signal that it is a priority. You may wish
to consider insurance companies that provide for regular preventive exams and other healthy lifestyles. Also, if you have a
choice you may wish to seek a place of employment that provides opportunities to do regular physical activity.

In 1960 very few adults performed regular physical activity in
their free time. The number of exercisers has increased dramatically since then. Exercise has become popular. This is reflected in the advertisements on television, in newspapers,
and in magazines. The trend toward regular exercise as the
"normal thing to do" is reinforcing to exercise adherence. Unfortunately the media can also foster unhealthy lifestyles. One
recent study indicated that young people were more often
able to identify a cartoon character associated with cigarettes
than they were political leaders in our country. This identifi-
cation is thought to contribute to smoking among children.

Other Facts About Physical Activity Adherence

Physical activity (or exercise) adherence means doing regular lifetime exercise. **Positive addiction** is another term
commonly used to describe this healthy lifestyle. The implication is that exercise is addicting, but unlike addictions
such as drugs and smoking, the consequences of the addiction are positive. Experts have not established that physical
activity can be addicting, though it is generally agreed that
some people develop very strong exercise habits (exceptional adherence) even to the point of activity neurosis.
Habitual exercisers regularly indicate that they have positive feelings, even feelings of euphoria, when they do regular, sustained exercise.

     Morgan and O'Connor (1988) have suggested several
possible explanations for the positive feelings associated with
exercise. They refer to these positive feelings as "positive
mood states." One theory is that the increase in body heat that
accompanies exercise could result in reduction in muscle tension. Another theory is that involvement in exercise provides a

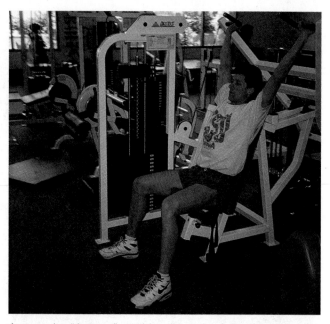

An exercise "time out" provides distraction from daily stressors.

"time out," or a period of time free from distractions. A regular exerciser gets away from the sources of stress and tension.
This distraction may account for positive mood states. Researchers find little support for the "endorphin theory" popularized in many jogging books and magazines. This explanation suggests that regular exercise elevates endorphins, or
substances in the brain, thought to be responsible for the positive feeling runners have referred to as the "runner's high."

The factors that help people adhere to healthy lifestyles are
sometimes referred to as the determinants. The determinants of physical activity as outlined in the Surgeon General's Report are essentially the same as the predisposing
enabling and reinforcing factors described earlier in this
concept. Predisposing, enabling, and reinforcing factors are
presented in the previous section of this concept.

The Facts About Self-Management Skills

When we think of skills we often think of things such as
sports skills and other physical skills. As noted above,
physical skills are important to adherence to physical activity. There are many other skills that can be learned to help
you adhere to healthy lifestyles. Table 21.1 lists several of
these important self-management skills. Like physical

Table 21.1
Self-Management Skills

Self-Management Skills	Examples for Physical Activity	Examples for other lifestyles
Adopting Coping Skills This involves developing a new way of thinking about things. People with this skill can see situations in more than one way and learn to think more positively about life situations.	A person avoids physical activity because he/she does not have the physical skills equal to peers. Coping skills allows this person to tell him or herself that self-comparisons are more important and chooses to be active anyway (see concept 4).	A person is stressed at work. The worries of the job are brought home. One coping strategy would be to take a "time out" to read or go for a walk to "get away" from work stress.
Balancing Attitudes This involves learning to balance positive and negative attitudes. To adhere to a healthy lifestyle it is important to develop positive attitudes and reduce the negative attitudes (see concept 1).	A person does not do activity because he or she lacks support from friends, has no equipment, and does not like to get sweaty. These are negatives. Shifting the balance to positive things such as fun, good health, and looking good can help promote activity.	A person who is ill avoids seeing a physician because he/she fears what the doctor might find. The person must learn that the positives of early detection outweigh the negatives.
Developing Goal Setting Skills This involves learning how to establish things that you want to achieve in the future. It is important that goals be realistic and achievable. Learning to set process goals is important for beginners (see concept 17).	A person wants to get stronger. If he/she has learned sound goal setting skills he/she will set a goal of doing strength exercise for a period of time. Specific strength or fitness goals will be longer term goals and should be achievable in the time established to meet them.	A person wants to lose body fat. If he/she sets a goal of losing 50 pounds success is unlikely. Setting a process goal of restricting 200 calories a day or expending 200 more a day for several weeks makes success more likely.
Developing Performance Skills This involves learning physical skills necessary for performance of a specific task such as performing a sport. These skills can help you feel confident and can help you enjoy activities.	A person avoids activity because of poor confidence in abilities. Practice and good instruction are the best way to develop these skills (see previous discussion in this concept).	A person is stressed and anxious in many life situations. Learning stress management skills such as relaxation skills can help a person cope. Stress management skills must be practiced to be effective (see concept 20).
Developing Self-Monitoring Skills Self-monitoring skills include record keeping skills. Many people think that they adhere to healthy lifestyles but they do not. They have a distorted view of what they actually do. Self-monitoring helps give you a true picture of your own behavior. Monitoring progress in meeting goals is also important.	A person thinks he/she is more active than other people. Monitoring time spent in activity can help a person get a true picture of his/her behavior. Learning to keep accurate records is a skill that can be developed with practice (see lab 14). Learning to keep records of progress is also important to adherence.	A person can't understand why he/she is not losing weight even though restricting calories. Keeping records may show that the person was eating more than he/she thought (see Lab 19B).
Finding Social Support This involves learning how to get the support of others for healthy lifestyles you want to adopt. You learn how to get this support from others. Support of an outside authority such as a doctor can help (see previous section).	A person wants to be active but peers and/or friends are not normally active and do not encourage you to be active. You can help yourself and others by soliciting the encouragement of others or actually encouraging their participation.	A person abuses alcohol. If friends and family also abuse alcohol the abuse will probably continue. In some cases it is best to find support elsewhere and then seek support of friends and family.
Overcoming Barriers This involves developing skills that allow you to overcome problems such as lack of facilities, lack of equipment, and inconvenience. People who develop skills to overcome barriers can learn to rearrange schedules, acquire personal equipment, and other skills that overcome these barriers.	A person lives 30 minutes from any fitness facilities and has no personal equipment that can be used to do exercise at home. This person can adapt by finding a new place to exercise, create inexpensive equipment that can be used at home, or plan a program that does not need facilities or equipment (see exercise concepts in this book).	The foods in a person's workplace are high in empty Calories and low in nutritional content. For this reason his/her nutrition is not what it could be. Skills in overcoming barrier's including planning and preparing your own food and selecting good foods (see concepts 14 and 19).

Table 21.1
Self-Management Skills (Continued)

Self-Management Skills	Examples for Physical Activity	Examples for other lifestyles
Learning Planning Skills This involves learning how to plan for yourself rather than having others do all the planning for you. Knowledge and practice in planning can help you develop these skills.	A person wants to start an activity program but doesn't know which activities to choose or when it is best to do them. Self-planning skills will help you plan your own activity program to meet personal needs.	A person wants to adopt other healthy lifestyles such as eating better. With knowledge and practice you can learn to use food labels and other information.
Learning Self-Assessment Skills This involves learning how to assess your own fitness, health and wellness. In addition it requires you to learn to interpret your own self-assessment results. With knowledge and practice these are skills you can learn.	A person wants to know his/her fitness strengths and weaknesses. The best procedure is to select good tests and self-administer them. Practicing the assessments at the end of many of the concepts in this book will help you self-assess and interpret results.	A person wants to assess other lifestyles. Using the procedures in this book many of these can be learned. Examples include stress and wellness assessment (concepts 18 and 20).
Managing Time This involves keeping records similar to self-monitoring. It relates to total time use rather than monitoring specific behaviors. Skillful monitoring of time can help you in planning and adhering to healthy lifestyles.	A person wants to be more active but says. "I am too busy." Monitoring time can help the person see how time is actually being used. This can help the person "find the time for activity."	A person wants more "quality time" with family and friends. Monitoring time can help a person re-allocate time to spend it in ways that are more consistent with personal priorities.
Learning Consumer Skills This involves gaining knowledge about products and services. It also may require rethinking untrue beliefs that may lead to poor consumer decisions (see concept 22).	A person avoids activity because previous decisions have resulted in purchase of "quack" devices that have made activity unenjoyable. Learning consumer decision skills will help you make better decisions.	A person takes in excessive calories leading to weight control problems. Decision-making skills would help read food labels and make better decisions about food.
Preventing Relapses This involves staying with a healthy behavior once you have adopted it. It is sometimes hard not to relapse to an old unhealthy behavior. There are skills such as avoiding high risk situations and learning how to say "no" that can help you avoid a relapse.	A person has been active for the last two weeks. The schedule is busy today and a relapse is possible. Some skills that will help the person to adhere are to set a schedule and stay with it (see concept 17), find support from others, have a planned statement to give for leaving work to go exercise.	People on a diet are at risk of a relapse. Learning how to refuse food in social situations is an example of a relapse prevention skill (see concept 14). Avoiding high risk situations is important.

skills, self-management skills do not happen automatically. To learn the skills listed in the table you may need the assistance of others and you will need to practice them. Information that will help you develop these skills is included throughout this text.

Suggested Readings

Dishman, R., and J. Sallis. "Determinants and Interventions for Physical Activity and Exercise." In Bouchard, C., et al. (Eds.), *Physical Activity, Fitness, and Health.* Champaign, IL: Human Kinetics Publishers, 1994.

King, A., et al. "Determinants of Physical Activity and Interventions in Adults." *Medicine and Science in Sports and Exercise* 24(1992):S221 (Supplement).

Sallis, J. "Influences on Physical Activity of Children, Adolescents, and Adults or Determinants of Active Living." *Physical Activity and Research Digest* 1(1994):1.

Sallis, J., et al. "Determinants of Physical Activity and Interventions in Youth." *Medicine and Science in Sports and Exercise* 24(1992):S248 (Supplement).

Surgeon General's Office. Surgeon General's Report on Physical Activity and Health. Washington, D.C.: U.S. Government Printing Office, (1996).

Score the Exercise Adherence Questionnaire as follows:

1. Give 2 points for every Very True answer, 1 point for each Somewhat True answer, and 0 points for each Not True answer.

2. Calculate your Predisposing Factors score by adding your points for items 1 through 7. This score indicates your general predisposition to start a physical activity program.

3. Calculate your Enabling Factors score by adding your points for items 8 through 11. This score indicates the extent to which you have the qualities necessary to continue a physical activity program once you have started one.

4. Calculate your Reinforcing Factors score by adding your points for items 12 through 15. This score indicates the encouragement and support you have for continuing your regular physical activity.

5. Calculate your Total Score by adding the three subtotals. This score gives you a general idea of your tendency to adhere to physical activity.

6. Use chart 21.2 to determine your ratings.

LAB RESOURCE MATERIALS

Chart 21.1 Physical Activity Adherence Questionnaire

The factors that predispose, enable, and reinforce physical activity adherence are listed below. Read each statement. Check the box under the most appropriate response for you.

	Very True	Somewhat True	Not True
PREDISPOSING FACTORS			
1. I am very knowledgeable about fitness and physical activity.	☐	☐	☐
2. I have a strong belief that physical activity is good for me.	☐	☐	☐
3. I enjoy doing regular exercise and physical activity.	☐	☐	☐
4. I am confident of my abilities in sports, exercise, and other physical activities.	☐	☐	☐
5. I am motivated to do physical activity without having to be encouraged by others or without receiving external rewards.	☐	☐	☐
6. I have been a regular exerciser most of my life.	☐	☐	☐
7. I like the way I look.	☐	☐	☐
			Subtotal _____
ENABLING FACTORS			
8. I possess good sports skills.	☐	☐	☐
9. I possess good general physical fitness.	☐	☐	☐
10. I have a place to exercise and equipment that I can use in or near my home.	☐	☐	☐
11. I am capable of setting my own physical activity goals and keeping track of my progress.	☐	☐	☐
			Subtotal _____
REINFORCING FACTORS			
12. I have the support of my family, especially my spouse, for doing my regular physical activity.	☐	☐	☐
13. I have many friends who enjoy the same kinds of physical activities that I do.	☐	☐	☐
14. I am successful in most physical activities that I try.	☐	☐	☐
15. I have a doctor and/or employer who encourages me to exercise.	☐	☐	☐
			Subtotal _____
			Total _____

Chart 21.2 Physical Activity Adherence Rating Scale

Classification	Predisposing Score	Enabling Score	Reinforcing Score	Total Score
Excellent	12–14	7–8	7–8	26–30
Very Good	10–11	6	6	22–25
Good	7–9	4–5	4–5	15–21
Fair	5–6	3	3	11–14
Poor	<5	<3	<3	<11

CONCEPT

·22·

Recognizing Quackery: Becoming an Informed Consumer

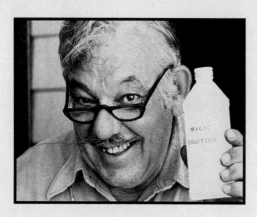

Concept 22

Caveat Emptor (Let the Buyer Beware) is a good motto for the consumer seeking advice or a program for developing or maintaining fitness, health, or wellness.

Introduction

People have always searched for the fountain of youth and the "easy," "quick," and "miraculous" route to health and happiness. This search has included the area of physical fitness, especially exercise and weight loss. Because of the popularity of these two subjects, the mass media have made it possible to convey as much *misinformation* as information. All people should seek the truth to protect their health as well as their pocketbooks. This concept discusses some myths and separates fact from fancy. Also see concepts 9, 12, and 19 for facts related to misconceptions.

Health Goal for the Year 2000

▬ Expand systems for dissemination of health information. (↑)

Note: (↑) indicates progress toward goal, (↓) indicates regression from goal, and (<>) indicates either no change or lack of new data since 1990.

Terms

▬ **AMA** Abbreviation for the American Medical Association.

▬ **FDA** Abbreviation for the Food and Drug Administration: a federal agency that recommends and enforces government regulations regarding certain foods and drugs.

▬ **Panacea** A cure-all; a remedy for all ills.

▬ **Passive Exercise** A type of exercise in which no voluntary muscle contraction occurs; some outside force moves the body part with no effort by the person.

▬ **Tonus** The most frequently misused and abused term in fitness vocabularies. It is "the resistance (tension) developed in a muscle as a result of passive stretch of the muscle. Tonus can not be determined by palpation or inspection of a muscle and has little or nothing to do with the voluntary strength of a muscle" (deLateur 1990).

Facts About Exercise

Exercise has many benefits, but it is not a **panacea**.

There are numerous benefits of exercise, many of which have been described throughout this book. However, some media accounts would have you believe the impossible. Those who contemplate beginning a fitness or weight reducing program are reminded of the following:

• The most satisfactory way to lose weight is to combine caloric reduction and exercise. There is *no fast and easy way*.

- Exercise will *not* change the size of bony structures (e.g., ankles).
- Exercise will *not* change the size of glands (e.g., breasts); however, chest/bust girth may be increased by strengthening chest muscles.
- Exercise does *not* break up fatty deposits, though it does burn calories, thus fat will eventually be burned.
- Exercise does *not* "ensure" good posture or good health, but it does help attain or maintain these attributes.
- There is *no* such thing as "effortless exercise."

Exercise, even of an active nature, is not effective in promoting physical fitness unless it meets the appropriate threshold of training.

Some popular literature suggests that only a few minutes of exercise a day are necessary to develop total physical fitness. Research, however, indicates that total fitness (cardiovascular fitness, strength, muscular endurance, flexibility, and desirable body composition) can be attained only through considerable effort. As mentioned previously, exercise must be of sufficient frequency (daily or every other day), intensity, and time (at least fifteen to thirty minutes *each* day you exercise) for it to be effective. Programs that promise complete fitness but do not meet the necessary levels for frequency, intensity, and time of exercise should be strongly questioned.

Contrary to some claims, hatha yoga is not a good program for developing physical fitness.

Some advocates of hatha yoga claim that regular practice of the asanas (positions) will bring about many benefits. There is *no* scientific evidence to support most of these claims. Hatha yoga will *not* help you lose weight, trim inches, remove flab, improve endurance, maintain proper circulation, strengthen glands and organs, or improve complexion as is claimed. Neither will it cure diseases or conditions such as arthritis, common cold, diabetes, gallstones, or menstrual disorders as claimed by some advocates.

Hatha yoga is considered useful for improving flexibility, although some positions are contraindicated (see concept 20). Hatha yoga is also useful in reducing stress reactions and in promoting neuromuscular relaxation. In some cases, it may be effective in lowering blood pressure in hypertensives. If a person has very weak muscles to begin with, mild (static) strengthening and muscular endurance may develop from assuming and holding the positions.

Getting rid of cellulite does not require a special exercise, diet, cream or device, as some books and advertisements insist.

Cellulite is ordinary fat with a fancy name. You do not need a special treatment or device to get rid of it. In fact, there is no special "remedy." Fat is fat. To decrease fat, reduce calories and exercise more.

"Spot reducing," or losing fat from a specific location on the body, is not possible. It is a fallacy.

When you exercise, calories are burned and fat is recruited from all over the body in a genetically determined pattern. You can not selectively exercise, bump, vibrate, or squeeze the fat from a particular spot. If you were flabby to begin with, local exercise could strengthen the local muscles, causing a change in the contour and the girth of that body part. But exercise affects the muscles, not the fat on that body part. General aerobic exercises are the most effective for burning fat, but you cannot control where the fat comes off.

Surgically sculpting the body with implants and liposuction to acquire physical beauty will not give you physical fitness and may be harmful.

Rather than doing it the hard way, an increasing number of people are having their "love handles" removed surgically and fake calf and pectoral muscles implanted to improve their physique. Liposuction is not a weight loss technique, but rather a contouring procedure. Like any surgery, it is not without risks. There have been fatalities and there is a risk of infection, hematoma, skin slough, and other conditions.

The muscle implants give a muscular appearance, but they do not make you stronger or more fit. The implants are not really muscle tissue, but rather silicon gel or saline such as that used in breast implants, or a hard substitute. Some complications can occur, such as infection and bleeding, but also, some physicians believe the calf implant may put pressure on the calf muscles and cause them to atrophy. A better way to improve physique and fitness is proper exercise.

The use of hand weights and wrist weights while walking, running, dancing, or bench-stepping can increase the energy cost but requires caution.

The practice of carrying small weights (1–3 pounds) while performing aerobic dance, walking, or other aerobic exercise has been found to increase the metabolic cost of the exercise. When the weight is simply carried, the effect is negligible, but when the arms are pumped (bending the elbow and raising the weight to shoulder height and then extending the elbow as the arm swings down) the energy output can increase enough to make a walk comparable to a slow jog. For the person who does not want to walk or jog faster or farther, it could be an effective way of burning more calories or increasing fitness. It may be better to use wrist weights than to carry a weight, since the act of gripping causes an increase in the diastolic blood pressure. The hand weights or wrist weights are more effective than ankle weights.

It has been suggested that for step-aerobics (bench-stepping), weights should be limited to intermediate and advanced steppers only and that they not exceed one or two pounds. Up to a point, the aerobic intensity can be increased by adding height to the bench (Fox and Broide 1991).

There are hazards to consider in using weights. Coronary patients and hypertensives should be aware that using weights increases both the systolic and diastolic blood pressures. Aerobic dance participants may find it wise to keep the weights below shoulder level if they aggravate the shoulder joint. Anyone with shoulder or elbow joint problems such as arthritis should use weights with caution.

Facts About Passive Exercise and Passive Devices

Passive exercise is not effective in weight reduction, spot reduction, increasing strength, or increasing endurance.

Passive exercise or devices come in a variety of forms.

- *Rolling machines*—These ineffective wooden or metal rollers, operated by an electric motor, roll up and down the body part to which they are applied. They do *not* remove, break up, or redistribute fat.
- *Vibrating belts*—These wide canvas or leather belts may be designed for the chin, hips, thighs, or abdomen. Driven by an electric motor, they jerk back and forth, causing loose tissue of the body part to shake. They do *not* have any beneficial effect on fitness, fat, or figure and they are potentially harmful if used on the abdomen (especially if used by women during pregnancy, menstruation, or while an IUD is in place). They might also aggravate a back problem.
- *Vibrating tables and pillows*—Some of these quack devices are actually called "toning tables." Contrary to advertisements, these passive devices will *not* improve posture, trim the body, reduce weight, nor will they develop muscle **tonus.** For some people, vibration can help induce relaxation.
- *Continuous Passive Motion Tables (CPM)*—The CPM table is motor driven, but unlike the vibrating table it moves body parts repeatedly through a range of motion. Tables are designed to do such things as passively extend the leg at the hip joint, raise the upper trunk in a sit-up-like motion, or rotate the legs while the client lies relaxed. Many of the same false claims are made for it as for the vibrating table. It also claims to remove cellulite, increase circulation and oxygen flow, and eliminate excess water retention. None of these claims is true, but the table might be justified in claiming to maintain the range of motion in certain body parts for people who cannot

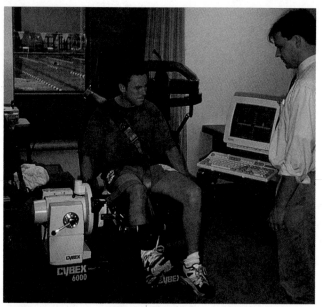

Doing machine exercises can help you recover from injury, but you must provide the movement —not the machine.

move themselves. A similar concept is incorporated in small, portable machines used in hospitals and rehabilitation centers to maintain range of motion in the leg of knee surgery patients, to maintain integrity of the cartilage, and decrease the incidence of thrombosis. Certainly the normal, healthy person has nothing to gain from using such a device.

- *Motor-driven cycles and rowing machines*—Like all mechanical devices that do the work for the individual, these motor-driven machines are *not* effective in a fitness program. They may help increase circulation, and some may even help maintain flexibility, but they are not as effective as active exercise. *Nonmotorized* cycles and rowing machines are very good equipment for use in a fitness program.
- *Massage*—Whether done by a masseur/masseuse or by a mechanical device, massage is passive, requiring no effort on the part of the individual. It can help increase circulation, induce relaxation, prevent or loosen adhesions, retard muscle atrophy, and serve other therapeutic uses when administered in the clinical setting for medical reasons, but massage has *no* useful role in a physical fitness program and will *not* alter your shape. There is no scientific evidence that it can hasten nerve growth, remove subcutaneous fat, or increase athletic performance.
- *Electrical muscle stimulators*—Neuromuscular electrical stimulators cause the muscle to contract involuntarily. In the hands of qualified medical personnel, muscle stimulators are valuable therapeutic devices. They can increase muscle strength and endurance selectively and aid in the treatment of edema. They can also help prevent atrophy in a patient who is unable to move, and they may decrease spasticity and contracture, but in a healthy person they do *not* have the same value as

exercise. The multiple muscle group stimulation as done in the so-called "toning clinics" or spas has been proven ineffective in muscle strengthening (Lake 1992). These devices can be harmful when used improperly and may induce heart attacks; complicate gastrointestinal, orthopedic, kidney, and other disorders; and aggravate epilepsy, hernias, and varicose veins. They should never be used by the layperson and have *no* place in a reducing or fitness program.

• *Weighted belts*—Claims have been made that these belts reduce waists, thighs, and hips when worn for several hours under the clothing. In reality, they do none of these things and have been reported to cause actual physical harm. When used in a progressive resistance program, wristlet, anklet, or laced-on weights can help produce an overload and, therefore, develop strength or endurance.

• *Inflated, constricting, or nonporous garments*—These garments include rubberized inflated devices ("sauna belts" and "sauna shorts") and paraphernalia that are airtight plastic or rubberized. Evidence indicates that their girth-reducing claims are *unwarranted*. If exercise is performed while wearing such garments, the exercise, *not* the garment, may be beneficial. You can *not* squeeze fat out of the pores *nor* can you melt it!

• *Body wrapping*—Some reducing salons, gyms, or clubs advertise that wrapping the body in bandages soaked in a "magic solution" will cause a permanent reduction in body girth. This so-called "treatment" is pure quackery. Tight, constricting bands can temporarily indent the skin and squeeze body fluids into other parts of the body, but the skin or body will regain its original size within minutes or hours. The solution used is usually something similar to epsom salts, which can cause fluid to be drawn from tissue. The fluid is water, not fat, and is quickly replaced. Body wrapping may be dangerous to your health; at least one fatality has resulted.

• *Elastic tights*—These are often worn by athletes such as cyclists for the purpose of decreasing chaffing of the skin. There have been some claims that the tights helped improve venous return and thus recovery from exercise. However, studies have shown that the recovery-response of those who wear tights is no different from that of nonwearers (Berry, et al., 1990).

Having a good tan is often associated with being fit and looking good, but getting tanned can be risky business.

Tanning salons may claim their lamps are safe because they emit only UV-A rays, but these rays can age the skin prematurely and make it look wrinkled and leathery. It may also increase the cancer-producing potential of UV-B rays and cause eye damage. Since there is no warning sign of redness, there is danger of overdosing. Thirty minutes of exposure to UV-A can suppress the immune system. Tanning devices can also aggravate certain skin diseases. The **FDA** advises against the

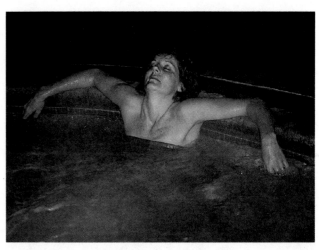

A hot tub may help you relax, but it does not improve fitness.

use of any suntan lamp. It is dangerous to use tanning accelerator lotions with the lamps because they can promote burning of the skin. Tanning pills are an even worse choice. They can cause itching, welts, hives, stomach cramps, and diarrhea, and can decrease night vision. Tanning in the sun is also hazardous because it damages the skin, making it age prematurely. It may cause skin cancer. It is best to use products with sun blockers if you must spend long periods in the sun.

Facts About Baths

Saunas, steambaths, whirlpools, and hot tubs are not effective in weight reduction or in the prevention and cure of colds, arthritis, bursitis, backaches, sprains, or bruises.

Baths do *not* melt off fat; fat must be metabolized. The heat and humidity from baths may make you perspire, but it is water, not fat, oozing from the pores.

The effect of such baths is largely psychological, although some temporary relief from aches and pains may result from the heat. The same relief can be had by sitting in a tub of hot water in your bathroom.

The so-called baths are potentially dangerous and should be used and maintained properly.

The following guidelines/precautions should be considered before using a sauna, steambath, whirlpool, or hot tub:

• Take a soap shower before and after entering the bath.
• Don't wear makeup or skin lotion/oil.
• Wait at least an hour after eating before bathing.
• Cool down after exercise before entering the bath to avoid overheating.
• Drink plenty of water before or during the bath to avoid dehydration.
• Don't wear jewelry.

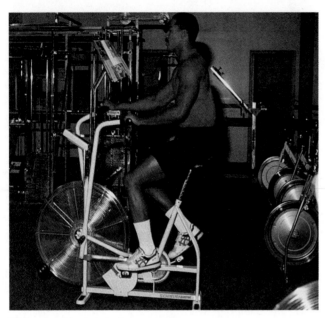

Visit a health club before you join.

- Don't sit on a metal stool; do sit on a towel in the steam or sauna bath.
- Don't bathe alone.
- Don't drink alcohol before bathing.
- Get out immediately if you become dizzy; feel hot, chilled, or nauseous; or get a headache.
- Get permission from your physician if you have heart disease, low or high blood pressure, a fever, kidney disease, or diabetes, are obese or pregnant, or are on medications (especially anticoagulants, stimulants, hypnotics, narcotics, or tranquilizers).
- Prolonged use can be hazardous for the elderly or for children.
- Don't exercise in a sauna or steam bath.
- Skin infections can be spread in a bath; make certain it is cleaned regularly and that the hot tub or whirlpool has proper pH and chlorination.
- Follow these recommendations on temperature and duration of stay:
  Sauna: should not exceed 190°F (88°C) and duration should not exceed ten to fifteen minutes.
  Steam Bath: should not exceed 120°F (49°C) and duration should not exceed six to twelve minutes.
  Whirlpool/Hot Tub: should not exceed 100°F (37°C) and duration should not exceed five to ten minutes.

Facts About Quacks

You can usually tell the difference between an expert and a quack because a quack does not use scientific methods.

A good example of this fact is seen in a study which attempted to obtain documentation supporting the claims of products claiming to enhance athletic performance. It was found that there was no published scientific evidence to support the promotional claims of 42 percent of the products. Thirty-two percent had some scientific documentation but were marketed in a misleading manner, and 21 percent were without any human clinical trials (*Annals of Pharmacotherapy,* 1993).

Some of the ways to identify quacks, frauds, and ripoffs are to look for these clues:

- They do not use the scientific method of controlled experimentation that can be verified by other scientists.
- To a large extent they use testimonials and anecdotes to support their claims rather than scientific methods. There is no such thing as a convincing testimonial. Anecdotal evidence is no evidence at all.
- They advise you to buy something you would not otherwise have bought.
- They have something to sell.
- They claim *everyone* can benefit from the product or service they are selling. There is no such thing as a simple, quick, easy, painless remedy/tonic or other concoction that is good for many ailments or useful for conditions for which medical science has not yet found a remedy ("Miracle Cures and Other Frauds," 1990).
- They promise "quick," "miraculous," results. There is no such thing as a perfect no-risk treatment.
- The claims for benefits are broad, covering a wide variety of conditions.
- They may offer a money-back guarantee. A guarantee is only as good as the company.
- They may claim the treatment or product is approved by the FDA. *Note:* Federal law does not permit the mention of the FDA in any way that suggests marketing approval.
- They may claim the support of experts, but the experts are not identified.
- The ingredients or materials in the product may not be identified.
- They may claim there is a conspiracy against them by "bureaucrats," "organized medicine," the FDA, the **AMA,** and other experts and governmental bodies. Never believe a doctor who claims the medical community is persecuting him/her or that the government is suppressing a wonderful discovery ("Miracle Cures and Other Frauds," 1990).
- Their credentials may be irrelevant to the area in which they claim expertise.
- They use scare tactics, such as "if you don't do this, you will die of a heart attack."
- They may appear to be a sympathetic friend who wants to share with you a "new discovery."
- They may quote from a scientific journal or other legitimate source, but they misquote or quote out of context to mislead you; or they may mix a little bit of truth with a lot of fiction.

- They may cite research or quote from individuals or institutions that have questionable reputations for scientific truth.
- They may claim it is a "new discovery" (usually it is said to have originated in Europe). There is never a great medical breakthrough that debuts in an obscure magazine or tabloid. There are no secret cures or magic formulae which have not been recognized by the scientific community, a picture on the cover of *Time* magazine, nomination for a Nobel prize, etc. ("Miracle Cures and Other Frauds," 1990).
- The product or organization named is often similar to that of a famous person or creditable institution (e.g., the "Mayo Diet" had no connection with the Mayo Clinic).
- They often sell products through the mail, which does not allow you to examine the product personally. There are no miracle products available only by mail order or from a single source.

> There are some common sense precautions one can take to avoid being a victim of a "rip-off."

The following suggestions can help protect you:

- Read the ad carefully, especially the small print.
- Do not send cash; use a check, money order, or credit card so you'll have a receipt.
- Do not order from a company with a P.O. box, unless you know the company.
- Do not let high-pressure sales tactics make you rush into a decision.
- Do not order from a company requiring use of an 800 telephone number and a credit card (they may be trying to avoid federal statutes).
- When in doubt, check out the company through your Better Business Bureau (BBB).
- If you have a complaint, write to the company first, but keep a copy of all receipts, checks, and correspondence.
- If that fails, write to the Direct Marketing Association. You may also report to the BBB, postmaster (if it was a mail order), state attorney general, and/or the Federal Trade Commission (FTC).

Facts About Equipment

> The consumer who plans to purchase exercise equipment should keep in mind certain guidelines to get the most for the money.

The following suggestions will help you select equipment:

- Unless you are wealthy or just like to collect gadgets, there is no need to buy a lot of exercise equipment. A complete fitness program can be carried out with *no*

equipment. If you learn to depend upon equipment, you may eventually feel that you cannot exercise unless you are at home or at a gym.
- If you do not like jogging or swimming, and you hate calisthenics, then the minimal equipment you may want to consider is a bicycle (regular or stationary), treadmill, or rowing machine for cardiovascular fitness; and a set of weights, pulleys, or isokinetic device for strength and endurance.
- Consult an expert if you want to know the effectiveness of a product. Individuals with college or university degrees in physical education, physical therapy, kinesiotherapy, and kinesiology should be able to give you good advice.
- Buy from a well-established, reputable company that will not disappear overnight and will back up warranties. Avoid mail-order products. If the product is not available in a retail store where it can be examined, you probably should not buy it.

Facts About "Health Clubs"

> It is not necessary to join a club, spa, or salon to develop fitness, but if you are considering joining such an establishment, make your choice with care.

The consumer should observe these precautions before becoming a member of a club, spa, or salon:

- Do not expect "miraculous" results as advertised.
- Be prepared to haggle over price and to resist a very hard sell for a long-term contract.
- Choose a no-contract, pay-as-you-go establishment if possible. Otherwise, choose the shortest term contract available.
- If there is a contract, read the fine print carefully and look for:
  1. the interest rate;
  2. "confession of judgment" clauses waiving your right to defend yourself in court;
  3. noncancelable clauses;
  4. "holder-in-due-course" doctrines allowing the establishment to sell your note to a collection agency;
  5. a waiver of the establishment's liability for injury to you on the premises.
- Consult with an independent expert if you have questions about the programs offered by the establishment.
- Do not accept diets, drugs, or food supplements from the club. Your physician will prescribe these if they are needed.
- You do not have to conform to the program the club suggests for you. Do not perform dangerous exercises, or passive exercises, or participate in fraudulent "treatments." Choose only those activities that meet the criteria explained in this book.

- Refuse to be pestered by solicitations for new members.
- Make a trial visit to the establishment during the hours when you would normally expect to use the facility to determine if it is open, if it is over-crowded, if the equipment is available, if the attendants are selling rather than assisting, and if you would enjoy the company of the other patrons.
- Determine the qualifications of the personnel, especially of the individual responsible for your program. Is he or she an expert as defined previously?
- Make certain the club is a well-established facility that will not disappear overnight.
- Check its reputation with the Better Business Bureau in your area.
- Investigate the programs offered by the Y, local colleges and universities, and municipal park and recreation departments. These agencies often have excellent fitness classes at lower prices than commercial establishments and usually employ qualified personnel. For weight loss, investigate franchised clubs, such as Weight Watchers or TOPS, or affiliate with a university or a hospital-based program.

Facts About Fitness Books, Magazines, and Articles

> All fitness books do not provide scientifically sound, accurate, and reliable information.

Because publishers are motivated by profit and publishing is a highly competitive field, the choice of material to be printed is often selected on the basis of how popular, famous, or attractive the author is, or how sensational or unusual his or her ideas are. Movie stars, models, TV personalities, and even Olympic athletes are rarely experts in biomechanics, anatomy and physiology, exercise, and other foundations of physical fitness. Having a good figure/physique, being fit, or having gone through a training program does not, in itself, qualify a person to advise others.

If you have read the facts presented in the other concepts, you should be able to distinguish between fact and fiction. To assist you further, however, there are ten guidelines listed in question form in the lab resource materials (Chart 22.1). These might help you evaluate whether or not a book, magazine, or article on exercise and fitness is valid, reliable, and scientifically sound. If the answer to each of the questions is not "yes," then you should be suspicious of the material. If in doubt, ask one or more experts, or write to the American Alliance of Health, Physical Education, Recreation and Dance (AAHPERD) or to the American College of Sports Medicine (ACSM) (see addresses in list of references at the end of this book). These organizations will refer your question to an appropriate expert.

Suggested Readings

Barrett, S. and Jarvis, W. Eds. *The Health Robbers: a Close Look at Quackery in America.* Buffalo, NY. Prometheus Books, 1993.

Berry, M. J., et al. "The Effects of Elastic Tights on the Post-Exercise Response." *Canadian Journal of Applied Sports Sciences* 15(1990):244.

Cardinal, B. J. "Rating the Clubs: A Health and Fitness Center Consumer Checklist." *American Fitness* Sept./Oct. 1994.

Consumer Reports. "Health clubs: The right choice." 61(1996):27.

Cornacchea, J. S. O., and Barrett, S. *Consumer Health,* 5th ed. C. V. Mosby, 1993.

deLateur, B. J., and J. F. Lehmann. "Therapeutic Exercise to Develop Strength and Endurance." In *Krusen's Handbook of Physical Medicine and Rehabilitation.* 4th ed. Kotke S. O. Lehman, Eds. Philadelphia: W. B. Saunders, 1990, pp. 480–95.

Fox, M., and D. Broide. *Molly Fox's Step On It.* New York: Avon Books, 1991.

"Health Spas, Exercise Clubs, etc." *Information For Prudent Consumers.* National Council Against Health Fraud. Loma Linda, CA 1994.

Lake, D. A. "Neuromuscular Stimulation: An Overview and Its Implications in the Treatment of Sports Injuries." *Sports Medicine* 13(1992):320–36.

Lightsey, D. M. "Deceptive Tactics Used in Marketing Purported Ergogenic Aids." *National Strength and Conditioning Association Journal.* 14:2 (1992):26.

"Miracle Cures and Other Frauds." *Johns Hopkins Medical Letter* 1(1990).

"Natural Products for Athletic Performance." *Annals of Pharmacotherapy* 27(1993):607.

"Shearing the Suckers." *Consumer Reports.* (February 1986):87.

LAB RESOURCE MATERIALS

Chart 22.1 Exercise/Device Evaluation*

	Yes	No			Yes	No
1. Is the article or book written by an expert as defined in this Concept?	☐	☐		7. Does it employ "active" exercise in which your own muscles contract?	☐	☐
2. Does the exercise/device employ the overload principle?	☐	☐		8. Are the benefits claimed for it reasonable?	☐	☐
3. Does it employ the progression principle?	☐	☐		9. Are the authors trying to help you (rather than selling a product)?	☐	☐
4. Does it employ the F.I.T. formula?	☐	☐		10. Do they refrain from using terms such as "quick," "miraculous," "tone," "remove fat," "new discovery," or other gimmick words?	☐	☐
5. Does it employ the principle of specificity?	☐	☐				
6. Is it a safe exercise?	☐	☐				

*If in doubt, you may seek an expert's opinion on some of these questions.

Chart 22.2 Health Club Ev.aluation

	Yes	No	Notes
1. Were claims for improvement in weight, figure/physique, or fitness realistic?	☐	☐	_____
2. Was a long-term contract (1–3 years) encouraged?	☐	☐	_____
3. Was the sales pitch high-pressure to make an immediate decision?	☐	☐	_____
4. Were you given a copy a the contract to read at home?	☐	☐	_____
5. Did the fine print include objectionable clauses?	☐	☐	_____
6. Did they recommend a physician's approval prior to joining?	☐	☐	_____
7. Did they sell diet supplements as a side line?	☐	☐	_____
8. Did they have passive equipment?	☐	☐	_____
9. Did they have cardiovascular training equipment or facilities (cycles, track, pool, aerobic dance)?	☐	☐	_____
10. Did they have unscientific claims for the equipment, exercise, baths, or diet supplements?	☐	☐	_____
11. Were the facilities clean?	☐	☐	_____
12. Were the facilities crowded?	☐	☐	_____
13. Were thee days and hours when facilities were open but would not be available to you?	☐	☐	_____
14. Were there limits on the number of minutes you could use a piece of equipment?	☐	☐	_____
15. Did the floor personnel closely supervise and assist clients	☐	☐	_____
16. Were the floor personnel qualified "experts"?	☐	☐	_____
17. Were the managers/owners qualified "experts"?	☐	☐	_____
18. Has the club been in business at this location for a year or more?	☐	☐	_____

CONCEPT
·23·

Planning Lifestyles for Optimal Health and Wellness

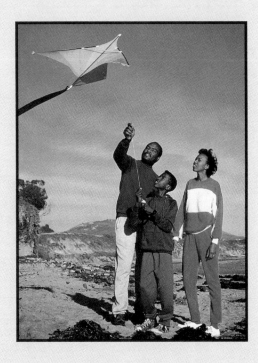

Concept 23

Lifestyle planning is necessary if optimal health and wellness are to be achieved.

Introduction

The nation's foremost health goal for the year 2000 is to increase the *optimally healthy* span of life for all of us. Living a long time, by itself, is not as important as living a healthy life that is full and rewarding. When they established the health goals for the year 2000, the nation's health leaders pointed out that health is more than preventing death and disease, it is also improved quality of life. Thus one's sense of well-being must also be considered.

Progress has been made in extending the life span of Americans since the goals for the year 2000 were established but we have not been effective in increasing the number of years of quality living. If the goals of increased quality of life is to be achieved, it is important that we practice healthy lifestyles. Unhealthful lifestyles account for more than one half of the early deaths in our society. Unhealthy environment is another significant source of early deaths and less than quality living. It is for this reason that practicing healthy lifestyles is so important. Suggestions for effective lifestyle planning are outlined in this concept.

Health Goals for the Year 2000

- Increase the life span of Americans. (↑)
- Increase the span of optimally healthy life. (<>)

Note: (↑) indicates progress toward goal, (↓) indicates regression from goal, and (<>) indicates either no change or lack of new data since 1990.

Terms

- **Behavioral Goal**   A statement of intent to perform a specific behavior. A behavioral goal is associated with changing a lifestyle. An example is: "I will reduce the fat consumed in my diet to 30 percent or less."
- **Outcome Goal**   A statement of intent to achieve a specific performance or standard associated with good health or wellness. An example is: "I will achieve a systolic blood pressure of 140 or less."

The Facts

There are certain areas of living that have great potential for improving wellness.

Some of the lifestyles identified in this book that have potential for improving health and wellness are outlined in table 28.1. Taking action to modify lifestyles in any of these areas that need attention can be useful for enhancing health and wellness.

Table 23.1

Healthy Lifestyles

- Exercising regularly
- Eating properly
- Controlling stress
- Avoiding destructive habits
- Practicing safe sex
- Adopting safety habits
- Learning first aid
- Adopting personal health behaviors
- Seeking and complying with medical advice
- Becoming an informed consumer
- Protecting the environment
- Managing time effectively

There are several steps that you can take to help change your lifestyle for better health and wellness.

Step 1—Identify areas of possible change

Consider possible lifestyle changes in the areas outlined in table 28.1. Are changes in any of these areas appropriate for you? (A checklist is provided in the Lab accompanying this concept.)

Step 2—Establish goals

Establishing goals can help you effectively change your lifestyle for health and wellness. There are several guidelines that can help you establish meaningful goals.

- Set goals that are attainable. It is easier to attain small goals. Each small success encourages you to persist in your long-term efforts to change your lifestyle.
- Set only a few goals at one time. Too many goals can lead to failure.
- For most people, **behavioral goals** are better than **outcome goals,** especially for the short term. A goal such as reducing your caloric intake by 200 calories every day is a behavioral goal. Trying to lose 20 pounds is an outcome goal. If you do the process (changing your lifestyle) on a consistent basis, you *will* meet your outcome goals.
- Make your goals specific. Specific goals help you evaluate to keep records and to determine if you have been successful in meeting your goals.
- Put your goals in writing. Making a written statement of goals allows you to keep records and can provide motivation for making lifestyle changes.

Step 3—Develop a plan for meeting your goals

Based on the areas of change identified in Step 1 and the goals established in Step 2, write out a plan for meeting your goals. Typically a plan includes a schedule (days and times) for performing the behavior outlined in your goals. For example, if you establish the goal of doing relaxation exercises for 15 minutes, five days a week, you should mark a calendar indicating the days you plan to do the exercises and the time of the day you plan to perform them. If your goal is to learn CPR, you should write down a date for calling to schedule a CPR class and a tentative date for going to the class.

Reminders can be useful in keeping with your plan. For example, if your plan calls for you to floss your teeth each night before you go to bed, you might tape a message to your mirror to remind you to do the flossing behavior.

Step 4—Keep records

Use your written plan to keep records. If you perform the lifestyle behavior as planned, make a check on the calendar. If you did not do the behavior as scheduled, reschedule it on your calendar. At the end of a specified period (a week or two), check to see if your plan is working. If, in the scheduled time, you have check marks for most of the days in your lifestyle plan, you will be well on the way to lifestyle change. You will be ready to develop a new plan (see Step 5). If you have only a few checks by the lifestyle behaviors in your plan, you will need to identify why you are not meeting your goals. The most common reasons for failure are:

- You established goals that were too hard or unrealistic.
- You established too many goals to accomplish during one short period of time.
- Your schedule may not have been well suited to your daily routine and may need modification.
- You lack commitment to the goals. If this is the case, you may need the assistance of a professional in meeting your goals.

Step 5—Evaluate and modify

If you were successful in performing most of the lifestyle behaviors that you wrote in your plan, go back to Step 2 and re-establish new short-term goals. Repeat Steps 3 and 4. After you have met your short-term goals several times, you may want to check to see if you are coming close to setting your long-term goals. By this time you will be well on your way to significant lifestyle change. Once you have made the new behaviors into "good habits," you may not need to continue to include them in your lifestyle plan. You may, at this time, want to start to work on meeting some new lifestyle goals.

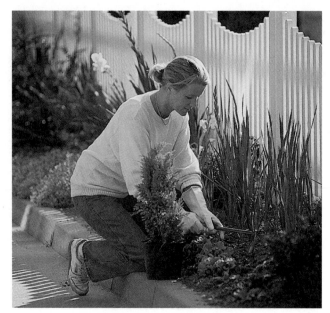

Making one lifestyle change, such as taking time for recreation, can lead to other changes.

If you have failed to live up to your plan, you may want to modify it to make it more realistic and to increase your chances of success. Go back to Step 1 and begin again. Try to determine why your previous plan was not successful.

> Sometimes lifestyle changes cannot be made without the assistance of others.

The support of friends and family can be very important in helping you to accomplish lifestyle changes. Friends and family play a significant role in exercise adherence. The same is true for other behaviors. For example, family members can help you reduce the fat calories in your diet by cooking special foods and not preparing high-fat meals. Friends can encourage friends to fasten their seat belts.

There are some lifestyle changes that may require the assistance of a professional. If your attempts to change your lifestyle meet with failure, don't set yourself up for repeated failure. Get help!

Most colleges have programs through their health center that provide free, confidential assistance or referral. Many businesses now have Employee Assistance Programs (EAP). The programs have counselors who will help you or your family members find help with a particular problem. The EAP staff are dedicated to help you *without revealing personal information to your employer*. These programs have a strong record for helping people with problems ranging from small to very serious, such as drug addiction or smoking cessation. Many other programs and support groups are now available to help you change your lifestyle. For example, most hospitals and many health organizations now have hotlines that provide you with referral services for establishing healthy lifestyles.

> One positive lifestyle change often leads to another.

If you make one significant lifestyle change to enhance wellness you are likely to make other changes. For example, people who begin a regular exercise program and adhere to it over a period of time are also likely to make modifications in diet and adopt effective stress-reduction procedures. Those who smoke are more likely to stop if they have been successful in becoming a regular exerciser or a healthy eater.

The wellness lifestyle seems to be contagious. The key is to start slowly to increase the chance of success. Remember, the ultimate goal for the year 2000 is increasing the span of optimally healthy life. This is best accomplished by altering lifestyles in a consistent and regular manner. The nation's health leaders believe that a commitment by each individual combined with scientific knowledge, professional skills, community support, and political effort will enable each of us to achieve our potential to live full, active lives.

Suggested Readings

Bruess, C., and G. Richardson. *Decisions for Health*. 4th ed. Dubuque, IA: Wm. C. Brown Publishers, 1995.

McGinnis, J. M., and P. R. Lee. "Healthy People 2000 at Mid Decade," *Journal of the American Medical Association*, 273(1995):1123.

Public Health Service. *Healthy People 2000: National Health Promotion and Disease Prevention Objectives*. Washington, DC: U.S. Government Printing Office, 1991.

LAB 1A

Physical Activity Questionnaire

Name _____ Section _____ Date _____

PURPOSE

The purposes of this laboratory are:

1. To evaluate your feelings concerning physical activity.
2. To determine the specific reasons why you do or do not participate in regular physical activity.

PROCEDURE

1. Read each of the fourteen items in the Physical Activity Questionnaire in the Lab Resource Materials.
2. After each statement, check one box indicating whether you strongly agree, agree, disagree, or strongly disagree with it. If you are unsure of your answer, check undecided.
3. When all fourteen items have been answered, use the scoring procedure in the Lab Resource Materials to score the Physical Activity Questionnaire.
4. Record your results.

RESULTS

1. After you have determined seven different physical activity questionnaire scores and your "balance of feelings" score, use the Physical Activity Questionnaire Rating Scale in the Lab Resource Materials to determine your rating for each score.
2. Check your rating for each of the seven reasons for exercising and your "balance of feelings" rating in the chart below.

	Excellent	Good	Fair	Poor	Very Poor
Health and fitness	☐	☐	☐	☐	☐
Fun and enjoyment	☐	☐	☐	☐	☐
Relaxation and tension release	☐	☐	☐	☐	☐
Challenge and achievement	☐	☐	☐	☐	☐
Social	☐	☐	☐	☐	☐
Appearance	☐	☐	☐	☐	☐
Competition	☐	☐	☐	☐	☐
Balance of feelings	☐	☐	☐	☐	☐

CONCLUSIONS AND IMPLICATIONS

Read concept 1 before completing this section. Experts indicate that people who have a "positive balance of feelings" about physical activity (have more positive feelings than negative ones) and who score well on several of the different scales are more likely to be active.

1. In a few sentences discuss your results on the Physical Activity Questionnaire (ratings for seven scores). Include comments on whether you think your ratings suggest that you will be active or inactive and whether your ratings are really indicative of your feelings.

2. In a few sentences discuss your "balance of feelings" rating. Include comments on whether you think your ratings suggest that you will be active or inactive and whether your ratings are really indicative of your feelings. Do you think that the scores on which you were rated "poor" or "very poor" might be reasons why you would avoid physical activity? Explain.

Chart 1.1 Physical Activity Questionnaire

The term "physical activity" in the following statements refers to all kinds of activities, including sports, formal exercises, and informal activities, such as jogging and cycling. Check your answers first, then read the directions for scoring, found in the Lab Resource Materials for Concept 1, on page 14.

	Strongly Agree	Agree	Undecided	Disagree	Strongly Disagree	Score
1. I should exercise regularly for my own good health and physical fitness.	☐	☐	☐	☐	☐	_____
2. One of the main reasons I do regular physical activity is because it is fun.	☐	☐	☐	☐	☐	_____
3. I enjoy taking part in physical activity because it helps me to relax and get away from the pressures of daily living.	☐	☐	☐	☐	☐	_____
4. The challenge of physical training is one reason why I participate in physical activity.	☐	☐	☐	☐	☐	_____
5. One of the things I like about physical activity is the participation with other people.	☐	☐	☐	☐	☐	_____
6. Regular exercise helps me look my best.	☐	☐	☐	☐	☐	_____
7. Competition is a good way to keep a game from being fun.	☐	☐	☐	☐	☐	_____
8. Doing regular physical activity can be as harmful to health as it is helpful.	☐	☐	☐	☐	☐	_____
9. Doing exercise and playing sports is boring.	☐	☐	☐	☐	☐	_____
10. Participating in physical activities makes me tense and nervous.	☐	☐	☐	☐	☐	_____
11. Most sports and physical activities are too difficult for me to enjoy.	☐	☐	☐	☐	☐	_____
12. I do not enjoy physical activities that require the participation of other people.	☐	☐	☐	☐	☐	_____
13. Doing regular physical activity does little to make me more physically attractive.	☐	☐	☐	☐	☐	_____
14. Competing against others in physical activities makes them enjoyable.	☐	☐	☐	☐	☐	_____

Physical Fitness Stunts

Name	Section	Date

This laboratory is not designed primarily to assess your fitness. These stunts are designed to help you better understand the nature of each component of physical fitness. Later in this book you will learn how to do accurate assessments for each fitness component. Read concept 1 before completing this lab.

PURPOSE

The purposes of this laboratory are:

1. To help you identify different components of physical fitness. Through participation in these stunts you can see the differences between the various aspects of physical fitness.
2. To help you gain insight into the importance of various physical fitness components.

PROCEDURE

Perform all of the physical fitness stunts as described in chart 1.3 in the Lab Resource Materials for concept 1 on pages 16–17. Record your results in the appropriate blank opposite each item.

RESULTS

As noted at the beginning of this lab, the stunts that you tried are not good tests of fitness, but attempting the stunts may help you see that fitness is not just one thing; it is many different things. Circle the number of different health-related and skill-related physical fitness stunts you passed.

Skill-related   1 2 3 4 5 6

Health-related   1 2 3 4 5

CONCLUSIONS AND IMPLICATIONS

1. Explain your performance on the health-related fitness stunts. In several sentences indicate whether you thought the stunts were good indicators of each fitness part and whether your performance on the stunts was reflective of your true health-related physical fitness.

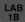

2. Explain your performance on the skill-related fitness stunts. In several sentences indicate whether you thought the stunts were good indicators of each fitness part and whether your performance on the stunts was reflective of your true skill-related physical fitness.

3. In several sentences predict the components of health-related physical fitness in which you think you will score well and which you do not think you will score so well when you take more accurate tests of fitness at a later time. Give reasons for your answer.

LAB 2

Assessing Heart Disease Risk Factors

Name _____   Section _____   Date _____

PURPOSE

The purpose of this lab is to assess your risk of developing coronary heart disease.

PROCEDURE

1. Complete the ten questions on the Heart Disease Risk Factor Questionnaire by circling the answer that is most appropriate for *you* (see back of this page).
2. Look at the top of the column for each of your answers. In the space provided at the right of each question, write down the number of risk points for that answer.
3. Determine your unalterable risk score by adding the risk points for questions 1, 2, and 3.
4. Determine your alterable risk score by adding the risk points for questions 4 through 10.
5. Determine your total heart disease risk score by adding the scores obtained in steps 3 and 4.
6. Look up your risk ratings on the Heart Disease Risk Rating Scale (chart 2.1).

RESULTS

Write your risk scores and risk ratings in the appropriate blanks below.

	Score	Rating
Unalterable risk	_____	_____
Alterable risk	_____	_____
Total heart disease risk	_____	_____

Chart 2.1 Heart Disease Risk Rating Scale			
Rating	**Unalterable Score**	**Alterable Score**	**Total Score**
Very high	9 or More	21 or More	31 or More
High	7–8	15–20	26–30
Average	5–6	11–14	16–25
Low	4 or Less	10 or Less	15 or Less

CONCLUSIONS AND IMPLICATIONS

The higher your score on the Heart Disease Risk Factor Questionnaire, the greater your heart disease risk. In several sentences discuss your risk for heart disease. Which of the risk factors do you need to control to reduce your risk of heart disease? Why?

Heart Disease Risk Factor Questionnaire

Circle the appropriate answer to each question.

Risk Points

	1	2	3	4	Score
Unalterable Factors					
1. How old are you?	30 or less	31–40	41–54	55+	_____
2. Do you have a history of heart disease in your family?	none	grandparent with heart disease	parent with heart disease	more than one with heart disease	_____
3. What is your sex?	female		male		_____
				Total Unalterable Risk Score	_____
Alterable Factors					
4. What is your percent of body fat?	F=20%↓ M=15%↓	25%↓ 20%↓	30%↓ 25%↓	35%↑ 30%↑	_____
5. Do you have a high-fat diet?	no	slightly high in fat	above normal in fat	eat a lot of meat, fried and fatty foods	_____
6. What is your blood pressure? (systolic, or upper, score)	120↓	121–140	141–160	160↑	_____
7. Do you have other diseases?	no	ulcer	*diabetes	both	_____
8. Do you exercise regularly?	4–5 days a week	3 days a week	less than 3 days a week	no	_____
9. Do you smoke?	no	cigar or pipe	less than ½ pack a day	more than ½ pack a day	_____
10. Are you under much stress?	less than normal	normal	slightly above normal	quite high	_____
				Total Alterable Risk Score	_____
				Grand Total Risk Score	_____

*Diabetes is a risk factor that is often not alterable.

From CAD Risk Assessor, William J. Stone, *Adult Fitness Programs*, 1987. Reprinted by permission of William J. Stone.

LAB 3A

Physical Activity Readiness

Name _____   Section _____   Date _____

■ Read concept 3 before completing this laboratory.

PURPOSE

The purpose of this lab is to help you determine your physical readiness for participation in a program of regular exercise.

PROCEDURE

1. Read the directions on the "PAR-Q & You" form shown in the Lab Resource Materials for this concept on page L-8.
2. Answer each of the seven questions on the form.
3. If you answered "yes" to one or more of the questions, follow the directions just below the PAR-Q questions regarding medical consultation.
4. If you answered "no" to all seven questions, follow the directions at the lower left-hand corner of the PAR-Q.
5. If you plan to participate in competitive sports or vigorous training, answer the five questions in chart 3.2 (Physical Readiness for Sports or Vigorous Training in the Lab Resource Materials).

RESULTS

PHYSICAL ACTIVITY READINESS QUESTIONNAIRE (PAR-Q)

Circle the number of "yes" answers that you had for the Physical Activity Readiness Questionnaire.

| 0 | 1 | 2 | 3 | 4 | 5 | 6 | 7 |

PHYSICAL READINESS FOR SPORTS OR VIGOROUS TRAINING

Circle the number of "yes" answers that you had for the Physical Readiness for Sports or Vigorous Training questionnaire from chart 3.2.

| 0 | 1 | 2 | 3 | 4 | 5 |

CONCLUSIONS AND IMPLICATIONS

In several sentences, discuss your readiness for physical activity. Base your comments on your PAR-Q (chart 3.1) results and the additional questions in chart 3.2 in the Lab Resource Materials as well as on the types of physical activities you plan to perform in the future.

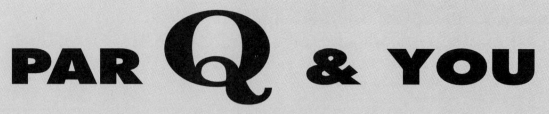

PAR Q & YOU

Regular physical activity is fun and healthy, and increasingly more people are starting to become more active every day. Being more active is very safe for most people. However, some people should check with their doctor before they start becoming much more physically active.

If you are planning to become much more physically active than you are now, start by answering the seven questions in the box below. If you are between the ages of 15 and 69, the PAR-Q will tell you if you should check with your doctor before you start. If you are over 69 years of age, and you are not used to being very active, check with your doctor.

Common sense is your best guide when you answer these questions. Please read the questions carefully and answer each one honestly: check YES or NO.

YES	NO	
☐	☐	1. Has your doctor ever said that you have a heart condition <u>and</u> that you should only do physical activity recommended by a doctor?
☐	☐	2. Do you feel pain in your chest when you do physical activity?
☐	☐	3. In the past month, have you had chest pain when you were not doing physical activity?
☐	☐	4. Do you lose your balance because of dizziness or do you ever lose consciousness?
☐	☐	5. Do you have a bone or joint problem that could be made worse by a change in your physical activity?
☐	☐	6. Is your doctor currently prescribing drugs (for example, water pills) for your blood pressure or heart condition?
☐	☐	7. Do you know of <u>any other reason</u> why you shoud not do physical activity?

If
You
Answered

Yes →

YES to one or more questions

Talk with your doctor by phone or in person BEFORE you start becoming much more physically active or BEFORE you have a fitness appraisal. Tell your doctor about the PAR-Q and which questions you answered YES.

- You may be able to do any activity you want—as long as you start slowly and build up gradually. Or, you may need to restrict your activities to those which are safe for you. Talk with your doctor about the kinds of activities you wish to participate in and follow his/her advice.
- Find out which community programs are safe and helpful for you.

No →

NO to all questions

If you answered NO honestly to <u>all</u> PAR-Q questions, you can be reasonably sure that you can:
- start becoming much more physically active—begin slowly and build up gradually. This is the safest and easiest way to go.
- take part in a fitness appraisal—this is an excellent way to determine your basic fitness so that you can plan the best way for you to live actively.

DELAY BECOMING MUCH MORE ACTIVE:
- if you are not feeling well because of a temporary illness such as a cold or a fever—wait until you feel better; or
- if you are or may be pregnant—talk to your doctor before you start becoming more active.

Please note: If your health changes so that you then answer YES to any of the above questions, tell your fitness or health professional. Ask whether you should change your physical activity plan.

<u>Informed Use of the PAR-Q</u>: The Canadian Society for Exercise Physiology, Health Canada, and their agents assume no liability for persons who undertake physical activity, and if in doubt after completing this questionnaire, consult your doctor prior to physical activity.

You are encouraged to copy the PAR-Q but only if you use the entire form

*Developed by the British Columbia Ministry of Health.

Produced by the British Columbia Ministry of Health and the Department of National Health & Welfare

Physical Activity Readiness
Questionnaire • PAR-Q
(revised 1994)

Note: It is important that you answer all questions honestly. The PAR-Q is a scientifically and medically researched pre-exercise selection device. It complements exercise programs, exercise testing procedures, and the liability considerations attendant with such programs and testing procedures. PAR-Q, like any other preexercise screening device, will misclassify a small percentage of prospective participants, but no preexercise screening method can entirely avoid this problem.

L A B 3B

The Warm-up and Cool-down

Name   Section   Date

■ Read concept 3 before completing this lab.

PURPOSE

The purpose of this lab is to familiarize you with a sample group of exercises that can be used as a warm-up or cool-down for aerobic types of workout.

PROCEDURE

Perform the exercises entitled, "A Sample Warm-up and Cool-down for an Aerobic Workout" (see pages 35–37 of concept 3).

RESULTS

1. In which of the stretches did you feel the most tightness? Check the amount of "tightness" you felt for each stretch exercise (on the chart below).

	None	Moderate	Severe
Calf stretcher	☐	☐	☐
Back-saver toe touch	☐	☐	☐
Leg hug	☐	☐	☐
Side stretch	☐	☐	☐
Zipper	☐	☐	☐

2. Did you notice an increase in heart rate during the cardiovascular warm-up? Yes ☐ No ☐

CONCLUSIONS AND IMPLICATIONS

1. In several sentences discuss the sample warm-up. Include a discussion of whether the warm-up is adequate for you (if so give reasons) or whether you would have to supplement the warm-up with additional exercises (if so what exercises would you add and why). *Note:* Those who plan sports and/or other more vigorous physical activities will need to include activities to warm-up the specific muscle groups to be used.

2. In several sentences discuss the sample cool-down. Include a discussion of whether the cool-down is adequate for you (if so give reasons) or whether you would have to supplement the cool-down with additional exercises (if so what exercises would you add and why).

LAB 5A

Evaluating Cardiovascular Fitness

Name _____ Section _____ Date _____

PURPOSE

The purposes of this laboratory are:
1. To acquaint you with several methods for evaluating cardiovascular fitness.
2. To help you evaluate and rate your own cardiovascular fitness.

PROCEDURE

Perform one or more of the four cardiovascular fitness tests described in the Lab Resource Materials. Determine your ratings on the test(s) using the rating charts provided.

RESULTS

Record the information obtained from taking the cardiovascular fitness test(s) (one or more) in the space provided.

Twelve-Minute Run

(Distance)_____ miles

Rating _____ (Chart 5.1 on page 65)

Rockport Walking Test

(Time) _____ minutes

Heart rate _____ bpm

Rating _____ (Charts 5.5 and 5.6, page 67 and 68)

The Step Test

Heart rate _____ bpm

Rating _____ (Chart 5.2, page 66)

The Bicycle Test

Workload _____ kpm

Heart rate _____ bpm

Weight _____ lbs

Weight in kg* _____

ml/O$_2$/kg _____

Rating _____
(Chart 5.4, page 67)

*Weight in lbs ÷ 2.2

CONCLUSIONS AND IMPLICATIONS

1. In several sentences explain why you selected the test or tests you chose. If you only selected one test explain why.

2. In several sentences explain your results. Discuss your perception of the accuracy of the test results. Also discuss whether you think you might have gotten different results if you had taken another test, and if so, why.

3. In several sentences discuss your current level of cardiovascular fitness and steps that you should take in the future to maintain or improve it.

LAB 5B

Counting the Target Heart Rate

Name _____   Section _____   Date _____

PURPOSE

The purposes of this laboratory session are:

1. To learn to count carotid pulse.
2. To learn to count radial pulse.
3. To understand the threshold of training and target zone concepts.
4. To establish a personal minimal cardiovascular threshold of training.
5. To establish a personal target zone for cardiovascular fitness.
6. To determine the specific jogging speed necessary to elevate your heart rate to threshold of training and target zones.

PROCEDURE

1. Practice counting the number of pulses felt for a given period of time at both the carotid and radial locations. Use a clock or watch to count for fifteen, thirty, and sixty seconds. To establish your heart rate in beats per minute, multiply your fifteen-second count by four, and your thirty-second count by two.
2. Practice locating your carotid and radial pulses quickly. This is important when trying to count your pulse after exercise.
3. Practice counting the pulse of another person using both the wrist and carotid locations (do not use your thumb).
4. One partner should run a quarter-mile, then the other partner should count her or his heart rate at the end of the run (use carotid pulse). Try to run at a rate you think will keep the rate of the heart above the threshold of training and in the target zone. Use fifteen-second pulse counts and multiply by four to get heart rate in beats per minute (bpm). Record the bpm in the Results section.
5. Repeat, alternating roles, the second person running and the first person counting heart rate. Record the results.
6. Repeat the test so each person runs a second time. Record the results.

RESULTS

Record the various **resting** pulse counts for carotid and radial pulses. Spaces are provided for a self-measurement and measurements made of your pulse by a partner. You do *not* need to record your partner's measurements.

Carotid Pulse (self)	**Heart Rate per Minute**	**Carotid Pulse (by a partner)**	**Heart Rate per Minute**
_____ 15 seconds × 4	_____	_____ 15 seconds × 4	_____
_____ 30 seconds × 2	_____	_____ 30 seconds × 2	_____
_____ 60 seconds × 1	_____	_____ 60 seconds × 1	_____
Radial Pulse (self)	**Heart Rate per Minute**	**Radial Pulse (by a partner)**	**Heart Rate per Minute**
_____ 15 seconds × 4	_____	_____ 15 seconds × 4	_____
_____ 30 seconds × 2	_____	_____ 30 seconds × 2	_____
_____ 60 seconds × 1	_____	_____ 60 seconds × 1	_____

What is your threshold of training? _____ bpm. Chart 5.8 is available in Lab Resource Materials to assist you.

What is your target zone? _____ bpm

What was your heart rate for the first run? (fifteen seconds)   _____ × 4 = _____ bpm

What was your heart rate for the second run? (fifteen seconds) _____ × 4 = _____ bpm

How fast do you have to run to get your heart rate above threshold and into the target zone? Check the following:

First run speed (just right) ☐   Faster than the first run ☐   Slower than the first run ☐

Second run speed (just right) ☐   Faster than the second run ☐   Slower than the second run ☐

Which resting pulse did you find easiest to locate on yourself? (circle one)   Carotid   Radial   No difference

Which resting pulse did you find easiest to locate on your partner? (circle one)   Carotid   Radial   No difference

Which of the two locations for counting the pulse do you think you would prefer to use when counting exercise heart rate? (circle one)   Carotid   Radial

CONCLUSIONS AND IMPLICATIONS

In several sentences discuss your results including which method you would use to count heart rate and why. Also discuss methods you currently use to elevate your heart rate to the target zone during a typical week.

LAB 5B SUPPLEMENT*

You may want to keep track of your exercise heart rate over a week's time or longer to see if you are reaching the target zone in your workouts. Shade your target zone with a highlight pen and plot your exercise heart rate for each day of the week (see sample).

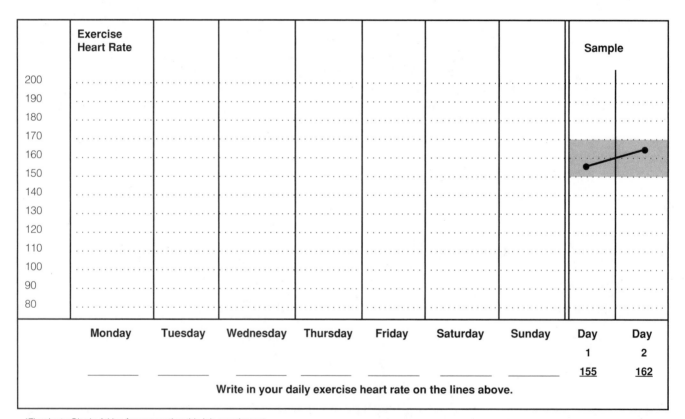

Exercise Heart Rate							Sample	
Monday	Tuesday	Wednesday	Thursday	Friday	Saturday	Sunday	Day 1	Day 2
							155	162

Write in your daily exercise heart rate on the lines above.

*Thanks to Ginnie Atkins for suggesting this lab supplement.

LAB 5C

Ratings of Perceived Exertion (RPE)

Name _____ Section _____ Date _____

PURPOSE

The purpose of this laboratory session is to learn to accurately perceive the intensity of exercise so that you can reduce the number of times that you must stop and count your heart rate during exercise workouts.

PROCEDURE

1. Find your threshold of training and target heart rates (chart 5.8 or see lab 5.B, page L-13) and record it in the Results section below.
2. Perform the following exercise bouts:
   a. Walk for 3 minutes at a brisk pace.
   b. Jog for 3 minutes at a slow pace.
   c. Jog for 3 minutes at a pace that you feel will elevate your heart rate to your threshold level.
3. After each exercise bout, count your heart rate. Record the heart rates in the Results section.
4. After each exercise bout, rate the intensity of the exercise using the Ratings of Perceived Exertion Scale (chart 5.C). Rate the intensity of the exercise by number but use the reference words to help you. Record your ratings for each exercise bout in the Results section.
5. Repeat the jog again at a faster pace. After the run, count your heart rate and make a rating of perceived exertion. Try to elevate the heart rate well into the target zone.

RESULTS

Threshold heart rate _____ (bpm)   Target heart rate zone _____ (bpm)

Activity	Heart Rate (bpm)	Rating of Perceived Exertion (Numerical Rating)
Walk	_____	_____
Slow jog	_____	_____
Threshold jog	_____	_____
Jog 2	_____	_____

CONCLUSIONS AND IMPLICATIONS

Ratings of perceived exertion were originally planned to correspond to heart rates. Adding a zero to a numerical rating would produce the expected heart rate for that rating. However, people perceive exertion differently depending on age, level of training, and experience in exercise, so ratings do not always correspond to heart rate values. The important thing to learn is the RPE number that corresponds to your threshold of training heart rate and the RPE that represents the upper limit heart rate of your target zone. Typically, numerical RPE ratings for exercise in the target zone will range from 12 to 16. With practice (such as you have done here), you can learn to make accurate ratings. More practice than is provided in this lab is necessary. Answering the questions below may help you learn to make accurate ratings of perceived exertion.

	Yes	No
1. Did the walk or slow jog elevate your heart rate to threshold level?	☐	☐
2. Was your RPE number less than 12 for the walk and slow jog?	☐	☐
3. Did the threshold run get your heart rate near your threshold heart rate?	☐	☐
4. Was your RPE number for threshold heart rate near 12–14?	☐	☐
5. Did your final run get your heart rate well into your target heart rate zone?	☐	☐
6. Was your RPE number in the final run in the range of 12–16?	☐	☐

Chart 5.C Ratings of Perceived Exertion (RPE)

Scale	Verbal Rating
6	
7	Very, very light
8	
9	Very light
10	
11	Fairly light
12	
13	Somewhat hard
14	
15	Hard
16	
17	Very hard
18	
19	Very, very hard
20	

From G. Borg, "Psychological Bases of Perceived Exertion" in *Medicine and Science in Sports and Exercise*, 14:377, 1982, © by The American College of Sports Medicine.

In several sentences discuss whether you think you would use ratings of perceived exertion. Discuss reasons why you may or may not use this technique including advantages or disadvantages you see with using the procedure.

Note: If the two runs did not elevate the heart rate into the target zone, it will be difficult to learn to make accurate ratings of perceived exertion.

Jogging/Running

Name _____   Section _____   Date _____

PURPOSE

The purposes of this laboratory session are:

1. To give you an opportunity to experience one type of jogging program that can be used to develop and maintain cardiovascular fitness.
2. To acquaint you with basic jogging techniques.

PROCEDURE

1. Work with a partner and evaluate each other on jogging techniques.
   a. Stand twenty yards in front of your partner while he/she jogs toward you; watch his/her arm and leg swing and foot placement.
   b. Jog along ten yards behind your partner while he/she is jogging and watch for arm and leg swing and foot placement.
   c. Stand ten yards to one side as your partner jogs past you; watch for body position and foot placement.
   d. Change places with your partner and repeat this procedure.
2. Check the appropriate Correct or Incorrect boxes in chart 6.1.
3. Using proper jogging technique, jog for fifteen minutes at your own individual cardiovascular threshold of training.

RESULTS

Record your target zone heart rate here _____ bpm

Record your heart rate after the jog _____ bpm

Have your partner evaluate your jogging technique and then record your results in chart 6.1.

Chart 6.1 Jogging Technique			
Body Segment	Check Appropriate Boxes Below		Technique
	Correct	Incorrect	
Foot placement	☐	☐	Heel hits ground first
	☐	☐	Rock forward, push off ball of foot
	☐	☐	Toes point straight ahead
	☐	☐	Feet under knees, do not swing side to side
Length of stride	☐	☐	Stride is several inches longer than regular step
Arm movement	☐	☐	Elbows bent at 90°
	☐	☐	Arms swing front to back, not side to side
	☐	☐	Arms and legs move in opposition
	☐	☐	Hands and arms are relaxed
Body position	☐	☐	Upper body nearly erect
	☐	☐	Head and chest are up

CONCLUSIONS AND IMPLICATIONS

In several sentences give an overall evaluation of your jogging technique.

In several sentences indicate whether jogging is an appropriate activity for you. Indicate your reasons for your answer.

LAB 6B

Aerobic and Anaerobic Exercises

Name _____ Section _____ Date _____

PURPOSE

The purposes of this laboratory session are:
1. To give you an opportunity to experience an aerobic or anaerobic exercise program.
2. To familiarize you with an exercise program that can be continued as part of your life's normal routine.

PROCEDURE

1. Select a sample program for some form of aerobic or anaerobic exercise and try it out. It can be earning points according to Cooper's aerobics program, dance aerobics, or performing a sample of any of the other forms of aerobic or anaerobic exercise discussed in this concept. For example, you may want to try a walking program, an interval training program, a rope jumping routine, or a circuit weight program.
2. If you would like to repeat this lab more than once doing a different activity each time, space is provided in the Results section for four descriptions.

RESULTS

Name the activity (or activities) in which you participated, and briefly describe and evaluate your experience.

Activity name _____

Time spent _____ minutes

Description and evaluation

Activity name _____

Time spent _____ minutes

Description and evaluation

Activity name _____

Time spent _____ minutes

Description and evaluation

CONCLUSIONS AND IMPLICATIONS

Did you like the activity or activities you performed? Yes ☐ No ☐

Do you think you would choose to make one or more of these activities part of your regular activity program? Yes ☐ No ☐

In several sentences explain the reasons for your two answers above including why you would or would not include the activity in your activity program.

In several sentences, discuss the lifestyle, aerobic or anaerobic activities you think you would most likely include in your personal activity program. Include the reasons for selecting the activities.

LAB 7

Evaluating Flexibility

Name   Section   Date

■ Read concept 7 before completing this lab.

PURPOSE

The purpose of this laboratory experience is to evaluate your flexibility in several joints.

PROCEDURE

1. Take the flexibility tests as outlined in the Lab Resource Materials (concept 7, pp. 85–86).
2. Record your scores in the Results section.
3. Use chart 7.1 in the Lab Resource Materials for concept 7 to determine your ratings on the test, then record your ratings in the Results section.

RESULTS

What were your flexibility scores?

Test 1		Test 2		Test 3		Test 4	
Left	**Right**	**Left-up**	**Right-up**	**Left**	**Right**	**Left**	**Right**
_____	_____	_____	_____	_____	_____	_____	_____

Flexibility *Ratings* on Selected Joints				
	High Performance	**Good Fitness**	**Marginal**	**Poor**
Test 1				
Left	☐	☐	☐	☐
Right	☐	☐	☐	☐
Test 2				
Left-up	☐	☐	☐	☐
Right-up	☐	☐	☐	☐
Test 3				
Left	☐	☐	☐	☐
Right	☐	☐	☐	☐
Test 4				
Left	☐	☐	☐	☐
Right	☐	☐	☐	☐

Do any of these muscle groups need stretching? Check one box for each muscle group.

	Yes	No
Back of the thighs and knees (hamstrings)	☐	☐
Calf muscles	☐	☐
Lower back (lumbar region)	☐	☐
Front of right shoulder	☐	☐
Back of right shoulder	☐	☐
Front of left shoulder	☐	☐
Back of left shoulder	☐	☐
Most of the body	☐	☐
Trunk muscles	☐	☐

Note: Read concept 8 and Lab 8 for exercises to improve your flexibility.

CONCLUSIONS AND IMPLICATIONS

In several sentences discuss your current flexibility and your flexibility needs for the future. Include comments about your current state of flexibiltiy, need for improvement in specific areas, and special flexibility needs for sports or other special activities.

Chart 7.1 Flexibility Rating Scale for Tests 1,2,3,4										
	Men					**Women**				
Classification	**Test 1**	**Test 2**		**Test 3**	**Test 4**	**Test 1**	**Test 2**		**Test 3**	**Test 4**
		Right Up	**Left Up**				**Right Up**	**Left Up**		
High performance zone	16+	5+	4+	111+	20+	17+	6+	5+	111+	20.5 or >
Good fitness zone	13–15	1–4	1–3	80–110	16–19.5	14–16	2–5	2–4	80–110	17–20
Marginal zone	10–12	0	0	60–79	13.5–15.5	11–13	1	1	60–79	14.5–16.5
Low zone	<9	<0	<0	<60	13 or less	<10	<1	<1	<60	14 or <

Flexibility Exercises

Name _____ Section _____ Date _____

■ Read concept 8 before performing this lab. Also review concept 7.

PURPOSE

The purposes of this laboratory experience are:

1. To give you an opportunity to experience different flexibility exercises.
2. To acquaint you with a flexibility program that can be continued throughout your life.
3. To help you distinguish between the types of flexibility exercises.

PROCEDURE

1. Review the stretching exercises in concept 8.
2. Perform each of the exercises to your threshold (or slightly below if you have not been exercising regularly). (See concept 7 for your threshold level.)
3. Answer the questions in the Results section.

RESULTS

Complete the checklist on the following page.

CONCLUSIONS AND IMPLICATIONS

In several sentences discuss the areas of the body in which you most need to do muscle stretching based on your results (see next page). Place a check beside several exercises (at least five) you think you would include in your exercise program. Place a check in the appropriate box if you did or did not experience muscle tightness when doing the exercise. List reasons for your exercise choices on the chart.

Name of Exercise	Tightness Yes No	Exercise Choice	Reason for Choosing the Exercise
Flexibility Exercises			
1. Lower leg stretcher	☐ ☐	_____	_____
2. Sitting stretcher	☐ ☐	_____	_____
3. One-leg stretcher	☐ ☐	_____	_____
4. Leg hug	☐ ☐	_____	_____
5. Pectoral stretch	☐ ☐	_____	_____
6. Billig's exercise	☐ ☐	_____	_____
7. Lateral trunk stretcher	☐ ☐	_____	_____
8. Hip and thigh stretcher	☐ ☐	_____	_____
9. Arm stretcher	☐ ☐	_____	_____
10. Shin stretcher	☐ ☐	_____	_____
11. Hamstring stretcher	☐ ☐	_____	_____
12. Trunk twister	☐ ☐	_____	_____
13. Rectus femoris stretcher	☐ ☐	_____	_____
14. Lateral thigh and hip stretch	☐ ☐	_____	_____
15. Arm pretzel	☐ ☐	_____	_____
16. Spine twist	☐ ☐	_____	_____
17. Neck rotation	☐ ☐	_____	_____
18. Wand exercise	☐ ☐	_____	_____
19. Calf stretcher	☐ ☐	_____	_____
20. Back-saver toe touch	☐ ☐	_____	_____
Stunts and Sport-Specific Ballistic Exercises			
1. Two-hand ankle wrap	☐ ☐	_____	_____
2. Wand step-through	☐ ☐	_____	_____
3. Wring the dishrag	☐ ☐	_____	_____
4. Trunk motions	☐ ☐	_____	_____
5. Arm and trunk motions	☐ ☐	_____	_____

Evaluating Muscle Strength: One Repetition Maximum (1RM)

Name _____   Section _____   Date _____

■ Read concept 9 before proceeding with this lab.

PURPOSE

The purposes of this lab are:

1. To evaluate your muscle strength using one repetition maximum for various strength exercises.
2. To determine the best amount of weight to use for various strength exercises.

PROCEDURE

One repetition maximum (1RM) refers to the maximum amount of weight you can lift for a specific exercise. Testing yourself to determine how much you can lift only one time using traditional methods can be fatiguing and even dangerous. The procedure you will perform here allows you to estimate 1RM based on the number of times you can lift a weight that is less than 1RM.

Evaluating Strength Using Estimated One RM

1. Use a weight machine for the leg press and bench press for the evaluation part of this lab.
2. Estimate how much weight you can lift two or three times. Be conservative; it is better to start with too little weight than too much. This procedure will *not* work if you select a weight heavier than you can lift ten times. If you lift a weight more than ten times, the procedure should be done again on another day when you are rested.
3. Using correct form (see page 135 concept 11), perform a leg press with the weight you have chosen. Perform as many times as you can up to 10.
4. Use chart 9.1 in the Lab Resource Materials page 112 (or on the back of this page), to determine your 1RM for the leg press. Find the weight used in the left-hand column and then find the number of repetitions you performed across the top of the chart.
5. Your 1RM score is the value where the weight row and the repetitions column intersect.
6. Repeat this procedure for the bench press using the technique described on page 128.
7. Record your 1RM scores for the leg press and bench press in the results section.
8. Next divide your 1RM scores by your body weight in pounds to get a "strength per pound of body weight" (str/lb/body wt.) score for each of the two exercises.
9. Finally determine your strength rating for your upper body strength (bench press) and lower body (leg press) using chart 9.2, page 116. Record in the results section. If time allows, assess IRM for other exercises (see Lab 11A).

RESULTS

Bench Press: Wt. selected _____   Reps _____   Estimated 1RM _____
    (chart 9.1, on back of sheet)

    Strength per lb. body weight _____   Rating _____
    (1RM ÷ body weight)   (chart 9.2, page 116)

Leg Press: Wt. selected _____   Reps _____   Estimated 1RM _____
    (chart 9.1, on back of sheet)

    Strength per lb. body weight _____   Rating _____
    (1RM ÷ body weight)   (chart 9.2, page 116)

Chart 9.1 Predicted 1 RM Based on Reps-to-Fatigue

Wt	Repetitions 1	2	3	4	5	6	7	8	9	10	Wt	Repetitions 1	2	3	4	5	6	7	8	9	10
30	30	31	32	33	34	35	36	37	38	39	170	170	175	180	185	191	197	204	211	219	227
35	35	37	38	39	40	41	42	43	44	45	175	175	180	185	191	197	203	210	217	225	233
40	40	41	42	44	46	47	49	50	51	53	180	180	185	191	196	202	209	216	223	231	240
45	45	46	48	49	51	52	54	56	58	60	185	185	190	196	202	208	215	222	230	238	247
50	50	51	53	55	56	58	60	62	64	67	190	190	195	201	207	214	221	228	236	244	253
55	55	57	58	60	62	64	66	68	71	73	195	195	201	206	213	219	226	234	242	251	260
60	60	62	64	65	67	70	72	74	77	80	200	200	206	212	218	225	232	240	248	257	267
65	65	67	69	71	73	75	78	81	84	87	205	205	211	217	224	231	238	246	254	264	273
70	70	72	74	76	79	81	84	87	90	93	210	210	216	222	229	236	244	252	261	270	280
75	75	77	79	82	84	87	90	93	96	100	215	215	221	228	235	242	250	258	267	276	287
80	80	82	85	87	90	93	96	99	103	107	220	220	226	233	240	247	255	264	273	283	293
85	85	87	90	93	96	99	102	106	109	113	225	225	231	238	245	253	261	270	279	289	300
90	90	93	95	98	101	105	108	112	116	120	230	230	237	244	251	259	267	276	286	296	307
95	95	98	101	104	107	110	114	118	122	127	235	235	242	249	256	264	273	282	292	302	313
100	100	103	106	109	112	116	120	124	129	133	240	240	247	254	262	270	279	288	298	309	320
105	105	108	111	115	118	122	126	130	135	140	245	245	252	259	267	276	285	294	304	315	327
110	110	113	116	120	124	128	132	137	141	147	250	250	257	265	273	281	290	300	310	321	333
115	115	118	122	125	129	134	138	143	148	153	255	255	262	270	278	287	296	306	317	328	340
120	120	123	127	131	135	139	144	149	154	160	260	260	267	275	284	292	302	312	323	334	347
125	125	129	132	136	141	145	150	155	161	167	265	265	273	281	289	298	308	318	329	341	353
130	130	134	138	142	146	151	156	161	167	173	270	270	278	286	295	304	314	324	335	347	360
135	135	139	143	147	152	157	162	168	174	180	275	275	283	291	300	309	319	330	341	354	367
140	140	144	148	153	157	163	168	174	180	187	280	280	288	296	305	315	325	336	348	360	373
145	145	149	154	158	163	168	174	180	186	193	285	285	293	302	311	321	331	342	354	366	380
150	150	154	159	164	169	174	180	186	193	200	290	290	298	307	316	326	337	348	360	373	387
155	155	159	164	169	174	180	186	192	199	207	295	295	303	312	322	332	343	354	366	379	393
160	160	165	169	175	180	186	192	199	206	213	300	300	309	318	327	337	348	360	372	386	400
165	165	170	175	180	186	192	198	205	212	220	305	305	314	323	333	343	354	366	379	392	407

This chart is used as modified with permission from the *Journal of Physical Education, Recreation & Dance,* January, 1993, p. 89. *JOPERD* is a publication of the American Alliance for Health, Physical Education, Recreation and Dance, 1900 Association Drive, Reston, VA 22091.

CONCLUSIONS AND IMPLICATIONS

In several sentences discuss your current strength, whether you believe it is adequate for good health, and whether you think that your "strength per pound of body weight" scores are really representative of your true strength.

LAB 9B

Evaluating Muscular Strength and Power

Name _____ Section _____ Date _____

■ Read concept 9 before completing this lab.

PURPOSE

The purposes of this lab are:

1. To evaluate your isotonic and isometric strength in selected muscle groups.
2. To evaluate leg muscle power.
3. To have fun.

PROCEDURE

I. Isotonic Strength
    1. Use an appropriate warm-up before attempting these stunts.
    2. Choose a partner to assist you in performing and scoring.
    3. Attempt the stunt groups found in the Lab Resource Materials for concept 9, pp. 110–113. Within each grouping, *start with the stunt that you believe is the most difficult one that you can pass*. If you pass that one, try the next most difficult one in the same grouping. If you cannot pass it, try the next lower stunt, and so on.
    4. You receive the score of the most difficult stunt you can perform in each grouping.
    5. Record your scores and your rating (chart 9.3, page 116) in the Results section of this report.
II. Isometric Strength
    1. Follow the directions in the Lab Resource Materials for concept 9, page 113.
    2. If time and equipment permit, take three measures of grip strength on each hand and record the best score on each, along with your total score and rating (charts 9.4 and 9.5, pages 116 and 117).
III. Leg Power
    1. Follow the directions in the Lab Resource Materials for concept 9, page 113.
    2. If time and equipment permit, take two trials and record your best score and your rating (charts 9.6 and 9.7, page 117).

RESULTS

Isotonic Strength		Isometric Strength		Leg Power	
Test I	_____	Right Grip	_____		
Test II	_____	Left Grip	_____	Best Score	_____
Test III	_____				
Test IV	_____				
Total Score	_____	Total Score	_____		
Rating	_____	Rating	_____	Rating	_____

On which measure did you score the best? Isometric strength ☐ Isotonic strength ☐ Leg power ☐

On which measure did you score the poorest? Isometric strength ☐ Isotonic strength ☐ Leg power ☐

In several sentences discuss your strength as measured by the isotonic and isometric measures. To what extent do you believe that these tests give you an accurate picture of your true strength? If you have taken other strength tests you may compare those results to the results of these tests.

In several sentences, discuss your leg power. To what extent is leg power important to you and are you satisfied with your current rating? Discuss.

Evaluating Muscular Endurance

Name _____ Section _____ Date _____

■ Read concept 10 before proceeding with this lab.

PURPOSE

The purposes of this laboratory session are:

1. To evaluate the dynamic muscular endurance of two muscle groups and the static endurance of the arms and trunk muscles.
2. To get acquainted with some exercises to improve endurance.

PROCEDURE

1. Perform the curl-up, push-up, and flexed-arm support tests described in the Lab Resource Materials (page 123).
2. Record your test scores in the Results section. Determine and record your rating from charts 10.1, 10.2, and 10.3 in the Lab Resource Materials for concept 10 (page 124).

RESULTS

Record your scores below.

Curl-up_____ Push-up_____ Flexed-arm support (seconds)_____

Check your ratings below.

	High Performance	Good Fitness	Marginal	Poor
Curl-up	☐	☐	☐	☐
Push-up	☐	☐	☐	☐
Flexed-arm support	☐	☐	☐	☐

On which of the tests of muscular endurance did you score the lowest? Curl-up ☐ Push-up ☐ Flexed-arm support ☐

On which of the tests of muscular endurance did you score the best? Curl-up ☐ Push-up ☐ Flexed-arm support ☐

CONCLUSIONS AND IMPLICATIONS

In several sentences, discuss your current level of muscular endurance and whether this level is enough to meet your health, work, and leisure time needs in the future.

LAB
10

Resistance Training for Strength

Name   Section   Date

■ Read concepts 9, 10, and 11 before proceeding with this lab.

LAB 11A

PURPOSE

The purpose of this lab are:
Assess your 1RM for various strength exercises to allow you to determine appropriate weights to use.
To experience a sample strength workout using free weights or a weight machine.

PROCEDURE

1. Determine your 1RM scores for each of the machine exercises listed below and record the 1RM scores (chart 11.1 below). Use the procedures described in Lab 9A.
2. Using your 1RM scores as a basis, select a percentage of 1RM to use for your strength training program. If you are a beginner, use 50 to 65 percent of 1RM, if you have been doing some strength training use 65 to 80 percent of 1RM, and if you are experienced select 80 to 90 percent. Record your selected percentage in chart 11.1.
3. Multiply your 1RM for each exercise by the percentage you selected to determine the weight you will use for each exercise. Example: if your 1RM is 100 lbs. and you choose 65% of 1RM you will use 65lbs. for this exercise. As time allows perform one to three sets of 6 to 10 repetitions of each of the exercises. **Note:** if you have to determine 1RM today it is best to perform the exercises on another day.
4. If weight machines are not available you may substitute the free weight exercises in chart 11.2. If you have a weight machine you may still want to try a free weight program. On another day assess your 1RM and appropriate weights for free weights. Determine 1RM for these exercises on one day and perform them on another. **Note:** This is a sample exercise program. When you actually plan your own program, you may decide to use different exercises and different percentages of 1RM (see concept 9).

RESULTS

Chart 11.1 Sample Machine Exercise Program				
Name	**Number**	**1RM**	**%1RM Selected**	**Weight Used**
Hamstring curl	Ex 31, page 138	_____	_____	_____
Bench press	Ex 28, page 137	_____	_____	_____
Leg press	Ex 25, page 135	_____	_____	_____
Biceps curl	Ex 23, page 135	_____	_____	_____
Triceps curl	Ex 27, page 136	_____	_____	_____
Ankle press	Ex 29, page 137	_____	_____	_____
Seated rowing	Ex 24, page 135	_____	_____	_____

Chart 11.2 Sample Free Weight Program

Name	Number	1RM	%1RM Selected	Weight Used
Shoulder shrug	Ex 15, page 131	_____	_____	_____
Military press	Ex 16, page 131	_____	_____	_____
Half squat	Ex 17, page 132	_____	_____	_____
Biceps curl	Ex 18, page 132	_____	_____	_____
Triceps curl	Ex 19, page 133	_____	_____	_____
Heel raise	Ex 20, page 133	_____	_____	_____
Upright row	Ex 21, page 134	_____	_____	_____

CONCLUSIONS AND IMPLICATIONS

LAB 11A

In several sentences, discuss the strength program you performed. If you made modifications in the program describe them. Indicate what you liked about the program and you disliked, as well as what you might change when you plan your own program.

Circuit Resistance Training for Muscular Endurance

Name _____ Section _____ Date _____

- Read concepts 9, 10, and 11, before proceeding with this lab.

PURPOSE

The purposes of this lab are:
1. To become familiar with a program of Circuit Resistance Training for muscular endurance.
2. To have fun.

PROCEDURE

1. Perform an appropriate warm-up and stretch.
2. Perform the exercises listed below. (*Note:* You or your instructor may prefer to substitute other resistance machine stations or use calisthenics.) If desired, you may also include a cardiovascular station such as jog-in-place or rope-jump. If there is a shortage of equipment, the instructor may wish to assign each person a partner and have the partner jump rope while the other person works on the machine, and then trade places before moving on to each new station.

Arm	**Leg**	**Trunk**
1. lat pull-down, Ex 26, page 136	2. knee extensions, Ex 30, page 138	3. crunch, Ex 7, page 128
4. seated rowing, Ex 24, page 135	5. ankle press, Ex 29, page 137	6. upper back lift, Ex 9, page 129
7. bench press, Ex 28, page 137	8. leg press, Ex 25, page 135	9. fist squeeze, Ex 33, page 140

3. Rotate in the order listed above or as designated by your instructor, alternating arm, leg, and trunk exercises.
4. On the first set (circuit), perform twenty reps at 30 to 40 percent 1 RM, or 20% of 1RM for forty-five seconds (this allows approximately two seconds for each repetition). Use the procedure described in Lab 11A to determine your percentage of 1RM. Record your 1RM, % of 1RM and weight used in chart 11.2.
5. On the signal at the end of the forty-five seconds, move to the next station, adjust the resistance and get ready in fifteen seconds.
6. Continue around the circuit, performing forty-five seconds work and fifteen seconds rest periods. Perform a second circuit and increase your reps at each station to twenty-five. If time permits, perform a third circuit of twenty-five reps.
7. Perform an appropriate cool-down and stretch.

RESULTS

Chart 11.2 Sample Circuit Resistance Training for Muscular Endurance			
Name	**1RM**	**%1RM**	**Wt. Used**
lat pull-down	_____	_____	_____
knee extensions	_____	_____	_____
crunch	reps _____	_____	_____
seated rowing	_____	_____	_____
ankle press	_____	_____	_____
upper back lift	reps _____	_____	_____
bench press	_____	_____	_____
leg press	_____	_____	_____
fist squeeze	reps _____	_____	_____

		Yes	No
1.	Were you able to complete twenty to twenty-five reps in forty-five seconds?	☐	☐
2.	Were you able to change stations in fifteen seconds?	☐	☐
3.	Was this your first experience with circuit resistance training?	☐	☐
4.	Did you like the workout?	☐	☐

CONCLUSIONS AND IMPLICATIONS

In several sentences, describe your reactions to circuit resistance training for muscular endurance as a potential program for use to develop your own fitness.

LAB
11B

In several sentences, describe any changes you might make in the program to make it better fit your needs.

LAB 12

Questionable Exercises

Name _____   Section _____   Date _____

■ Read concept 12 before completing this lab.

PURPOSE

To experience some "good" exercises that can accomplish the purpose of some "questionable" exercises.

PROCEDURE

1. Look at the illustrations of questionable exercises in concept 12, then review the exercises suggested as good alternatives.
2. For each questionable exercise listed, there is one (or more) good alternative to accomplish the same purpose without harm to the individual. Perform the good exercises listed.

RESULTS

Record your results below.

1. Place a check by all of the risky exercises you have done in the past or that you have seen others perform.
2. In the second column opposite the types of risky exercises checked, list safer alternative exercises.

"Questionable" Exercises		Good "Alternative" Exercises
1. repetitive hyperextension of the lower back	☐	1. _____
2. back-arching abdominal stretch	☐	2. _____
3. donkey kick	☐	3. _____
4. double leg lift or straight leg sit-up	☐	4. _____
5. windmill exercise	☐	5. _____
6. hyperextending the neck (rear neck circle)	☐	6. _____
7. neck and upper back hyperflexion	☐	7. _____
8. hands behind the head sit-up or crunch	☐	8. _____
9. hyperextending the knee (standing toe touches or seated two-leg toe touches)	☐	9. _____
10. leg stretches at ballet bar or on hurdle	☐	10. _____
11. hyperflexing the knee ("quadricep stretch")	☐	11. _____
12. deep squatting exercises	☐	12. _____
13. hero or hurdler's stretch with leg to side	☐	13. _____
14. hands over knee pull-down	☐	14. _____
15. arm circles with palms down	☐	15. _____

CONCLUSIONS AND IMPLICATIONS

Use several sentences to write a statement about risky exercises. Indicate how frequently you have used them in the past and how you hope to avoid them in the future.

LAB
12

Evaluating Body Composition

Name _____   Section _____   Date _____

PURPOSE

The purposes of this laboratory session are:
1. To learn to use skinfold calipers to assess body fatness.
2. To assess your waist-to-hip ratio using circumference measurements.
3. To determine desirable weight.
4. To determine body mass index (BMI).
5. To compare different methods of assessing body composition.

PROCEDURE

1. Read the directions for making skinfold and/or body circumference measurements (Lab Resource Material, pages 168–172).
2. If possible, observe a demonstration of the proper procedures for measuring skinfolds and body circumferences at each of the different body locations. In the future, you may wish to help a person of the same or opposite sex take measurements, so you may wish to learn how to make all the measurements.
3. Work with a partner if possible. Take several measurements on your partner at each of the different skinfold and body circumference locations. Allow your partner to make the appropriate measurements on you.
4. If possible, have an expert make measurements on you and your partner so that you can compare your measurements.
5. Record each of the measurements in the Results section on the back of this page.
6. Calculate your body fatness from skinfolds by summing the appropriate skinfold values (chest, abdominal, and thigh for men; triceps, iliac crest, and thigh for women). Using your age and the sum of the appropriate skinfolds, determine your body fatness using the charts in the Lab Resource Materials (charts 13.1 and 13.2, pages 170–171).
7. Rate your fatness using the Fatness Rating Scale in the Lab Resource Materials (chart 13.3, page 172).
8. If different types of calipers are available to you, practice making measurements with each type so that comparisons of results can be made.
9. Use chart 13.4, page 172, or divide your waist score by your hip score to calculate your waist-to-hip ratio from body circumferences. Rate yourself using the Waist-to-Hip Rating Scale in the Lab Resource Materials (chart 13.5, page 173).
10. Measure height and weight.
11. Determine your "healthy weight range" using chart 13.6, page 173 in the Lab Resource Materials. You may want to use your elbow breadth (chart 13.6, page 173) to help you.
12. Determine your BMI using chart 13.7, page 173 and determine your rating using chart 13.8, page 173.
13. Determine your "desirable weight range" based on your current weight and your current percentage of body fat using charts 13.9 for males and 13.10 for females. Locate your current body weight in the left column and your percent of fat across the top of the chart. Your desirable weight range is located at the point where the row and column intersect.
14. Remember that body composition measurements are confidential information. Care should be taken not to discuss another person's results. Results are intended to be useful information to the people being tested. Take the skinfold testing seriously.

Record your scores and ratings.

Skinfolds by Partner

Male (chart 13.1)	Female (chart 13.2)
Chest _____ mm	Tricep _____ mm
Abdominal _____ mm	Iliac Crest _____ mm
Thigh _____ mm	Thigh _____ mm
Sum _____	Sum _____
Percent Body Fat _____	Percent Body Fat _____
Rating _____	Rating _____

Skinfolds by Instructor (if possible)

Male (chart 13.1)	Female (chart 13.2)
Chest _____ mm	Triceps _____ mm
Abdominal _____ mm	Iliac Crest _____ mm
Thigh _____ mm	Thigh _____ mm
Sum _____	Sum _____
Percent Body Fat _____	Percent Body Fat _____
Rating _____	Rating _____

Waist to Hip Ratio: Partner or Self Measure

Waist Circumference_____ in./mm

Hip Circumference _____ in./mm

Waist-to-Hip Ratio _____ (chart 13.4, page 172)

Rating _____ (chart 13.5, page 173)

Healthy Weight Range

Healthy Weight Range _____ lbs. (chart 13.6, page 173)

Body Mass Index: Partner or Self Measure

Weight _____ lbs. or kg. (lb. ÷ 2.2)

Height _____ in. or meters (inches × .0254)

Body Mass Index _____ (chart 13.7, page 174)

Rating _____ (chart 13.8, page 174)

Desirable Weight Range from % Fat

Desirable Weight Range _____ lbs. (charts 13.9/13.10, pages 175–176)

CONCLUSIONS AND IMPLICATIONS

In two or three paragraphs discuss your body composition. Is it what you would like it to be? Use your personal data in answering the question. Note discrepancies among different measures. Explain which measure you consider to be most useful to you.

LAB 14

Keeping Records for Fat Control

Name _____   Section _____   Date _____

PURPOSE

1. To learn to keep records of calories consumed.
2. To learn to keep records of calories expended.
3. To learn to keep records of fat and weight changes.
4. To learn to chart behavior (diet and exercise) and fat and weight changes over time.

PROCEDURE

1. Write your daily calorie intake goal (the number of calories you would like to consume each day) and your daily calorie expenditure goal (the number of calories you would like to expend each day) in the diet log chart.
2. Keep a dietary log for one day to learn how it is done (use chart 14.1). Record the food eaten, the time eaten, and the calories in the food. Use the calorie chart diet log in chart 14.1 on the back of this page.
3. Keep an exercise log for one day to learn how it is done (use chart 14.2). Record the activity, the length of time each activity was done, and the calories expended in each activity on chart 14.2 on the back of this page.
4. Record your current weight in the Results section. Also record your goal weight for fourteen days from now.
5. Record your current percent fat in the Results section. Also record your goal percent fat for fourteen days from now.
6. This one-day record-keeping effort will get you started. If you really want to lose fat, you should make extra copies of logs and keep records for fourteen days. If you do this for fourteen days, determine your weight and percent fat to see if you met your goals.

LAB
14

RESULTS

Starting weight   _____   Goal weight   _____

Starting fat %   _____   Goal fat %   _____

OPTIONAL RESULTS

Weight after fourteen days _____ Percent fat after fourteen days _____

Number of days your exercise goals were met _____ Number of days your dietary goals were met _____

Chart 14.1 Diet Log		
Food Eaten and Amount	Calories	Time of Day
Total Calories	_____	
Daily Calorie Goal	_____	

Chart 14.2 Exercise Log		
Activity	Time (min.)	Calories
Total Calories		_____
Daily Calorie Goal		_____

LAB
14

CONCLUSIONS AND IMPLICATIONS

In several sentences, discuss how record keeping may or may not be useful to you.

Evaluating Skill-Related Physical Fitness

Name _____ Section _____ Date _____

PURPOSE

The purpose of this lab is to help you evaluate your own skill-related fitness, including agility, balance, coordination, power, speed, and reaction time. This information may be of value in planning your personal fitness program and in deciding which sports may be best, based on your own skill-related fitness.

PROCEDURE

1. Read the directions for each of the skill-related fitness tests presented in the Lab Resource Materials, pages 194–196.
2. Take as many of the tests as possible, given the time and equipment available.
3. Be sure to warm up before and to cool down after the tests.
4. It is all right to practice the tests before trying them. However, you should decide ahead of time which trial you will use to test your skill-related fitness.
5. After completing the tests, write your scores in the appropriate places in the Results section.
6. Determine your rating for each of the tests from the rating charts in the Lab Resource Materials, pages 194–196.

RESULTS

Place a check in the box for each of the tests you completed.

Agility (Illinois run) ☐

Balance (Bass test) ☐

Coordination (stick test) ☐

Power (vertical jump) ☐

Reaction time (stick drop test) ☐

Speed (three-second run) ☐

Record your score and rating (from charts 15.1–6 in the Lab Resource Materials) in the following spaces.

	Score	Rating	
Agility	_____	_____	(chart 15.1, page 194)
Balance	_____	_____	(chart 15.2, page 195)
Coordination	_____	_____	(chart 15.3, page 195)
Power	_____	_____	(chart 15.4, page 195)
Reaction time	_____	_____	(chart 15.5, page 196)
Speed	_____	_____	(chart 15.6, page 196)

CONCLUSIONS AND IMPLICATIONS

In two or three paragraphs discuss the results of your skill-related fitness tests. Comment on the areas in which you did well or did not do well, the meaning of these findings, and the implications of the results with specific reference to the activities you will include in your future physical activity programs.

LAB 16A

Healthy Back Test

Name _____ Section _____ Date _____

■ Read concept 16 before completing this lab.

PURPOSE

The purpose of this laboratory session is to determine if you have some muscle imbalance and potential for back problems.

PROCEDURE

1. Secure a partner and administer the Healthy Back Tests to each other. (Details appear in chart 16.1, page 214 of the Lab Resource Materials for concept 16.) Record results of tests in the Results section of this laboratory. If you failed a test, indicate the muscles involved.
2. Determine your ratings by referring to chart 16.2 below.

RESULTS

Test	Pass	Fail	If you failed, what were the tight muscles involved?
1. Back to wall	☐	☐	_____
2. Straight-leg lift	☐	☐	_____
3. Thomas test	☐	☐	_____
4. Ely's test	☐	☐	_____
5. Ober's test	☐	☐	_____
6. Press-up	☐	☐	_____
7. Knee roll	☐	☐	_____
Total	_____	_____	

Chart 16.2 Healthy Back Test Ratings	
Classification	**Number of Tests Passed**
Excellent	7
Very good	6
Good	5
Fair	4
Poor	1–3

CONCLUSIONS AND IMPLICATIONS

In several sentences discuss your need to do exercises for care of the back. Include in your discussion whether you think your muscles are fit enough to prevent back problems, the areas in which you are most likely to experience problems, and steps you might take to prevent future back problems. Use your test results to answer.

Evaluating Posture

Name _____   Section _____   Date _____

■ Read concept 16 before completing this lab.

PURPOSE

The purposes of this laboratory session are as follows:
1. To learn to recognize postural deviations and thus become more posture conscious.
2. To determine your posture limitations in order to institute a preventive and corrective program.

PROCEDURE

1. Wear as little clothing as possible (bathing suits are recommended) and remove shoes and socks.
2. Work in groups of two or three, with one person acting as the "subject" while partners serve as "examiners," then alternate roles. *Note:* The instructor may prefer to conduct all examinations by individual screening exams or posture photographs.
   a. Stand by a vertical plumb line.
   b. Use chart 16.3 below. Check any deviations and indicate their severity as follows:
      0—none; 1—slight; 2—moderate; 3—severe.
   c. Total the score and determine your posture rating from the Posture Rating Scale (chart 16.4) below.
3. If time permits, perform back and posture exercises assigned by your instructor from pages 206 to 213.

RESULTS

Record your posture score _____.

Record your posture rating from the Posture Rating Scale (chart 16.4) below _____.

Chart 16.3 Posture Evaluation

Side View	Points	Back View	Points
Head forward	_____	Tilted head	_____
Sunken chest	_____	Protruding scapulae	_____
Round shoulders	_____	Symptoms of scoliosis	
		Shoulders uneven	_____
Kyphosis	_____	Hips uneven	_____
Lordosis	_____	Lateral curvature of spine (Adam's position)	_____
Abdominal ptosis	_____	One side of back high (Adam's position)	_____
Hyperextended knees	_____		
Body lean	_____	Total score _____	

Chart 16.4 Posture *Rating Scale*

Classification	Total Score
Excellent	0–2
Very good	3–4
Good	5–7
Fair	8–11
Poor	12 or more

CONCLUSIONS AND IMPLICATIONS

Were you aware of the deviations that were found? Yes ☐   No ☐

List the deviations that were moderate or severe.

In several sentences describe your current posture status. Include in this discussion your overall assessment of your current posture, whether you think you will need special exercises in the future, and the reasons why your posture rating is good or not so good

Preventive and Therapeutic Exercises for Posture, Neck, and Back

Name   Section   Date

■ Read concept 16 before completing this lab.

PURPOSE

1. Under the direction and supervision of the instructor, perform the exercises described in concept 16.
2. In the following list, place a check beside the exercise that you think you would most likely include in your program.
3. In the Conclusions and Implications section, explain why you choose the exercise.

RESULTS

Check at least three exercises from concept 16 that you are most likely to perform.

1. Wand Exercise ☐   **Sitting Tucks**

Postural Stretch

2. Side Bender ☐
3. Isometric Neck Exercises ☐
4. Neck Rotation Exercises ☐
5. Back-Saver Hamstring Stretch ☐
6. Hip and Thigh Stretcher ☐
7. Low Back Stretcher ☐
8. Single Knee-to-Chest ☐
9. Double Knee-to-Chest ☐
10. Calf Stretcher ☐

Lower Leg Stretch

11. Half-Squat (Wts.) ☐
12. Pelvic Tilt ☐
13. Reverse Curl ☐
14. Crunch (Curl-Up) ☐
15. Crunch with Twist/Bench ☐

16. Standing Crunch ☐
17. Arm Lift ☐
18. Seated Rowing ☐
19. Upper Trunk Lift ☐
20. Lower Trunk Lift ☐
21. Press-Up ☐
22. Bridging ☐
23. Wall Slide ☐
24. Spine Trunk Twist ☐

CONCLUSIONS AND IMPLICATIONS

In several sentences explain why you chose the exercises you chose, and discuss your plan for preventing posture, neck, and back problems in the future.

Planning Your Personal Physical Activity Program

Name _____   Section _____   Date _____

PURPOSE

The purpose of this lab is to plan a personal activity program using the seven steps outlined in this concept.

PROCEDURE AND RESULTS

Answer the questions and fill in the charts following the seven steps outlined below.

STEP 1.   Establish the Reasons for Your Program
In the space provided, write your principal reasons for wanting to start a physical activity program (provide 3 to 8).

1. _____   5. _____

2. _____   6. _____

3. _____   7. _____

4. _____   8. _____

STEP 2.   Identify Your Personal Fitness Needs

In chart 17.1, darken the boxes of your self-test rating for each of the skill-related physical fitness tests you have taken. (Refer to the appropriate rating charts to determine your ratings.) If you did not take a test, darken the "No Results" box. Also, record your results on the healthy back test and the posture test in chart 17.1.

In chart 17.2 darken the boxes of your self-test rating for each of the health related physical fitness tests you have taken. (Refer to the appropriate rating charts to determine your ratings.) If you did not take a test, darken the "No Results" box.

In chart 17.3, darken one box for each component of fitness. Record only *one* rating for each part of health related physical fitness by averaging ratings from chart 17.2. If you took more than one test for a particular fitness component, use your own judgment in determining your average rating. Use ratings 1–4 for cardiovascular fitness, 5–8 for flexibility, 9–12 for strength, 13–15 for muscular endurance, and 16–17 for fatness. Record one average rating for skill-related fitness using ratings 1–6 from chart 17.1. Record one average rating for fitness of the back and posture using ratings 7–8 from chart 17.1. Connect the darkened boxes to create your own personal fitness profile. The completed profile will give you important information for planning your program. Check the "No Results" box if you did no tests in an area.

Chart 17.1 *Ratings* for Other Fitness Self-Tests					
	Rating				
Fitness Tests	**High Performance Zone**	**Good Fitness Zone**	**Marginal Zone**	**Low Zone**	**No Results**
1. Agility (chart 15.1, page 194)	☐	☐	☐	☐	☐
2. Balance (chart 15.2, page 195)	☐	☐	☐	☐	☐
3. Coordination (chart 15.3, page 195)	☐	☐	☐	☐	☐
4. Power (chart 15.4, page 195)	☐	☐	☐	☐	☐
5. Reaction Time (chart 15.5, page 196)	☐	☐	☐	☐	☐
6. Speed (chart 15.6, page 196)	☐	☐	☐	☐	☐
7. Fitness of the Back (chart 16.2, page 215)	☐	☐	☐	☐	☐
8. Posture (chart 16.4, page 215)	☐	☐	☐	☐	☐

Chart 17.2 *Ratings* for Health Related Fitness Self-Tests

Fitness Tests	High Performance Zone	Good Fitness Zone	Marginal Zone	Low Zone	No Results
1. Cardiovascular: Twelve-Minute Run (chart 5.1, page 65)	☐	☐	☐	☐	☐
2. Cardiovascular: Step Test (chart 5.2, page 66)	☐	☐	☐	☐	☐
3. Cardiovascular: Bicycle Test (chart 5.4, page 67)	☐	☐	☐	☐	☐
4. Cardiovascular: Walking Test (chart 5.5 & 5.6, pages 67 & 68)	☐	☐	☐	☐	☐
5. Flexibility: Sit and Reach (chart 7.1, page 87)	☐	☐	☐	☐	☐
6. Flexibility: Shoulder Flexibility (chart 7.1, page 87)	☐	☐	☐	☐	☐
7. Flexibility: Hamstring/ Hip Flexibility (chart 7.1, page 87)	☐	☐	☐	☐	☐
8. Flexibility: Trunk Rotation (chart 7.1, page 87)	☐	☐	☐	☐	☐
9. Strength: Isotonic Stunts (chart 9.3, page 116)	☐	☐	☐	☐	☐
10. Strength: 1RM Upper Body (chart 9.2, page 116)	☐	☐	☐	☐	☐
11. Strength: 1RM Lower Body (chart 9.2, page 116)	☐	☐	☐	☐	☐
12. Isometric Strength (total): (chart 9.4 & 9.5, pages 116–117)	☐	☐	☐	☐	☐
13. Muscular Endurance: Curl-Up (chart 10.1 & 10.2, page 124)	☐	☐	☐	☐	☐
14. Muscular Endurance: 90 degree push-up (chart 10.1 & 10.2, page 124)	☐	☐	☐	☐	☐
15. Muscular Endurance: Flexed Arm Support (chart 10.3, page 124)	☐	☐	☐	☐	☐
16. Fatness Rating: Skinfold (chart 13.3, page 172)	☐	☐	☐	☐	☐
17. Body Mass Index: (chart 13.9, page 174)	☐	☐	☐	☐	☐

LAB 17

Chart 17.3 A Profile of Personal Fitness Needs

Fitness Component	High Performance Zone	Good Fitness Zone	Marginal Zone	Low Zone	No Results
Cardiovascular	☐	☐	☐	☐	☐
Endurance	☐	☐	☐	☐	☐
Strength	☐	☐	☐	☐	☐
Flexibility	☐	☐	☐	☐	☐
Fat control	☐	☐	☐	☐	☐
Skill-related fitness	☐	☐	☐	☐	☐
Posture and fitness of the back	☐	☐	☐	☐	☐

STEP 3. **Establish Your Physical Activity and Fitness Goals**

    A. Short-Term Goals

        Physical Activity Goals: Provide information about your proposed activity goals. Give the length of time for your proposed workout (in minutes) and the number of workouts per day and per week.

        Length of workout _____ minutes

        Workouts per day _____

        Workout days per week _____

        Weeks of program _____ no more than four

        Fitness Goals: Beginners should omit this section. If you have been exercising regularly, write the specific goals you expect to accomplish in the number of weeks specified in your physical activity goals. Example: Perform ten pull-ups or perform twenty-five crunches. Consider goals for each component of fitness.

        1. _____   4. _____

        2. _____   5. _____

        3. _____   6. _____

    B. Long-Term Goals

        Physical Activity Goals: Designate the number of months for which you are making a commitment to do the plan you designed in this lab.

        Months _____ (no more than twelve)

        Fitness Goals: Write your specific performance goals for the number of months specified above. Indicate expected scores on fitness tests. For example: Run one and one-half miles in twelve minutes or attain 21 percent body fatness.

        1. _____   4. _____

        2. _____   5. _____

        3. _____   6. _____

STEP 4. **Select Your Activities**

Complete chart 17.4. In the top part of the chart, list the activities you currently do on a regular basis that you would like to continue. In the middle section, indicate some new activities that would be especially good for developing your fitness goals or meeting a weakness or special need (see chart 17.4). Finally, in the bottom section of the chart, list some new activities you would especially like to try because you enjoy them (even if they do not meet your special fitness needs). After each, note the component of fitness developed by the activity. You should have at least one activity for each of the health-related fitness components. You should be especially careful to include exercise for the components of fitness for which you have low ratings. You may want to consider activities that match your skill-related fitness abilities (see chart 17.1).

STEP 5. **Prepare a Personal Weekly Physical Activity Schedule**

Complete chart 17.5. For each day of the week, write in the activities you plan to do on that particular day. Select the activities from chart 17.4. A special place is provided for your warm-up and cool-down activities. In this section, write in the activities you will do to warm up and cool down each day. (Sections for flexibility and strength/muscular endurance exercises are also provided. Use these spaces to list specific exercises for these parts of fitness. Another section is provided for "special exercises" that you may do on a regular basis.) These may include exercises for the back, or just a set of calisthenics or exercises you plan to do. Once you list these activities, you need only refer to them in your daily schedule by the name of the section (example: flexibility exercises) rather than write them on each day's schedule. Table 17.1 (see concept 17, page 218) is a sample program that you might want to consult before preparing your personal schedule.

STEP 6. **Keep Physical Activity and Fitness Records**

Record keeping can help you stick with your physical activity program and can help you attain your fitness goals. Use a one-month calendar or chart 17.6 to keep track of your regular physical activity and fitness changes. Follow these steps in using the calendar.

- Write the month at the top and the dates on the calendar beginning on the day you expect to begin your program (yellow).
- Place an X in the appropriate box of the dates you expect to do your program (green).
- Write fitness goals on the calendar on the day you expect to accomplish them.
- Place an X in the appropriate box each time you do your activities as planned (blue).
- Test your fitness on dates with goals. Set new goals for the future.
- Prepare a new record-keeping calendar when the current one expires.

Chart 17.4 Personal Physical Activities

Current Activities
(List activities in which you currently participate.)

Activity	Fitness Components Developed by Activity
1. _____	_____
2. _____	_____
3. _____	_____
4. _____	_____
5. _____	_____

Proposed New Activities for Fitness
(List new activities for meeting fitness needs.)

Activity	Fitness Components Developed by Activity
1. _____	_____
2. _____	_____
3. _____	_____
4. _____	_____
5. _____	_____

New Activities Just for Fun
(List new activities that you think you might especially enjoy, but that may not be good for developing fitness.)

Activity
1. _____
2. _____
3. _____

LAB
17

STEP 7.   Evaluate and Modify Your Program

After you have tried your program, either in class or on your own, evaluate it. *Remember, even the best program needs periodic reevaluation and modification.*

Select activities that you enjoy and that are best for meeting your own personal goals.

Chart 17.5 Weekly Physical Activity Program

Daily Schedules
(List the activities and times of day for each activity.)

Monday	Tuesday	Wednesday

Thursday	Friday	Saturday

Sunday	Flexibility Exercises			Strength and Muscular Endurance Exercises		
	Exercise	Time	Reps	Exercise	Sets	Reps

Warm-Up and Cool-Down Activities	Other Special Exercises

Chart 17.6 Record-Keeping Calendar

Sunday	Monday	Tuesday	Wednesday	Thursday	Friday	Saturday
Date	Date	Date	Date	Date	Date	Date
Goals:	Goals:	Goals:	Goals:	Goals:	Goals:	Goals:
Date	Date	Date	Date	Date	Date	Date
Goals:	Goals:	Goals:	Goals:	Goals:	Goals:	Goals:
Date	Date	Date	Date	Date	Date	Date
Goals:	Goals:	Goals:	Goals:	Goals:	Goals:	Goals:
Date	Date	Date	Date	Date	Date	Date
Goals:	Goals:	Goals:	Goals:	Goals:	Goals:	Goals:

Assessing Personal Wellness

Name _____ Section _____ Date _____

PURPOSE

The purpose of this laboratory experience is to make you aware of your own perceptions of personal wellness.

PROCEDURE

1. Answer the questions in the Self-Perceptions of Wellness Questionnaire on the back of this page.
2. Score the questionnaire using the procedures outlined in the Lab Resource Materials on page 229.
3. Record your scores in the spaces provided in the Results section.
4. Determine your ratings for each wellness score using the Wellness Rating Scale (chart 18.3) on the back of this page.

RESULTS

Write your scores and ratings in the appropriate blanks below.

Wellness Dimension (Perceptions)	Score	Rating	
Emotional wellness	_____	_____	(question 1)
Intellectual wellness	_____	_____	(question 2)
Physical wellness	_____	_____	(question 3)
Social wellness	_____	_____	(question 4)
Spiritual wellness	_____	_____	(question 5)
General wellness	_____	_____	(question 6)
Total wellness	_____	_____	(all questions)

CONCLUSIONS AND IMPLICATIONS

In several sentences evaluate your own wellness. Include comments on the accuracy of the five wellness ratings recorded in the Results section (one for each dimension of wellness).

Chart 18.1 Wellness *Rating Scale*

	Individual Wellness Dimensions	Total Wellness
Excellent	4	21–24
Good	3	18–20
Marginal	2	12–17
Low	1	11 or less

Chart 18.2 Self-Perceptions of Wellness Questionnaire

Directions
There are four possible responses for each question. Place an X in **one** of the four boxes for *each* question.

Sample Question: A person who likes ice cream a lot would mark the box as indicated below.

Some people like ice cream very much. **but** Other people do not like ice cream at all.

Especially true for me	True for me		Not true for me	Especially not true for me
☒	☐		☐	☐

1. Some people are happy most of the time. **but** Other people feel depressed much of the time.

Especially true for me	True for me		Not true for me	Especially not true for me
☐	☐		☐	☐

2. Some people are well informed about health and wellness. **but** Other people are ignorant of the facts concerning their health and well-being.

Especially true for me	True for me		Not true for me	Especially not true for me
☐	☐		☐	☐

3. Some people are physically fit. **but** Other people are not so fit physically.

Especially true for me	True for me		Not true for me	Especially not true for me
☐	☐		☐	☐

4. Some people have a lot of friends and are very involved socially. **but** Other people do not have many friends and are often lonely.

Especially true for me	True for me		Not true for me	Especially not true for me
☐	☐		☐	☐

5. Some people feel fulfilled spiritually. **but** Other people are not so fulfilled spiritually.

Especially true for me	True for me		Not true for me	Especially not true for me
☐	☐		☐	☐

6. Some people have a very positive outlook on life—they are optimistic. **but** Other people have a more negative outlook on life—they are pessimistic.

Especially true for me	True for me		Not true for me	Especially not true for me
☐	☐		☐	☐

LAB 18

Selecting Nutritious Foods

Name   Section   Date

PURPOSE

The purposes of this lab are:
1. To learn to select a nutritious diet.
2. To determine the nutritive value of favorite foods.
3. To compare a nutritious food's values to a favorite food's values.

PROCEDURE

1. Select a breakfast, lunch, and dinner from the Foods list in Appendix D. Include between-meal snacks with the nearest meal. If you cannot find foods you would normally choose, select those most similar to choices you might make.
2. Select a breakfast, lunch, and dinner from foods you feel would make the most nutritious meals. Include between-meal snacks with nearest meal.
3. Record the foods you list in the "favorite foods" and "nutritious foods" in chart 19.1. Record the calories for proteins, carbohydrates, and fats for each of the foods you choose.
4. Total each column for the "favorite" and the "nutritious" meal.
5. Determine the percentages of your total calories that are protein, carbohydrate, and fat by dividing each column total by the total number of calories consumed.
6. Answer the questions in the Conclusions section below.

RESULTS

Record results in Chart 19.1 and summarize below. Calculate percent of calories from each source by dividing total calories into calories from each food source (protein, fat, or carbohydrate).

	Favorite Foods		Nutritious Foods	
Source	**Calories**	**% of Total Calories**	**Calories**	**% of Total Calories**
Protein	_____	_____	_____	_____
Fat	_____	_____	_____	_____
Carbohydrate	_____	_____	_____	_____
Total	_____	100%	_____	100%

CONCLUSIONS AND IMPLICATIONS

In several sentences discuss differences you found between your nutritious diet and your favorite diet. Discuss the quality of your nutritious diet as well as other things you learned from doing this lab.

Chart 19.1 "Favorite" versus "Nutritious" Food Choices for Three Daily Meals

Breakfast Favorite Food No. and Name	Food Choices Cal.	Pro. Cal.	Car. Cal.	Fat Cal.	Breakfast Nutritious Food No. and Name	Food Choices Cal.	Pro. Cal.	Car. Cal.	Fat Cal.
Totals					Totals				

Lunch Favorite Food No. and Name	Food Choices Cal.	Pro. Cal.	Car. Cal.	Fat Cal.	Lunch Nutritious Food No. and Name	Food Choices Cal.	Pro. Cal.	Car. Cal.	Fat Cal.
Totals					Totals				

Dinner Favorite Food No. and Name	Food Choices Cal.	Pro. Cal.	Car. Cal.	Fat Cal.	Dinner Nutritious Food No. and Name	Food Choices Cal.	Pro. Cal.	Car. Cal.	Fat Cal.
Totals					Totals				
Daily Totals (Calories)					Daily Totals (Calories)				
Daily % of Total Calories					Daily % of Total Calories				

LAB 19B

Nutrition Analysis

Name _____   Section _____   Date _____

PURPOSE

The purposes of this laboratory are:
1. To determine the nutritional quality of your diet.
2. To determine your average daily caloric intake.
3. To determine necessary changes in eating habits.

PROCEDURE

1. a. Record your dietary intake for two days using the Daily Diet Record sheet. Record intake for one weekday and one weekend day.
   b. Include the actual foods eaten, the amount (size of portion in teaspoons, tablespoons, cups, ounces, or other standard units of measurement). Be sure to include all drinks (coffee, tea, soft drinks, etc.)
   c. Include *all* foods eaten including sauces, gravies, dressings, toppings, spreads, etc.
   d. Determine your calorie consumption for each of the two days. Use the Calorie Guide to Common Foods (Appendix C) to assist you.
   e. List the number of servings from each food group by each food choice.
   f. Estimate the proportion of complex carbohydrate, simple carbohydrate, protein, and fat in each meal and in snacks.

2. a. Answer the questions in chart 19.2 (see back of this page) using information from each of the dietary record sheets.
   b. Score one point for each "yes" answer on chart 19.2.
   c. Use chart 19.3 to rate your dietary habits. Circle the appropriate rating.

RESULTS

Record the number of calories consumed for each of the two days.

Day 1 _____   Day 2 _____

CONCLUSIONS AND IMPLICATIONS

In several sentences discuss your diet as recorded in this lab. Explain any changes in your eating habits that may be necessary. Comment on whether the days you surveyed are typical of your normal diet.

Chart 19.2 Dietary Habits Questionnaire

Yes	No	
☐	☐	1. Do you eat regular meals?
☐	☐	2. Do you eat a good breakfast daily?
☐	☐	3. Do you eat lunch regularly?
☐	☐	4. Does your diet contain about 55%–60% carbohydrates with a high concentration of fiber?
☐	☐	5. Are less than one-fourth of the carbohydrates you eat simple carbohydrates?
☐	☐	6. Does your diet contain 10%–15% protein?
☐	☐	7. Does you diet contain less than 30% fat?
☐	☐	8. Do you limit the amount of saturated fat in your diet?
☐	☐	9. Do you limit salt intake to acceptable amounts?
☐	☐	10. Do you get adequate amounts of vitamins in your diet without a supplement?
☐	☐	11. Do you eat regularly from all food groups?
☐	☐	12. Do you drink adequate amounts of water?
☐	☐	13. Do you get adequate minerals in your diet without a supplement?
☐	☐	14. Do you limit your caffeine and alcohol consumption to acceptable levels?
☐	☐	15. Is your average calorie consumption for the two-day period reasonable for your body size and for the amount of calories you normally expend?

_____ Total number of "Yes" answers

Chart 19.3 Dietary Habits _Rating Scale_

Score	Rating
14–15	Very Good
12–13	Good
10–11	Marginal
9 or less	Poor

Evaluating Your Stress Level

Name   Section   Date

■ Read concept 20 before proceeding with this lab.

PURPOSE

The purpose of this lab is to evaluate your stress during the past year and determine its implications. Research shows that when people become too stressed, they are more susceptible to certain diseases such as heart disease, ulcers, allergies, hypertension, and insomnia. There are also some physiological implications, as this lab will show. People with high stress need to recognize its causes and effects, and find ways of coping with or reducing stress.

PROCEDURE

1. Look at the Life Experience Survey in the Lab Resource Materials (pp. 253–255). Indicate with a check whether the experience (if it occurred in the past year) occurred during the first six months or the last six months. Circle the score representing the impact the experience had on you.
2. Add all of the negative numbers and record your score (distress) in the Results section below. Add the positive numbers and record your score (eustress) in the Results section below. Use all of the events in the last year.
3. Find your scores on the Rating Scale (chart 20.1 below) and record your ratings.
4. Interpret the results by answering the questions, and discussing the conclusions and implications in the space provided.
5. You may also want to calculate your distress and eustress scores over the last six months rather than the last year. The more recent the event, the greater the likelihood that it will be stressful.

Chart 20.1 Rating Scale for Life Experiences and Stress	Sum of Negative Scores (Distress)	Sum of Positive Scores (Eustress)
May need counseling	14+	
Above average stress	9–13	>10
Average	6–9	9–10
Below average stress	<6	<8

RESULTS

Sum of negative scores   _____   (distress)

Sum of positive scores   _____   (eustress)

Rating on negative scores   _____

Rating on positive scores   _____

The higher the negative score, the greater the distress and the more likely you are to:

1. have high anxiety;
2. have some personal maladjustments, psychological problems, and/or neuroticism;
3. be depressed;
4. feel less capable of exerting control over your environment; and
5. have academic problems; lower GPA.

A high positive score (eustress) suggests that your life's experiences are enriching your quality of life.

CONCLUSIONS AND IMPLICATIONS

In several sentences discuss your current stress level and what, if anything, needs to be done about it. Use your stress rating in your discussion.

LAB
20A

Evaluating Neuromuscular Tension

Name _____ Section _____ Date _____

■ Read concept 20 before proceeding with this lab.

PURPOSE

The purpose of this laboratory session is to learn to recognize signs of excess tension in yourself and in others by symptomatic mannerisms and by manually testing your ability to relax. If time permits, perform the relaxation exercises in concept 20 before executing the lab. A trained person can diagnose neuromuscular hypertension by observation and by manual testing. While there is insufficient time in this course to master either the technique of relaxing or the techniques of evaluation, it is possible to learn the procedures for both.

PROCEDURE

1. Choose a partner. Designate one partner as the subject and the other as the tester. Alternate roles.
2. The subject should lie supine in a comfortable position and consciously try to relax as described in concept 20. This may be done alone, or the instructor may wish to direct the entire group in this procedure.
3. The tester should kneel beside the subject's right hand and remain very still and quiet while the subject is concentrating.
4. After five minutes have elapsed, the tester should observe the subject for signs of tension in Part A of chart 20.2 and check "yes" or "no" for symptoms of visual tension.
5. Quietly and gently, the tester should grasp the subject's right wrist with his or her fingers, and slowly raise it about three inches from the floor, letting it hinge at the elbow, then let the hand drop. Observe the signs of tension outlined in Part B of chart 20.2. *Caution:* Make no movement or sound to disturb your partner's concentration and relaxation. Check the chart to indicate manual symptoms of tension (see next page).
6. You may wish to repeat this after another minute or two.
7. Arouse the subject at the end of the testing and total the number of "yes" checks.
8. Find the rating in chart 20.3 and record it below.
9. Change places and repeat the evaluation with a new subject and tester.
10. Draw conclusions and discuss the implications by answering the questions that follow.

RESULTS

What is your tension score? _____

What is your tension-relaxation rating? _____

Check one box for each of the following questions.

Yes	No	
☐	☐	Were you aware of your own tension?
☐	☐	Was it more difficult to relax than you expected?
☐	☐	Did your awareness of your partner make it more difficult to concentrate?
☐	☐	Can you concentrate on your breathing without altering its rhythm?
☐	☐	Could you learn to release muscular tension and help manage your stress with additional practice?
☐	☐	Could you learn to release tension while sitting or standing with your eyes open?
☐	☐	Do you think your score today is typical of your normal tension level?

Chart 20.2 Signs of Tension Observed by Tester

A.	Visual Symptoms	No	Yes
	Frowning	☐	☐
	Twitching	☐	☐
	Eyelids fluttering	☐	☐
	Breathing:		
	shallow	☐	☐
	rapid	☐	☐
	irregular	☐	☐
	Mouth tight	☐	☐
	Swallowing	☐	☐

B.	Manual Symptoms	No	Yes
	Assistance (subject helps lift arm)	☐	☐
	Resistance (subject resists movement)	☐	☐
	Posturing (subject holds arm in raised position)	☐	☐
	Perseveration (subject continues upward movement)	☐	☐

Total number of "yes" checks _____

Chart 20.3 Tension-Relaxation *Rating Scale*

Classification	Total Score
Excellent (relaxed)	0
Very good (mild tension)	1–3
Good (moderate tension)	4–6
Fair (tense)	7–9
Poor (marked tension)	10–12

LAB
20B

CONCLUSIONS AND IMPLICATIONS

In several sentences describe the implications this concept has for you in terms of your daily life (e.g., sleeping, studying, taking exams, performing on stage, etc.)?

Relaxing Tense Muscles

Name   Section   Date

■ Read concept 20 before completing this lab.

PURPOSE

The purpose of this lab is to learn how to relax tense muscles.

PROCEDURE

Part I

Perform each of the Relaxation Exercises that follow.

Part II

1. Sit in a chair or lie on your back in a quiet, nondistracting atmosphere while you are learning this relaxation technique. (Later you will want to be able to use the technique in public, everyday situations, while you are at work, or any time you are under stress.) Get as comfortable as possible.
2. Do the Contract-Relax Exercise Routine for Relaxation. Contract the muscles to a moderate level of tension (do not use maximum contractions) as you inhale for five to seven seconds. Study where you are feeling the tension. Try to keep the tension isolated to the designated muscle group without allowing it to spill over to other muscles. Use the dominant side of the body first; repeat on the nondominant side.
3. Next, release the tension completely, instantly relaxing the muscles, and exhale. Extend the feeling of relaxation throughout your muscles for twenty to thirty seconds before contracting again. Think of relaxing expressions like "warm," "calm," "peaceful," and "serene."
4. If time permits, you should practice each muscle group two to five times (until tension is gone) before going to the next group. In a class, you may have time for only one trial. For home practice, do the routine twice a day for fifteen minutes.

LAB
20C

RESULTS, CONCLUSIONS, AND IMPLICATIONS

Did you find the relaxation exercises effective? Yes ☐ No ☐
Do you think you would find them useful as part of your normal daily routine or as a "quick fix" for stress? Yes ☐ No ☐
Did you find the contract-relax exercise routine relaxing? Yes ☐ No ☐
Do you think you would find them useful as part of your normal daily routine or as a "quick fix" for stress? Yes ☐ No ☐

In several sentences, discuss whether or not you feel that relaxation exercises will be a part of your wellness program.

Relaxation Exercises

1. **Neck Stretch** Roll the head slowly in a half circle from 9:00 to 8:00 to 7, 6, 5, 4, and 3, then reverse from 3 to 9. Close your eyes and feel the stretch. Do *not* make a full circle by tipping the head back. Repeat several times.

2. **Shoulder Lift** Hunch the shoulders as high as possible (contract) and then let them drop (relax). Repeat several times. Inhale on the lift; exhale on the drop.

3. **Trunk Stretch and Drop** Stand and reach as high as possible; tiptoe and stretch every muscle, then collapse completely, letting knees flex and trunk, head, and arms dangle. Repeat two or three times. Inhale on the stretch and exhale on the collapse.

4. **Trunk Swings** Following the "trunk stretch and drop," remain in the "drop" position and with a minimum of muscular effort, set the trunk swinging from side to side by shifting the weight from one foot to the other, letting the heels come off the floor alternately. Keep the entire body (especially the neck) limp.

5. **Tension Contrast** With arms extended overhead, lie on your side. Tense the body as stiff as a board, then let go, and relax, letting the body fall either forward or backward in whatever direction it loses balance. Continue letting go for a few seconds after falling and allow yourself to feel like you are still sinking. Repeat on the other side.

CONTRACT-RELAX EXERCISE ROUTINE FOR RELAXATION*

1. Hand and forearm—Contract your right hand, making a fist; hold 3 counts; relax and keep letting go 6–10 counts. Repeat, then do left fist, then both fists.

2. Biceps—Flex both elbows and contract your biceps; hold 3 counts; relax and continue relaxing 6–10 counts. Repeat.

3. Triceps—Same as biceps except extend both elbows, contract the triceps on the back of the arm. Repeat.

4. Relax both hands, forearms, and upper arms.

5. Forehead—Raise your eyebrows and wrinkle your forehead; hold 3 counts; relax and continue relaxing 6–10 counts.

6. Cheeks and nose—Make a face; wrinkle your nose and squint; hold 3 counts; relax and continue relaxing 6–10 counts.

7. Jaws—Clench your teeth 3 counts; relax 6–10 counts.

8. Lips and tongue—With teeth apart, press lips together and press tongue to roof of mouth; hold 3 counts; relax 6–10 counts.

9. Neck and throat—Push head backward while tucking chin, pushing against floor or pillow if lying; if sitting, push against high chair-back; hold 3 counts; relax for 6–10 counts.

10. Relax forehead, cheeks, nose, jaws, lips, tongue, neck, and throat. Relax hands, forearms, and upper arms.

11. Shoulder and upper back—Hunch shoulders to ears; hold 3 counts; relax 6–10 counts.

12. Relax lips, tongue, neck, throat, shoulders, and upper back.

13. Abdomen—Suck in abdomen; hold 3 counts; relax 6–10 counts.

14. Lower back—Contract and arch the back; hold 3 counts; relax 6–10 counts.

15. Thighs and buttocks—Squeeze your buttocks together and push your heels into the floor (if lying) or against a chair rung (if sitting); hold 3 counts; relax 6–10 counts.

16. Relax shoulders and upper back, abdomen, lower back, thighs, and buttocks.

17. Calves—Pull instep and toes toward shins; hold 3 counts; relax 6–10 counts.

18. Toes—Curl toes; hold 3 counts; relax 6–10 counts.

19. Relax every muscle in your body.

Note: Eventually, you should progress to a combination of muscle groups and gradually eliminate the "contract" phase of the program. Refer to Jacobson's (1978) or Greenberg's (1996) books.

LAB 21

The Physical Activity Adherence Questionnaire

Name _____ Section _____ Date _____

PURPOSE

The purposes of this laboratory are:
1. To help you understand the factors that lead to physical activity adherence.
2. To help you see which of these factors may keep you from adhering to physical activity.
3. To help you see which factors you might change to improve your chances of adhering to physical activity.

PROCEDURE

1. Read each of the fifteen items in the Physical Activity Adherence Questionnaire, chart 21.1 on the back of this page.
2. After each statement, check the box indicating whether you think the item is Very True, Somewhat True, or Not True of you.
3. When you have answered all fifteen items, use the scoring procedures in the Lab Resource Materials (page 264) to score the questionnaire.

RESULTS

After you have scored the questionnaire, record your scores for each of the three scales and your total score in the spaces provided below. Use chart 21.2 in the Lab Resource Materials on the back of this page to determine your rating for each score. Write the ratings in the appropriate blanks.

	Score	Rating
Predisposing factors	_____	_____
Enabling factors	_____	_____
Reinforcing factors	_____	_____
Total	_____	_____

LAB 21

CONCLUSIONS AND IMPLICATIONS

In several sentences, discuss your ratings on the physical activity adherence questionnaire. Also discuss the predisposing, enabling, and reinforcing factors that you may need to alter to increase your prospects for lifetime activity.

Chart 21.1 Physical Activity Adherence Questionnaire

The factors that predispose, enable, and reinforce physical activity adherence are listed below. Read each statement. Check the box under the most appropriate response for you.

	Very True	Somewhat True	Not True
PREDISPOSING FACTORS			
1. I am very knowledgeable about fitness and physical activity.	☐	☐	☐
2. I have a strong belief that physical activity is good for me.	☐	☐	☐
3. I enjoy doing regular exercise and physical activity.	☐	☐	☐
4. I am confident of my abilities in sports, exercise, and other physical activities.	☐	☐	☐
5. I am motivated to do physical activity without having to be encouraged by others or without receiving external rewards.	☐	☐	☐
6. I have been a regular exerciser most of my life.	☐	☐	☐
7. I like the way I look.	☐	☐	☐
		Subtotal	_____
ENABLING FACTORS			
8. I possess good sports skills.	☐	☐	☐
9. I possess good general physical fitness.	☐	☐	☐
10. I have a place to exercise and equipment that I can use in or near my home.	☐	☐	☐
11. I am capable of setting my own physical activity goals and keeping track of my progress.	☐	☐	☐
		Subtotal	_____
REINFORCING FACTORS			
12. I have the support of my family, especially my spouse, for doing my regular physical activity.	☐	☐	☐
13. I have many friends who enjoy the same kinds of physical activities that I do.	☐	☐	☐
14. I am successful in most physical activities that I try.	☐	☐	☐
15. I have a doctor and/or employer who encourages me to exercise.	☐	☐	☐
		Subtotal	_____
		Total	_____

Chart 21.2 Physical Activity Adherence Rating Scale

Classification	Predisposing Score	Enabling Score	Reinforcing Score	Total Score
Excellent	12–14	7–8	7–8	26–30
Very Good	10–11	6	6	22–25
Good	7–9	4–5	4–5	15–21
Fair	5–6	3	3	11–14
Poor	<5	<3	<3	<11

Evaluating Exercises and Exercise Devices from the Literature

Name _____ Section _____ Date _____

■ Read concept 22 before proceeding with this lab.

PURPOSE

The purpose of this lab is to practice evaluating exercises found in popular literature.

PROCEDURE

1. Read a popular book or magazine and find what you believe to be a poor exercise or device that claims to improve your health, fitness, figure, or posture. If possible, attach a copy of the description of the exercise/device to this lab sheet.
2. Use chart 22.1A to evaluate the *literature's description of an* exercise/device. Check "yes" or "no" for each item. Then record your scores in the Results section.
3. Write the name of the book, magazine, or newspaper from which your article was taken as well as the date of the article and the name of the author (chart 22.1A). Describe the exercise/device you evaluated in the space provided in chart 22.1A on the back of this lab sheet.

RESULTS

1. Give the literature and exercise/device you are evaluating one point for each "yes" answer on questions 1, 8, 9, and 10.   (Score A) _____
2. Give it one point for each "yes" answer on questions 2, 3, 4, 5, 6, and 7.   (Score B) _____
3. Total of score 1 and score 2.   (Total Score) _____

Chart 22.1A Exercise/Device Evaluation*

	Yes	No		Yes	No
1. Is the article or book written by an expert as defined in this Concept?	☐	☐	7. Does it employ "active" exercise in which your own muscles contract?	☐	☐
2. Does the exercise/device employ the overload principle?	☐	☐	8. Are the benefits claimed for it reasonable?	☐	☐
3. Does it employ the progression principle?	☐	☐	9. Are the authors trying to help you (rather than selling a product)?	☐	☐
4. Does it employ the F.I.T.T. formula?	☐	☐	10. Do they refrain from using terms such as "quick," "miraculous," "tone," "remove fat," "new discovery," or other gimmick words?	☐	☐
5. Does it employ the principle of specificity?	☐	☐			
6. Is it a safe exercise?	☐	☐			

*If in doubt, you may seek an expert's opinion on some of these questions.

1. A high Score A total (3 or 4) in the Results section indicates that the authors of the exercise or device know what they are talking about.
2. A high Score B total (5 or 6) indicates that it is consistent with good exercise theory.
3. A high Total Score (8 to 10) suggests that it is sound for at least some aspects of fitness.

Chart 22.3A Exercise/Device Description
Name of book or magazine:
Name of author:
Date of book or magazine:
I evaluated an: exercise ☐   exercise device ☐
Describe the exercise or exercise device in the space provided.

CONCLUSIONS AND IMPLICATIONS

Use several sentences to write an assessment of the exercise or exercise device you described. Use the results obtained from chart 22.1 in writing your answer.

LAB
22A

Evaluating A Health/Wellness or Fitness Club

Name _____ Section _____ Date _____

■ Read concept 22 before proceeding with this lab.

PURPOSE

The purpose of this lab is to practice evaluating a "health" club. (Various combinations of the words health, wellness, and fitness are often used for these clubs.)

PROCEDURE

1. Visit a club and pretend to be interested in becoming a member. (*Note:* Only one or two class members should go to each club to avoid suspicion.)
2. Listen carefully to all that is said and ask lots of questions (without exposing your real motives).
3. Look carefully all around you as you are given the tour of the facilities; ask what the exercises or the equipment does for you or ask leading questions such as, "Will this take inches off my hips?", etc.
4. As soon as you leave the club, jot some notes before you forget what you heard and saw or complete this report immediately. Do not take notes while you are in the club. Space is provided for notes in the Health Club Evaluation Chart (chart 22.2B).

Chart 22.2B Health Club Evaluation

	Yes	No	Notes
1. Were claims for improvement in weight, figure/physique, or fitness realistic?	☐	☐	_____
2. Was a long-term contract (1–3 years) encouraged?	☐	☐	_____
3. Was the sales pitch high-pressure to make an immediate decision?	☐	☐	_____
4. Were you given a copy of the contract to read at home?	☐	☐	_____
5. Did the fine print include objectionable clauses?	☐	☐	_____
6. Did they recommend a physician's approval prior to joining?	☐	☐	_____
7. Did they sell diet supplements as a side line?	☐	☐	_____
8. Did they have passive equipment?	☐	☐	_____
9. Did they have cardiovascular training equipment or facilities (cycles, track, pool, aerobic dance)?	☐	☐	_____
10. Did they make unscientific claims for the equipment, exercise, baths, or diet supplements?	☐	☐	_____
11. Were the facilities clean?	☐	☐	_____
12. Were the facilities crowded?	☐	☐	_____
13. Were there days and hours when facilities were open but would not be available to you?	☐	☐	_____
14. Were there limits on the number of minutes you could use a piece of equipment?	☐	☐	_____
15. Did the floor personnel closely supervise and assist clients?	☐	☐	_____
16. Were the floor personnel qualified "experts"?	☐	☐	_____
17. Were the managers/owners qualified "experts"?	☐	☐	_____
18. Has the club been in business at this location for a year or more?	☐	☐	_____

1. Check the evaluation list on chart 22.2B by checking the "yes" or "no" answers, and add any special notes opposite each item.
2. Score the chart as follows:

   A. Give one point for each "no" answer for items 1, 2, 3, 4, 5, 7, 8, 10, 13, and 14,
   and place the score in the blank. Total A _____

   B. Give one point for each "yes" answer for items 6, 9, 11, 12, and 17, and
   place the score in the blank. Total B _____

   Total A and B above and place the score in the blank. Total A and B _____

   C. Give one point for each "yes" answer on 14, 15, and 16, and
   place the score in the blank. Total C _____

3. A total score of 12–15 points on items *A* and *B* suggests the club rates at least "fair" compared to other clubs.

4. A score of 3 on item *C* indicates that the personnel are qualified and suggests that you could expect to get accurate technical advice from the staff.

5. Regardless of the total scores, you would have to decide the importance of each item in chart 22.2B to you personally, as well as evaluate other considerations such as cost, location, personalities of the clients and the personnel, and so on, to decide if this would be a good place for you or your friends to join.

CONCLUSIONS AND IMPLICATIONS

In the space below, use several sentences to discuss your conclusion about the quality of this club and whether you think it would fit your needs if you wanted to belong.

LAB
22B

Planning for Lifestyle Changes

Name   Section   Date

PURPOSE

The purpose of this lab is to make plans for lifestyle change using the five steps outlined in the concept.

PROCEDURE

Answer the questions and fill in the spaces following the five steps outlined below.

1. Identify Areas of Possible Change

Place an X in the box beside the areas in chart 23.1 in which you would like to make changes. Physical activity is not included because you planned for it in Lab 17.

Chart 23.1 Areas of Possible Lifestyle Change	
☐ Eating properly	☐ Adopting personal health behaviors
☐ Controlling stress	☐ Seeking and complying with medical advice
☐ Avoiding destructive habits	☐ Becoming an informed consumer
☐ Practicing safe sex	☐ Protecting the environment
☐ Adopting safety habits	☐ Managing time effectively
☐ Learning first aid	☐ Other (designate) _____

2. Establish Your Goals

In chart 23.2, write your goals for the next month. Write the date by which the goal is to be accomplished. Do not include physical activity or fitness goals.

Chart 23.2 Lifestyle Goals			
Goal	Date to Be Met	Goal	Date to Be Met

3. Write Your Plan in Chart 23.3

If appropriate, write a specific plan for meeting your goals. For example, if you plan to learn first-aid write the days of the week and the time of the day that you will take a class.

Chart 23.3 Plans for Lifestyle Change

4. Keep Records

You can use the monthly calendar below or make one like it on a full sheet of paper to keep track of your goals and lifestyle changes. Write in the dates on the calendar (yellow) beginning on the day you plan to begin modifying your lifestyle. Write goals on the calendar. Place an X in the green boxes for dates goals are to be met or programs are to be planned. Place an X in the blue boxes each time you carry out your program or meet your goals.

5. Periodically Revise

Check to see how successful you have been in meeting your goals and revise your plan if necessary.

Chart 23.4 Lifestyle Record-Keeping Calendar

MONTH _____

Sunday	Monday	Tuesday	Wednesday	Thursday	Friday	Saturday	
Date	Date	Date	Date	Date	Date	Date	GOAL 1:
Goals:	Goals:	Goals:	Goals:	Goals:	Goals:	Goals:	
Date	Date	Date	Date	Date	Date	Date	GOAL 2:
Goals:	Goals:	Goals:	Goals:	Goals:	Goals:	Goals:	
Date	Date	Date	Date	Date	Date	Date	GOAL 3:
Goals:	Goals:	Goals:	Goals:	Goals:	Goals:	Goals:	
Date	Date	Date	Date	Date	Date	Date	GOAL 4:
Goals:	Goals:	Goals:	Goals:	Goals:	Goals:	Goals:	

APPENDIX A

Metric Conversion Chart

Approximate Conversions from Metric to Traditional Measures

Length
centimeters to inches: cm $\times$ .39 = in
meters to feet: m $\times$ 3.3 = ft
meters to yards: m $\times$ 1.09 = yd
kilometers to miles: km $\times$ 0.6 = mi

Mass (Weight)
grams to ounces: g $\times$ 0.0352 = oz
kilograms to pounds: kg $\times$ 2.2 = lbs

Area
square centimeters to square inches: $cm^2 \times 0.16 = in^2$
square meters to square feet: $m^2 \times 11.11 = ft^2$
square meters to square yards: $m^2 \times 1.02 = yd^2$

Volume
milliliters to fluid ounces: ml $\times$ 0.03 = fl oz
liters to quarts: 1 $\times$ 1.06 = qt
liters to gallons: 1 $\times$ 0.264 = gal

Approximate Conversions from Traditional to Metric Measures

Length
inches to centimeters: in $\times$ 2.54 = cm
feet to meters: ft $\times$ .3048 = m
yards to meters: yd $\times$ 0.92 = m
miles to kilometers: mi $\times$ 1.6 = km

Mass (Weight)
ounces to grams: oz $\times$ 28.41 = gm
pounds to kilograms: lbs $\times$ 0.45 = kg

Area
square inches to square centimeters: $in^2 \times 6.5 = cm^2$
square feet to square meters: $ft^2 \times 0.09 = m^2$
square yards to square meters: $yd^2 \times 0.76 = m^2$

Volume
fluid ounces to mililiters: fl oz $\times$ 29.573 = ml
quarts to liters: qt $\times$ 0.95 = 1
gallons to liters: gal $\times$ 3.8 = 1

APPENDIX B

Metric Conversions of Selected Charts and Tables

Chart 5.1 Twelve-Minute Run Test (Scores in Meters)				
Men (age)				
Classification	**17–26**	**27–39**	**40–49**	**50+**
High performance zone	2880+	2560+	2400+	2240+
Good fitness zone	2480–2779	2320–2559	2240–2399	2000–2239
Marginal zone	2160–2479	2080–2319	2000–2239	1760–1999
Low zone	< 2160	< 2080	< 2000	< 1760
Women (age)				
Classification	**17–26**	**27–39**	**40–49**	**50+**
High performance zone	2320+	2160+	2000+	1840+
Good fitness zone	2000–2319	1920–2159	1840–1999	1680–1839
Marginal zone	1840–1999	1680–1919	1600–1839	1520–1679
Low zone	< 1840	< 1680	< 1600	< 1520

Charts 9.2 and 9.3 Isometric Strength *Rating Scales*

Strength *Rating Scale* for Men (kg)

Classification	Left Grip	Right Grip	Total Score
High Performance zone	57+	61+	118+
Good fitness zone	45–56	50–60	95–117
Marginal zone	41–44	43–49	84–94
Low zone	< 41	< 43	< 84

Strength *Rating Scale* for Women (kg)

Classification	Left Grip	Right Grip	Total Score
High Performance zone	34+	39+	73+
Good fitness zone	27–33	32–38	59–72
Marginal zone	20–26	23–31	43–58
Low zone	< 20	< 23	< 43

Charts 2 and 3 are suitable for use by young adults between 18 and 30 years of age. After 30, an adjustment of 0.5 of 1 percent per year is appropriate because some loss of muscle tissue typically occurs as you grow older.

Chart 15.5 Reaction Time *Rating Scale*

Classification	Score in Inches	Score in Centimeters
Excellent	21+	53+
Very good	19–21	48–52
Good	16–18¾	41–47
Fair	13–15¾	33–40
Poor	< 13	< 33

Chart 15.6 Speed *Rating Scale*

Classification	Men		Women	
	Yards	Meters	Yards	Meters
Excellent	24+	22+	22+	20+
Very good	22–23	20–21.9	20–21	18–19.9
Good	18–21	16.5–19.9	16–19	14.5–17.9
Fair	16–17	14.5–16.4	14–15	13–14.4
Poor	< 16	< 14.5	< 14	< 13

Chart 15.4 Power *Rating Scale*

Classification	Men	Women
Excellent	68 cm+	60 cm+
Very good	53–67 cm	48–59 cm
Good	42–52 cm	37–47 cm
Fair	32–41 cm	27–36 cm
Poor	< 32 cm	< 27 cm

APPENDIX C

Calorie Guide to Common Foods*

Beverages

Coffee (black)	0
Coke (12 oz.)	137
Hot chocolate, milk (1 cup)	247
Lemonade (1 cup)	100
Limeade, diluted to serve (1 cup)	110
Soda, fruit flavored (12 oz.)	161
Tea (clear)	0

Breads and Cereals

Bagel (1 half)	76
Biscuit (2″ × 2″)	135
Bread, pita (1 oz.)	80
Bread, raisin (½″ thick)	65
Bread, rye	55
Bread, white enriched (½″ thick)	64
Bread, whole wheat (½″ thick)	55
Bun (hamburger)	120
Cereals, cooked (½ cup)	80
Corn flakes (1 cup)	96
Corn grits (1 cup)	125
Corn muffin (2½″ diam.)	103
Crackers, graham (1 med.)	28
Crackers, soda (1 plain)	24
English muffin (1 half)	74
Macaroni, with cheese (1 cup)	464
Muffin, plain	135
Noodles (1 cup)	200
Oatmeal (1 cup)	150
Pancakes (1–4″ diam.)	59
Pizza (1 section)	180
Popped corn (1 cup)	54
Potato chips (10 med.)	108
Pretzels (5 small sticks)	18
Rice (1 cup)	225
Roll, plain (1 med.)	118
Roll, sweet (1 med.)	178
Shredded wheat (1 med. biscuit)	79
Spaghetti, plain cooked (1 cup)	218
Tortilla (1 corn)	70
Waffle (4½″ × 5″)	216

Dairy Products

Butter, 1 pat (1½ tsp.)	50
Cheese, cheddar (1 oz.)	113
Cheese, cottage (1 cup)	270
Cheese, cream (1 oz.)	106
Cheese, Parmesan (1 tbsp.)	29
Cheese, Swiss natural (1 oz.)	105
Cream, sour (1 tbsp.)	31
Dairy Queen Cone (med.)	335
Frozen custard (1 cup)	375
Frozen yogurt, vanilla (1 cup)	180

Ice cream, plain (prem.) (1 cup)	350
Ice cream soda, choc. (large glass)	455
Ice milk (1 cup)	184
Ices (1 cup)	177
Milk, chocolate (1 cup)	185
Milk, half-and-half (1 tbsp.)	20
Milk, malted (1 cup)	281
Milk, skim (1 cup)	88
Milk, skim dry (1 tbsp.)	28
Milk, whole (1 cup)	166
Sherbet (1 cup)	270
Whipped topping (1 tbsp.)	14
Yogurt (1 cup)	150

Desserts and Sweets

Cake, angel (2″ wedge)	108
Cake, chocolate (2″ × 3″ × 1″)	150
Cake, plain (3″ × 2½″)	180
Chocolate, bar	200–300
Chocolate, bitter (1 oz.)	142
Chocolate, sweet (1 oz.)	133
Chocolate, syrup (1 tbsp.)	42
Cocoa (1 tbsp.)	21
Cookies, plain (1 med.)	75
Custard, baked (1 cup)	283
Doughnut (1 large)	250
Gelatin, dessert (1 cup)	155
Gelatin, with fruit (1 cup)	170
Gingerbread (2″ × 2″ × 2″)	180
Jams, jellies (1 tbsp.)	55
Pie, apple (¹/₇ of 9″ pie)	345
Pie, cherry (¹/₇ of 9″ pie)	355
Pie, chocolate (¹/₇ of 9″ pie)	360
Pie, coconut (¹/₇ of 9″ pie)	266
Pie, lemon meringue (¹/₇ of 9″ pie)	302
Sugar, granulated (1 tsp.)	27
Syrup, table (1 tbsp.)	57

Fruit

Apple, fresh (med.)	76
Applesauce, unsweetened (1 cup)	184
Avocado, raw (½ peeled)	279
Banana, fresh (med.)	88
Cantaloupe, raw (½, 5″ diam.)	60
Cherries (10 sweet)	50
Cranberry sauce, unsweetened (1 tbsp.)	25
Fruit cocktail, canned (1 cup)	170
Grapefruit, fresh (½)	60
Grapefruit juice, raw (1 cup)	95
Grape juice, bottled (½ cup)	80
Grapes (20–25)	75
Nectarine (1 med.)	88
Olives, green	72

Olives, ripe (10)	105
Orange, fresh (med.)	60
Orange juice, frozen diluted (1 cup)	110
Peach, fresh (med.)	46
Peach, canned in syrup (2 halves)	79
Pear, fresh (med.)	95
Pears, canned in syrup (2 halves)	79
Pineapple, crushed in syrup (1 cup)	204
Pineapple (½ cup fresh)	50
Prune juice (1 cup)	170
Raisins, dry (1 tbsp.)	26
Strawberries, fresh (1 cup)	54
Strawberries, frozen (3 oz.)	90
Tangerine (2½″ diam.)	40
Watermelon, wedge (4″ × 8″)	120

Meat, Fish, Eggs

Bacon, drained (2 slices)	97
Bacon, Canadian (1 oz.)	62
Beef, hamburger chuck (3 oz.)	316
Beef, pot pie	560
Beef steak, sirloin or T-bone (3 oz.)	257
Beef and vegetable stew (1 cup)	185
Chicken, fried breast (8 oz.)	210
Chicken, fried (1 leg and thigh)	305
Chicken, roasted breast (2 slices)	100
Chili, without beans (1 cup)	510
Chili, with beans (1 cup)	335
Egg, boiled	77
Egg, fried	125
Egg, scrambled	100
Fish and chips (2 pcs. fish; 4 oz. chips)	275
Fish, broiled (3″ × 3″ × ½″)	112
Fish stick	40
Frankfurter, boiled	124
Ham (4″ × 4″)	338
Lamb (3 oz. roast, lean)	158
Liver (3″ × 3″)	150
Luncheon meat (2 oz.)	135
Pork chop, loin (3″ × 5″)	284
Salmon, canned (1 cup)	145
Sausage, pork (4 oz.)	510
Shrimp, canned (3 oz.)	108
Tuna, canned (½ cup)	185
Veal, cutlet (3″ × 4″)	175

Nuts and Seeds

Cashews (1 cup)	770
Coconut (1 cup)	450
Peanut butter (1 tbsp.)	92
Peanuts, roasted, no skin (1 cup)	805
Pecans (1 cup)	752
Sunflower seeds (1 tbsp.)	50

*Note: For a complete listing of foods, the reader is referred to: *Nutritive Value of Foods,* U.S. Department of Agriculture, Washington, D.C., Home and Gardens Bulletin, No. 72. (Available in most libraries, university bookstores, and Home Economics departments.)

Sandwiches

(2 slices of bread—plain)

Bologna	214
Cheeseburger (small McDonald's)	300
Chicken salad	185
Egg salad	240
Fish filet (McDonald's)	400
Ham	360
Ham and cheese	360
Hamburger (small McDonald's)	260
Hamburger, Burger King Whopper	600
Hamburger, Big Mac	550
Hamburger (McDonald's Quarter Pounder)	420
Peanut butter	250
Roast beef (Arby's Regular)	425

Sauces, Fats, Oils

Catsup, tomato (1 tbsp.)	17
Chili sauce (1 tbsp.)	17
French dressing (1 tbsp.)	59
Margarine (1 pat)	50
Mayonnaise (1 tbsp.)	92
Mayonnaise-type (1 tbsp.)	65
Vegetable, sunflower, safflower oils (1 tbsp.)	120

Soup, Ready to Serve (1 cup)

Bean	190
Beef noodle	100
Cream	200
Tomato	90
Vegetable	80

Vegetables

Alfalfa sprouts (½ cup)	19
Asparagus (6 spears)	22
Bean sprouts (1 cup)	37
Beans, green (1 cup)	27
Beans, lima (1 cup)	152
Beans, navy (1 cup)	642
Beans, pork and molasses (1 cup)	325
Broccoli, fresh cooked (1 cup)	60
Cabbage, cooked (1 cup)	40
Cauliflower (1 cup)	25
Carrot, raw (med.)	21
Carrots, canned (1 cup)	44
Celery, diced raw (1 cup)	20
Coleslaw (1 cup)	102
Corn, sweet, canned (1 cup)	140
Corn, sweet (med. ear)	84
Cucumber, raw (6 slices)	6
Lettuce (2 large leaves)	7
Mushrooms, canned (1 cup)	28
Onions, french fried (10 rings)	75
Onions, raw (med.)	25
Peas, field (½ cup)	90
Peas, green (1 cup)	145
Pickles, dill (med.)	15
Pickles, sweet (med.)	22
Potato, baked (med.)	97
Potato, french fried (8 stick)	155
Potato, mashed (1 cup)	185
Radish, raw (small)	1
Sauerkraut, drained (1 cup)	32
Spinach, fresh, cooked (1 cup)	46
Squash, summer (1 cup)	30
Sweet pepper (med.)	15
Sweet potato, candied (small)	314
Tomato, cooked (1 cup)	50
Tomato, raw (med.)	30

■ APPENDIX D ■

Calories of Protein, Carbohydrates, and Fats in Foods*

Food No./Food Choice	Total Calories	Protein Calories	Carbohydrate Calories	Fat Calories
Breakfast				
1. Scrambled Egg (1 lg)	111	29	7	75
2. Fried Egg (1 lg)	99	26	1	72
3. Pancake (1–6^W)	146	19	67	58
4. Syrup (1 T)	60	0	60	0
5. French Toast (1 slice)	180	23	49	108
6. Waffle (7-inch)	245	28	100	117
7. Biscuit (medium)	104	8	52	44
8. Bran Muffin (medium)	104	11	63	31
9. White Toast (slice)	68	9	52	7
10. Wheat Toast (slice)	67	14	52	6
11. Peanut Butter (1 T)	94	15	11	68
12. Yogurt (8 oz. plain)	227	39	161	27
13. Orange Juice (8 oz.)	114	8	100	6
14. Apple Juice (8 oz.)	117	1	116	0
15. Soft Drink (12 oz.)	144	0	144	0
16. Bacon (2 slices)	86	15	2	70
17. Sausage (1-link)	141	11	0	130
18. Sausage (1 patty)	284	23	0	261
19. Grits (8 oz.)	125	11	110	4
20. Hash Browns (8 oz.)	355	18	178	159
21. French Fries (reg.)	239	12	115	112
22. Donut Cake	125	4	61	60
23. Donut Glazed	164	8	87	69
24. Sweet Roll	317	22	136	159
25. Cake (medium slice)	274	14	175	85
26. Ice Cream (8 oz.)	257	15	108	134
27. Cream Cheese (T)	52	4	1	47
28. Jelly (T)	49	0	49	0
29. Jam (T)	54	0	54	0
30. Coffee (cup)	0	0	0	0
31. Tea (cup)	0	0	0	0
32. Cream (T)	32	2	2	28
33. Sugar (t)	15	0	15	0
34. Corn Flakes (8 oz.)	97	8	87	2
35. Wheat Flakes (8 oz.)	106	12	90	4
36. Oatmeal (8 oz.)	132	19	92	21
37. Strawberries (8 oz.)	55	4	46	5
38. Orange (medium)	64	6	57	1
39. Apple (medium)	96	1	86	9
40. Banana (medium)	101	4	95	2
41. Cantaloupe (half)	82	7	73	2
42. Grapefruit (half)	40	2	37	1
43. Custard Pie (slice)	285	20	188	77
44. Fruit Pie (slice)	350	14	259	77
45. Fritter (medium)	132	11	54	67
46. Skim Milk (8 oz.)	88	36	52	0
47. Whole Milk (8 oz.)	159	33	48	78
48. Butter (pat)	36	0	0	36
49. Margarine (pat)	36	0	0	36

Food No./Food Choice	Total Calories	Protein Calories	Carbohydrate Calories	Fat Calories
Lunch				
1. Hamburger (reg. FF)	255	48	120	89
2. Cheeseburger (reg. FF)	307	61	120	126
3. Doubleburger (FF)	563	101	163	299
4. ¼ lb. Burger (FF)	427	73	137	217
5. Doublecheese Burger (FF)	670	174	134	362
6. Doublecheese Baconburger (FF)	724	138	174	340
7. Hot Dog (FF)	214	36	54	124
8. Chili Dog (FF)	320	51	90	179
9. Pizza, Cheese (slice FF)	290	116	116	58
10. Pizza, Meat (slice FF)	360	126	126	108
11. Pizza, Everything (slice FF)	510	179	173	158
12. Sandwich, Roast Beef (FF)	350	88	126	137
13. Sandwich, Bologna	313	44	106	163
14. Sandwich, Bologna-Cheese	428	69	158	201
15. Sandwich, Ham-Cheese (FF)	380	91	133	156
16. Sandwich, Peanut Butter	281	39	118	124
17. Sandwich, PB and Jelly	330	40	168	122
18. Sandwich, Egg Salad	330	40	109	181
19. Sandwich, Tuna Salad	390	101	109	180
20. Sandwich, Fish (FF)	432	56	147	229
21. French Fries (reg. FF)	239	12	115	112
22. French Fries (lg. FF)	406	20	195	191
23. Onion Rings (reg. FF)	274	14	112	148
24. Chili (8 oz.)	260	49	62	148
25. Bean Soup (8 oz.)	355	67	181	107
26. Beef Noodle Soup (8 oz.)	140	32	59	49
27. Tomato Soup (8 oz.)	180	14	121	45
28. Vegetable Soup (8 oz.)	160	21	107	32
29. Small Salad, Plain	37	6	27	4
30. Small Salad, French Dressing	152	8	50	94
31. Small Salad, Italian Dressing	162	8	28	126
32. Small Salad, Bleu Cheese	184	13	28	143
33. Potato Salad (8 oz.)	248	27	159	62
34. Cole Slaw (8 oz.)	180	0	25	155
35. Macaroni and Cheese (8 oz.)	230	37	103	90
36. Taco Beef (FF)	186	59	56	71
37. Bean Burrito (FF)	343	45	192	106
38. Meat Burrito (FF)	466	158	196	112
39. Mexican Rice (FF)	213	17	160	36
40. Mexican Beans (FF)	168	42	82	44
41. Fried Chicken Breast (FF)	436	262	13	161
42. Broiled Chicken Breast	284	224	0	60
43. Broiled Fish	228	82	32	114
44. Fish Stick (1 stick FF)	50	18	8	24
45. Fried Egg	99	26	1	72
46. Donut	125	4	61	60
47. Potato Chips (small bag)	115	3	39	73
48. Soft Drink (12 oz.)	144	0	144	0

*Notes:
1. FF by a food indicates that it is typical of a food served in a fast food restaurant.
2. Your portions of foods may be larger or smaller than those listed here. For this reason you may wish to select a food more than once (i.e., two hamburgers) or select only a portion of a serving (i.e., divide the calories in half for a half portion).
3. An oz. equals an ounce or 28.4 grams.
4. T = Tablespoon and t = teaspoon.
The principal reference for the calculation of values used in this appendix were the *Nutritive Value of Foods,* published by the United States Department of Agriculture, Washington, D.C., Home and Gardens Bulletin, No. 72, although other published sources were consulted, including Jacobson, M., and S. Fritschner, *The Fast-Food Guide* (an excellent source of information about fast foods), New York, Workman Publishing Company, 1986.

Food No./Food Choice	Total Calories	Protein Calories	Carbohydrate Calories	Fat Calories
49. Apple Juice (8 oz.)	117	1	116	0
50. Skim Milk (8 oz.)	88	36	52	0
51. Whole Milk (8 oz.)	159	33	48	78
52. Diet Drink (12 oz.)	0	0	0	0
53. Mustard (t)	4	0	4	0
54. Catsup (t)	6	0	6	0
55. Mayonnaise (T)	100	0	0	100
56. Fruit Pie	350	14	259	77
57. Cheese Cake	400	56	132	212
58. Ice Cream (8 oz.)	257	15	108	134
59. Coffee (8 oz.)	0	0	0	0
60. Tea (8 oz.)	0	0	0	0

Dinner

Food No./Food Choice	Total Calories	Protein Calories	Carbohydrate Calories	Fat Calories
1. Hamburger (reg. FF)	255	48	120	89
2. Cheeseburger (reg. FF)	307	61	120	126
3. Doubleburger (FF)	563	101	163	299
4. ¼ lb. Burger (FF)	427	73	137	217
5. Doublecheese Burger (FF)	670	174	134	362
6. Doublecheese Baconburger (FF)	724	138	174	412
7. Hot Dog (FF)	214	36	54	124
8. Chili Dog (FF)	320	51	90	179
9. Pizza, Cheese (slice FF)	290	116	116	58
10. Pizza, Meat (slice FF)	360	126	126	108
11. Pizza, Everything (slice FF)	510	179	173	158
12. Steak (8 oz.)	880	290	0	590
13. French Fried Shrimp (6 oz.)	360	133	68	158
14. Roast Beef (8 oz.)	440	268	0	172
15. Liver (8 oz.)	520	250	52	218
16. Corned Beef (8 oz.)	493	242	0	251
17. Meat Loaf (8 oz.)	711	228	35	448
18. Ham (8 oz.)	540	178	0	362
19. Spaghetti, No Meat (13 oz.)	400	56	220	124
20. Spaghetti, Meat (13 oz.)	500	115	230	155
21. Baked Potato (medium)	90	12	78	0
22. Cooked Carrots (8 oz.)	71	12	59	0
23. Cooked Spinach (8 oz.)	50	18	18	14
24. Corn (one ear)	70	10	52	8
25. Cooked Green Beans (8 oz.)	54	11	43	0
26. Cooked Broccoli (8 oz.)	60	19	26	15
27. Cooked Cabbage	47	12	35	0
28. French Fries (reg. FF)	239	12	115	112
29. French Fries (lg. FF)	406	20	195	191
30. Onion Rings (reg. FF)	274	14	112	148
31. Chili (8 oz.)	260	49	62	148
32. Small Salad, Plain	37	6	27	4
33. Small Salad, French Dressing	152	8	50	94
34. Small Salad, Italian Dressing	162	8	28	126
35. Small Salad, Bleu Cheese	184	13	28	143
36. Potato Salad (8 oz.)	248	27	159	62
37. Cole Slaw (8 oz.)	180	0	25	155
38. Macaroni and Cheese (8 oz.)	230	37	103	90
39. Taco Beef (FF)	186	59	56	71
40. Bean Burrito (FF)	343	45	192	106
41. Meat Burrito (FF)	466	158	196	112
42. Mexican Rice (FF)	213	17	160	36
43. Mexican Beans (FF)	168	42	82	44
44. Fried Chicken Breast (FF)	436	262	13	161

Food No./Food Choice	Total Calories	Protein Calories	Carbohydrate Calories	Fat Calories
45. Broiled Chicken Breast	284	224	0	60
46. Broiled Fish	228	82	32	114
47. Fish Stick (1 stick FF)	50	18	8	24
48. Soft Drink (12 oz.)	144	0	144	0
49. Apple Juice (8 oz.)	117	1	116	0
50. Skim Milk (8 oz.)	88	36	52	0
51. Whole Milk (8 oz.)	159	33	48	78
52. Diet Drink (12 oz.)	0	0	0	0
53. Mustard (t)	4	0	4	0
54. Catsup (t)	6	0	6	0
55. Mayonnaise (T)	100	0	0	100
56. Fruit Pie (slice)	350	14	259	77
57. Cheese Cake (slice)	400	56	132	212
58. Ice Cream (8 oz.)	257	15	108	134
59. Custard Pie (slice)	285	20	188	77
60. Cake (slice)	274	14	175	85

Snacks

Food No./Food Choice	Total Calories	Protein Calories	Carbohydrate Calories	Fat Calories
1. Peanut Butter (1 T)	94	15	11	68
2. Yogurt (8 oz. plain)	227	39	161	27
3. Orange Juice (8 oz.)	114	8	100	6
4. Apple Juice (8 oz.)	117	1	116	0
5. Soft Drink (12 oz.)	144	0	144	0
6. Donut, Cake	125	4	61	60
7. Donut, Glazed	164	8	87	69
8. Sweet Roll	317	22	136	159
9. Cake (medium slice)	274	14	175	85
10. Ice Cream (8 oz.)	257	15	108	134
11. Soft Serve Cone (reg.)	240	10	89	134
12. Ice Cream Sandwich Bar	210	40	82	88
13. Strawberries (8 oz.)	55	4	46	5
14. Orange (medium)	64	6	57	1
15. Apple (medium)	96	1	86	9
16. Banana (medium)	101	4	95	2
17. Cantaloupe (half)	82	7	73	2
18. Grapefruit (half)	40	2	37	1
19. Celery Stick	5	2	3	0
20. Carrot (medium)	20	3	17	0
21. Raisins (4 oz.)	210	6	204	0
22. Watermelon (4″ × 6″ slice)	115	8	99	8
23. Chocolate Chip Cookie	60	3	9	48
24. Brownie	145	6	26	113
25. Oatmeal Cookie	65	3	13	49
26. Sandwich Cookie	200	8	112	80
27. Custard Pie (slice)	285	20	188	77
28. Fruit Pie (slice)	350	14	259	77
29. Gelatin (4 oz.)	70	4	32	34
30. Fritter (medium)	132	11	54	67
31. Skim Milk (8 oz.)	88	36	52	0
32. Diet Drink	0	0	0	0
33. Potato Chips (small bag)	115	3	39	73
34. Roasted Peanuts (1.3 oz.)	210	34	25	151
35. Chocolate Candy Bar (1 oz.)	145	7	61	77
36. Choc. Almond Candy Bar (1 oz.)	265	38	74	164
37. Saltine Cracker	18	1	1	16
38. Popped Corn	40	7	33	0
39. Cheese Nachos	471	63	194	214

■REFERENCES■

A Guide to Managing Stress. Daly City, CA: Krames Communications, n.d.

"A Modified Internal Rotation Stretching Technique for Overhand and Throwing Athletes." *Journal of Sports Physical Therapy* 21:4 April 1995.

"A Primer on Food Additives." *FDA Consumer* 22(1988):13.

"A Prudent Toast to Your Health." *Tufts University Diet & Nutrition Letter* (December 1989):3.

AAHPERD. *Technical Manual: Health Related Physical Fitness.* Reston, VA: AAHPERD, 1984.

About Inhalants. South Deerfield, MA: Channing L. Bete Co., Inc., 1992.

Adams, K., et al. "The Effect of Six Weeks of Squat, Plyometric and Squat-Plyometric Training on Power Production." *Journal of Applied Sport Science Research* 6(1992):36–41.

"Aerobicizers Getting More Than They Asked For?" *Journal of Physical Education, Recreation and Dance* 62(1991):16.

Aisenbrey, J., and J. L. DePaepe. "A Review of Osteoporosis Research: Implications for Exercise Education and Future Inquiry." *Clinical Kinesiology* 46(1992):2–12.

Alaimo, K. et al. "Dietary Intake of Vitamins, Minerals, and Fiber of Persons Ages 2 Months and Over in the United States." *Vital and Health Statistics: Advance Data* 258(1994):1.

"Alcohol and Cognition." *Alcohol Alert.* Washington, DC: National Institute on Alcohol Abuse and Alcoholism, 1989. Produced for the U.S. Department of Health and Human Services; Public Health Service; Alcohol, Drug Abuse, and Mental Health Administration.

Alcohol and Health. Seventh Special Report to the U.S. Congress from the Secretary of Health and Human Services, NIAAA. Rockville, MD: U.S. Department of Health and Human Services, 1990.

"Alcohol and Prescription Drugs." Reprint. *SRX—Medication Education for Seniors of San Francisco Health Department.* San Francisco, CA: Office of Senior Health Services, n.d.

"Alcohol and Tolerance." *Alcohol Alert.* Nov. 28 PH356 April, 1995, National Institute on Alcohol Abuse and Alcoholism.

"Alcohol Related Impairment." *Alcohol Alert.* No. 25 PH351 July, 1994, National Institute on Alcohol Abuse and Alcoholism.

Aleshire, P. "Fourteen in State Tell of Side Effects from Diet Aid L-Tryptophan." *The Arizona Republic,* November 15, 1989.

Allsen, P. E., and P. Witbeck. *Racquetball.* 6th ed. Dubuque, IA: Brown & Benchmark Publishers, 1996.

Almkinders, L. C. et al. "An In Vitro Investigation Into the Effects of Repetitive Motion and Nonsteroidal Antiinflammatory Medication on Human Tendon Fibroblasts," *American Journal of Sports Medicine* 23(1995):119.

Alon, G., et al. "Comparison of the Effects of Electrical Stimulation and Exercise on Abdominal Musculature." *Journal of Orthopaedic and Sports Physical Therapy* 8(1987):567.

Alpert, J. S., et al. "Athletic Heart Syndrome." *Physician and Sportsmedicine* 17(1989):103.

Alsop, K. "Potential Hazards of Abdominal Exercises." *Journal of Physical Education, Recreation and Dance* 42(1971):89.

Alter, M. J. *Sports Stretch.* Champaign, IL: Human Kinetics Publishers, 1990.

Alter, M. J. *The Science of Stretching.* 2nd ed. Champaign, IL: Human Kinetics Publishers, 1996.

Althoff, S. A., et al. "Back to the Basics—Whatever Happened to Posture." *Journal of Physical Education, Recreation and Dance* 59(1988):20.

Alvarado, D. "Survey of Exercises Determines Skating a High-Risk Activity." *The Arizona Republic* (June 11, 1992):D7.

"Alzado Tribute Called Off at Last Minute." *Los Angeles Times,* Jan. 12, 1992.

American Alliance of Health, Physical Education, Recreation and Dance. 1900 Association Drive, Reston, VA 22091.

American Cancer Society. *Cancer Facts and Figures—1994.* New York: The American Cancer Society, 1995.

American Cancer Society, "CPSII and Tobacco Control," *CPSII, Newsletter* 12(1995):1.

American College of Sports Medicine. *ACSM's Guidelines for Exercise Testing and Prescription,* 5th ed. Baltimore, MD: Williams and Wilkins, 1995.

American College of Sports Medicine. *ACSM's Guidelines for Exercise Testing and Prescription.* 5th ed. Philadelphia: Lea & Febiger, 1995.

American College of Sports Medicine. "Proper and Improper Weight Loss Programs." *Medicine and Science in Sports and Exercise* 15(1983):ix.

American College of Sports Medicine. *Resource Manual for Guidelines for Exercise Testing and Prescription.* (2nd ed.) Philadelphia: Lea and Febiger, 1993.

American College of Sports Medicine. "The Recommended Quantity and Quality of Exercise for Developing and Maintaining Cardiorespiratory and Muscular Fitness in Healthy Adults." *Medicine and Science in Sports and Exercise* 22(1990):2.

American Heart Association (Greater Long Beach Chapter). "Stress—Bona Fide A.H.A. Risk Factor." *Heart Lines* 41(1984):1.

American Heart Association. *1992 Heart Facts Reference Sheet.* Dallas: American Heart Association, 1992.

American Heart Association. "Active and Passive Tobacco Exposure. A Serious Pediatric Health Problem." (Scientific Statement) *Circulation* Nov. (1995).

American Heart Association. "A Statement on Exercise: Benefits and Recommendations for Physical Activity Programs for All Americans." *Circulation* 91(1995), 580.

American Institute of Stress. "Signs and Symptoms of Stress." In *Aviation Medical Bulletin.* Atlanta, GA: Harvey W. Watt and Co., March, 1991.

Anderson, M. B., and J. M. Williams. "A Model of Stress and Athletic Injury: Prediction and Prevention." *Journal of Sport and Exercise Psychology* 10(1988):294–306.

Anderson, T., and J. T. Kearney. "Effects of Three Resistance Training Programs on Muscular Strength and Absolute and Relative Endurance." *Research Quarterly for Exercise and Sport* 53(1982):1.

"Antisteroid Program Needed in Schools." *JOPERD* (Nov./Dec. 1993):14.

Antoni, M. H. "Psychoneuroimmunology and HIV-1." *Journal of Consulting and Clinical Psychology* 15(1990):38.

"Are Sports Drinks Better Than Water?" *Physician and Sportsmedicine* 20(1992):33.

Ascherio, A., et al. "Dietary Intake of Marine n–3 Fatty Acids, Fish Intake, and the Risk of Coronary Disease Among Men. " *The New England Journal of Medicine* 332(1995):977.

Ashton-Miller, J. A., and A. B. Schultz. "Biomechanics of the Human Spine and Trunk." *Exercise and Sports Sciences Reviews* 16(1988):169–204.

Aspinall, W. "Clinical Testing for Cervical Mechanical Disorders Which Produce Ischemic Vertigo." *Journal of Orthopaedic and Sports Physical Therapy* 11(Nov. 1989):176–82.

Astrand, P. O., and K. Rodahl. *Textbook of Work Physiology.* 3d ed. New York: McGraw-Hill, 1986.

"Athletes Find Health Food Supplements Big Trouble." *Toronto Star,* Nov. 15, 1995.

Auble, T. E., et al. "Aerobic Requirement for Moving Handweights through Various Ranges of Motion While Walking." *Physician and Sportsmedicine* 15(1987):133.

Avery, C. "Abdominal Obesity: Scaling Down This Deadly Risk." *Physician and Sportsmedicine* 19(1991):113.

Avis, H. *Drugs and Life.* 2d ed. Dubuque, IA: Wm. C. Brown Publishers, 1993.

Back Owners Manual. Daly City, CA: Krames Communications, 1990.

"Back Specialists Hit 'Inversion Fad.' " *Medical World News* 28(1983).

Back to Butter? *University of California at Berkeley Wellness Letter* 10(1994):1.

Baechle, T., and R. Earle. *Fitness Weight Training.* Champaign, IL: Human Kinetics Publishers, 1995.

Baily, D. A., et al. "Growth, Physical Activity and Bone Mineral Acquisition." *Exercise and Sport Sciences Reviews* 24(1996):233.

Baker, G. "Safety Consideration in Teaching the Overhead Lifts." *Strength and Conditioning* 16:1(1994):40.

Bammel, G., and L. Burrus-Bammel. *Leisure and Human Behavior.* 2d ed. Dubuque, IA: Wm. C. Brown Publishers, 1992.

Barnard, R. J. "The Heart Needs a Warm-Up Time." *Physician and Sportsmedicine* 4(1976):40.

Barrack, R. L., et al. "Joint Laxity and Proprioception in the Knee." *Physician and Sportsmedicine* 11(1983):130.

Barrett, S. *The Health Robbers.* 2d ed. Philadelphia: George F. Stickley Co., 1993.

Barrett, S., and Editors of Consumers Reports. *Health Schemes, Scams and Frauds.* Fairfield, OH: Consumer Report Books, 1991.

Barrett, S., and V. Herbert. "How Athletes are Exploited" in *The Vitamin Pushers.* Prometheus, 1994.

Barrett, S., and W. Jarvis. Eds. *The Health Robbers: A Close Look at Quackery in America.* Buffalo, NY: Prometheus Books, 1993.

Bartels, R. L. "Weight Training: How to Lift and Eat for Strength and Power." *Physician and Sportsmedicine* 20(1992):233–34.

Basmajian, J. V. *Therapeutic Exercise.* 5th ed. Baltimore: Williams & Wilkins, 1990.

Bazzoli, A. S. "Chronic Back Pain: A Common Sense Approach." *American Journal of Physical Medicine and Rehabilitation* 71(1992):53–54.

"Beating Depression." *U.S. News and World Report* 108 (1990):48.

Beighton, P. H. "Dominant Inheritance in Familial Generalized Articular Hypermobility." *Journal of Bone and Joint Surgery* 52B(1970):145–47.

Bember, M. G., et al. "The Effect of the Rate of Muscle Contraction on the Force-Time Curve Parameters of Male and Female Subjects." *Research Quarterly for Exercise and Sports* 61(1990):96–99.

Benda, C. "Stepping Into the Right Sock." *Physician and Sportsmedicine* 19(1991):125–28.

Benson, H. *Beyond the Relaxation Response.* New York: Berkeley Publishing Group, 1985.

Beringer, G. B., et al. "Beauty Parlor Stroke: When a Beautician Becomes a Physician." (Letter to the Editor) *Journal of the American Medical Association* 270(1993):1198.

Berlin, J., et al. "A Meta-analysis of Physical Activity in the Prevention of Heart Disease." *American Journal of Epidemiology* 132(1990):612.

Berry, M. J., et al. "The Effects of Elastic Tights on the Post-Exercise Response." *Canadian Journal of Applied Sports Sciences* 15(1990):244.

Bertera, R. "The Effects of Workplace Health Promotion on Absenteeism and Employee Costs in a Large Industrial Population." *American Journal of Public Health* 80(1990):1101.

"Beta Carotine Pills: Should You Take Them?" *University of California at Berkeley Wellness Letter* 12(April 1996):1.

Biddle, S. "Exercise and Psychosocial Health." *Research Quarterly for Exercise and Sport* 66(1995):292.

Bishop, K. N., et al. "The Effect of Eccentric Strength Training as Various Speeds on Concentric Strength of the Quadriceps and Hamstring Muscles." *Journal of Orthopaedic and Sports Physical Therapy* 13(1991):226–30.

Black, D. R., and M. E. Burckes-Miller. "Male and Female College Athletes: Use of Anorexia Nervosa and Bulimia Nervosa Weight Loss Methods." *Research Quarterly for Exercise and Sports* 59(1988):252.

Blackburn, S. E., and Blair, S. "Science, Medicine and Health: Risk of Sedentary Living." ARAPCS Newsletter 12(1990):1.

Blair, S., et al. "Bone Gain in Young Adult Women." *Journal of the American Medical Association* 268(1992):2403.

Blair, S., et al. "Physical Activity and Health: A Lifestyle Approach." *Medicine, Exercise, Nutrition and Health* 1(1992):54.

Blair, S., et al. "Physical Fitness and All-Cause Mortality." *Journal of the American Medical Association* 262(1989):2395.

Blair, S. N., and A. Oberman. "Epidemiological Analysis of Coronary Heart Disease." *Cardiology Clinics* 5(1987):271.

Blair, S. N., and R. S. Paffenbarger. "Physical Activity and Risk of Cancer." (ab.) *Medicine and Science in Sports and Exercise* 19(1987):418.

Blair, S. N., et al. "Changes in Physical Fitness and All-Cause Mortality." *Journal of the American Medical Association* 273(1995):1093.

Bland, J. *Disorders of the Cervical Spine: Diagnosis and Medical Management.* 2d ed. Philadelphia: W. B. Saunders Company, 1994.

Blumenthal, D. "A Simple Guide to Complex Carbohydrates." *FDA Consumer* 23(1989):13.

Bonham, B. J., et al. "Binge Drinking in College." *Journal of the American Medical Association* 273(1995):1903.

Boone, T., et al. "A Physiological Evaluation of the Sports Massage." *Athletic Training* 26(1991):51–54.

"Booze for Health: Let the Drinker Beware." San Rafael, CA: The Marin Institute for the Prevention of Alcohol and Other Drug Problems (Summer 1991):4.

Borms, J., et al. "Optional Duration of Static Stretching Exercises for Improvement of Coxo-Femoral Flexibility." *Journal of Sports Science* 16(1988):152–61.

Bouchard, C. "Heredity and Health-Related Fitness." *Physical Activity and Fitness Research Digest* 1(1993):1.

Bouchard, C. "Heredity and the Path to Overweight and Obesity." *Medicine and Science in Sports and Exercise* 23(1991):285.

Bouchard, C., et al. "Genetics of Aerobic and Anaerobic Performances." *Exercise and Sport Sciences Reviews* 20(1992):27.

Bouchard, C., et al., eds. *Physical Activity, Fitness, and Health.* Champaign, IL: Human Kinetics Publishers, 1994.

Bouchard, C., and J. Despres. Physical Activity and Health: Atherosclerotic, Metabolic and Hypertensive Diseases. *Research Quarterly for Exercise and Sport* 66(1995):268.

Bourey, R. E., et al. "Interactions of Exercise, Coagulation, Platelets, and Fibrinolysis: A Brief Review." *Medicine and Science in Sports and Exercise* 20(1988):439.

Bowles, W., et al. "Abrasive Particles in Tobacco Products: A Possible Factor in Dental Attrition." *Journal of the American Dental Association* 126(1995):327.

Boyce, R., and S. Jackson. "One-Arm Lifting for a Healthy Back." *Strategies* (Jan. 1991):19–22.

Bray, G. A. "Obesity: A Blueprint for Progress." *Contemporary Nutrition* 12(1987):1.

"Break the Habit, Not Bones." *Health Digest* (May/June 1992):7.

Brehm, B. Health Disease: A Women's Health Issue. *Fitness Management* 12(1996):18.

Brill, P. A., et al. "Recruitment, Retention, and Success in Worksite Health Promotion: Association with Demographic Characteristics." *American Journal of Health Promotion* 5(1991):215.

Brittenham, G. "Plyometric Exercise: A Word of Caution." *Journal of Physical Education, Recreation and Dance* (Jan. 1992):20–23.

Brodie, D. A., et al. "Joint Laxity in Selected Athletic Populations." *Medicine and Science in Sports and Exercise* 14(1982):190.

Brooks, G. A., et al. *Exercise Physiology.* 2d ed. Mountain View, CA: Mayfield Publishing Co., 1995.

Brower, K. J., et al. "Evidence for Physical and Psychological Dependence on Anabolic Androgenic Steroids in Eight Weight Lifters." *American Journal of Psychiatry* 147(1990):510–12.

Brown, B. S., et al. "Anaerobic Power Changes Following Short Term Task Specific, Dynamic and Static Loading." *Journal of Applied Sport Science Research* 2(1988):35–38.

Brown, R., and J. Henderson. *Fitness Running.* Champaign, IL: Human Kinetics Publishers, 1994.

Brown, S., et al. "Injury Prevention and Control: Prospects for the 1990s." *Annual Review of Public Health* 11(1990):251.

Brownell, K., J. Rodin, and J. Wilmore, eds. *Eating, Body Weight, and Performance in Athletes: Disorders of Modern Society.* Philadelphia: Lea & Febiger, 1992.

Brownell, K. D. *The LEARN Program for Weight Control.* Philadelphia: University of Pennsylvania, 1987.

Brownell, K., et al. "Matching Weight Control Programs to Individuals." *The Weight Control Digest* 1(1991):65.

Brownson, R., et al. "Physical Activity on the Job and Cancer in Missouri." *American Journal of Public Health* 81(1991):639.

Bruess, C., and G. Richardson. *Decisions for Health.* 4th ed. Dubuque, IA: Wm. C. Brown Publishers, 1995.

Brunick, T. "Choosing the Right Shoe." *Physician and Sportsmedicine* 18(1990):104.

Bryant, C., and J. A. Peterson. "Measuring Strength." *Fitness Management* (June 1995):32.

Bureau of Labor Statistics. *Annual Survey of Occupational Injuries and Illness.* Washington, DC: Department of Labor, 1989.

Buroker, K. C., and J. A. Schwane. "Does Post-Exercise Static Stretching Alleviate Delayed Muscle Soreness?" *Physician and Sportsmedicine* 17(1989):65.

Butterfield, G. "Letter to the Editor-in-Chief." *Medicine and Science in Sports and Exercise* 20(1988):415.

Byers, T. "Body Weight and Mortality." *New England Journal of Medicine* 334(1996):723.

Byers, T. "Dietary Trends in the United States." *Cancer* 72(1993):1015.

Cailliet, R. *Knee Pain and Disability.* 3d ed. Philadelphia: F. A. Davis, Co., 1992.

Cailliet, R. *Low Back Pain Syndrome.* 5th ed. Philadelphia: F. A. Davis, Co., 1994.

Cailliet, R. *Neck and Arm Pain.* 3d ed. Philadelphia: F. A. Davis, Co., 1991.

Cailliet, R. *Shoulder Pain.* 3d ed. Philadelphia: F. A. Davis, Co., 1995.

Cailliet, R. *Soft Tissue Pain and Disability.* 2d ed. Philadelphia: F. A. Davis, Co., 1988.

"Calcium: Vital for Women and Men." *Consumer Reports on Health* 6(1994):13.

Califano, J. A. Jr. "The Wrong Way to Stay Slim." *New England Journal of Medicine* 333(1995):1214.

"Can One Train Cardiorespiratory and Muscular Fitness Simultaneously?" (Editorial). *Canadian Journal of Sport Science* 16(1991):167–68.

"Can You Live Longer?" *Consumer Reports* 57(1992):7.

"Can Your Mind Heal Your Body?" *Consumer Reports* (Feb. 1993):107.

Cancer Facts and Figures—1995. Atlanta: American Cancer Society, 1995.

"Cancer Screening Guidelines." *Healthplex* 8(1992):17.

Cardinal, B. J. "Rating the Clubs: A Health and Fitness Center Consumer Checklist."*American Fitness* Sept./Oct. 1994.

Carmichael, C., and E. Burke. *Fitness Cycling.* Champaign, IL: Human Kinetics Publishers, 1994.

Carrol, C. R. *Drugs in Modern Society.* 3d ed. Dubuque, IA: Wm. C. Brown Publishers, 1993.

Carruthers, C. P., and C. D. Hood. "Alcoholics and Children of Alcoholics: The Role of Leisure in Recovery." *Journal of Physical Education, Recreation and Dance* (April 1992):48.

Casperson, C. J., et al. "Physical Activity, Exercise, and Physical Fitness: Concepts, Methods, and Application to Exercise Science." *Exercise and Sports Sciences Review* 17(1989):126.

Casperson, C. J., et al. "Physical Activity, Exercise, and Physical Fitness: Definitions and Distinctions for Health-Related Research." *Public Health Reports* 100(1985):126.

Cates, W. "The Other STD's: Do They Really Matter?" *Journal of the American Medical Association* 259(1988):3606.

Centers for Disease Control. "Cigarette Smoking Among Adults." Epidemiology Branch, Office on Smoking Health. National Center for Chronic Disease Prevention and Health Promotion. *Journal of the American Medical Association* 273(1995):369.

Centers for Disease Control. *HIV/AIDS Surveillance Report.* Atlanta, GA: U.S. Department of Health and Human Services, 1991.

Centers for Disease Control. *Morbidity and Mortality Weekly Report* 39(1990):110.

Centers for Disease Control. "Vigorous Physical Activity Among High School Students." *Morbidity and Mortality Weekly Report* 41(1992):1.

Centers for Disease Control. "Years of Potential Life Lost Before Age 65—United States 1987." *Morbidity and Mortality Weekly Report* 38(1989):27.

Centers for Disease Control and Prevention. "Frequent Alcohol Consumption Among Women of Childbearing Age." *Journal of the American Medical Association* 271(1994):1820.

Chadbourne, R. "A Hard Look at Running Surfaces." *Physician and Sportsmedicine* 18(1990):103.

Chambers, M. "Exercise: A Prescription for a Good Night's Sleep?" *Physician and Sportsmedicine* 19(1991):107.

Champs, M. "Pumping Down: How Fast Do Strength Trainers Lose It?" *American Fitness* (Sept./Oct. 1994):60.

Chandler, T. J., and M. H. Stone. "The Squat Exercise in Athletic Conditioning: A Review of the Literature." *National Strength and Conditioning Association Journal* 13(1991):52–60.

Chandler, T. J., et al. "The Effect of the Squat Exercise on Knee Stability." *Medicine and Science in Sports and Exercise* 21(June 1989):299–303.

Chandrasheckhar, Y., et al. "Exercise as a Coronary Protective Factor." *American Heart Journal* 122(1991):1723.

Changing Your Mind: Drugs that Alter Your Moods. Center City, MN: Hazelden Educational Materials, 1991.

Ching, L., et al. "Activity Level and Risk of Overweight in Male Health Professionals." *American Journal of Public Health* 86(1996):25.

Cho, A. K. "Ice: A New Dosage Form of an Old Drug." *Science* (August 10, 1990):631.

Chodak, G. W., et al. "Routine Screening for Prostate Cancer Using the Digital Rectal Examination." *Progress and Clinical and Biological Research* 269(1988):87.

Cinque, C. "Are Americans Fit? Survey Data Conflict." *Physician and Sportsmedicine* 14(1986):24.

Clark, N. "Fueling Up with Carbs: How Much Is Enough?" *Physician and Sportsmedicine* 19(1991):68.

Clark, N. "How to Gain Weight Healthfully." *Physician and Sportsmedicine* 19(1991):53.

Clark, N. "Protein Myths: The Meat of the Matter." *Sportcare and Fitness* 2(1989):53.

Clark, N. "Water: The Ultimate Nutrient." *Physician and Sportsmedicine* 23(1995):21.

Clarkson, P. "Minerals, Exercise Performance and Supplementation." *Journal of Sport Sciences* 9(1991):91.

Clements, M. "Sex in America Today." *Parade Magazine* (August 7, 1994):4.

Clouet, D., K. Asghar, and R. Brown. "Mechanisms of Cocaine Abuse and Toxicity." Rockville, MD: National Institute on Drug Abuse (1988):ix. Research Monograph 88, U.S. Department of Health and Human Services, Public Health Service.

Cocaine in the Workplace: What You Can Do. Daly City, CA: Krames Communications, 1986.

Cohen, J. S., et al. "Hypercholesterolemia in Male Power Lifters Using Anabolic-Androgenic Steroids." *Physician and Sportsmedicine* 16(1988):49.

Cohen, L. I., et al. "Lipoprotein (a) and Cholesterol in Body Builders Using Anabolic Androgenic Steroids." *Medicine and Science in Sports and Exercise* 28(1996):176.

Coleman, D., and J. Gurin. Eds. *Mind/Body Medicine.* Consumer Reports Books, Fairfield, OH: 1993.

Collingwood, T. R., et al. "Enlisting Physical Education for the War on Drugs." *Journal of Health, Physical Education, Recreation and Dance* 63(1992).

Colucci, D., et al. "Comparison of Static versus PNF Stretching on Shoulder ROM in Intercollegiate Baseball Players." *Athletic Training* 24(1989):116.

Commandre, F. A., et al. "Lumbar Spine, Sport and Actual Treatment." *Journal of Sports Medicine and Physical Fitness* 31(1992):129–35.

Condon, S. A., and R. S. Hutton. "Soleus Electromyographic Activity and Ankle Dorsiflexion Range of Motion during Four Stretching Procedures." *Physical Therapy* 67(1987):24–30.

Consumer Reports, "Health Clubs: The Right Choice." 61(1996):27.

Consumer Reports on Health. "What Can E Do for You?" *Consumer Reports on Health* 5(1993):33.

Cooper, E. "Statement on Physical Activity and Heart Disease." American Heart Association News Release. July 1, 1992, pp.1–2.

Cooper, K. H. *The Aerobics Program for Total Well-Being.* New York: M. Evans & Co., 1982.

Cooper, K. H. *Controlling Cholesterol.* New York: Bantam Books, 1988.

Cooper, K. H. *Dr. Kenneth H. Cooper's Antioxidant Revolution.* New York: Nelson, 1995.

Cooper, K. H. *Running Without Fear.* New York: M. Evans & Co., Inc., 1988.

Corbin, C. B., and R. Lindsey. *Fitness for Life.* 4th ed. Glenview, IL: Scott, Foresman and Co., 1997.

Corbin, C. B., and R. Pangrazi. "Are American Children and Youth Fat?" *Research Quarterly for Exercise and Sport* 63(1993):96.

Corbin, C. B., and R. Pangrazi. "The Health Benefits of Exercise." *Research Digest for Physical Activity and Fitness* 1(1993):1.

Corbin, C. B., and R. P. Pangrazi. Answers to Questions: How Much Physical Activity is Enough? *Journal of Physical Education Recreation and Dance* x(1996):xx.

Corbin, C. B., and R. P. Pangrazi. "What You Need to Know About the Surgeon General's Report on Physical Activity and Health." *Physical Activity and Fitness Research Digest* 2(1996):1.

Corbin, C. B., R. P. Pangrazi, and G. J. Welk. "Toward an Understanding of Appropriate Physical Activity Levels for Youth." *Physical Activity and Fitness Research Digest* 1(1994):1.

Corbin, D. E., and J. Metal-Corbin. *Reach for It: A Handbook of Health, Exercise and Dance Activities, for Older Adults.* 2d ed. Dubuque, IA: E. Bowers, 1990.

Cordain, L., et al. "The Effects of an Aerobic Running Program on Bowel Transit Time." *Journal of Sports Medicine* 26(1986):101.

Cornacchea, J., and S. Barrett. *Consumer Health* 5th ed. C. V. Mosby, 1993.

Cornelius, W. L. "Modified PNF Stretching: Improvement in Hip Flexion." *National Strength and Conditioning Association Journal* 12(1990):44–46.

Cornelius, W. L. "PNF Ankle Stretching: Partner/No-Partner Procedures." *National Strength and Conditioning Association Journal* 13(1991):59–63.

Couldry, W., et al. "Carotid vs. Radial Pulse Counts." *Physician and Sportsmedicine* 10(1982):67.

Cousins, N. *Head First—The Biology of Hope.* New York: Dutton, 1989.

Couzens, G. S. "Surgically Sculpting Athletic Physiques: Liposuction and Calf and Pectoral Implants." *Physician and Sportsmedicine* 20(1992):153–66.

Cowart, V. "Dietary Supplements." *Physician and Sportsmedicine* 20(1992):189.

Cowart, V. "If Youngsters Overdose with Anabolic Steroids, What's the Cost Anatomically and Otherwise?" *Journal of the American Medical Association* 261(1989):1856.

Cowart, V. S. "Can Exercise Help Women with PMS?" *Physician and Sportsmedicine* 17(1989):169.

"CPII adds to Breast Cancer Knowledge." *CPSII, Newsletter* 11(1994):1.

Crack Kills, Don't Do It. Skill Builder. St. Rose, LA: SYNDISTAR, Inc., n.d.

Csikszentmihalyi, M., and R. Graef. "Feeling Free." *Psychology Today* 12(1979):84.

Culhane, C. "Ice Spreads to West Coast Area." *U.S. Journal of Drug and Alcohol Dependence* 14 1(1990):16.

Cureton, K. J., et al. "Muscle Hypertrophy in Men and Women." *Medicine and Science in Sports and Exercise* 20(1988):338.

Curran, J. W., et al. "Epidemiology of HIV Infection and AIDS in the United States." *Science* 239(1988):610.

"'Date Rape Drug' Raises Fears in O.C." *Orange County Register,* Nov. 26, 1995.

Danner, S. A., et al. "A Short-Term Study of the Safety, Pharmacokinetics, and Efficacy of Ritonavir, an Inhibitor of HIV-1 Protease." *New England Journal of Medicine* 333(1995):1528.

Davis, A. A., and E. J. Carragee. "Sciatica: Treating a Painful Symptom." *Physician and Sportsmedicine* 20(Jan. 1992):126–35.

DeBenedette, V. "Health Club Tanning Booths: Risky Business." *Physician and Sportsmedicine* 15(1987):59.

DeBusk, R., et al. "Training Effects of Long Versus Short Bouts of Exercise in Healthy Subjects." *American Journal of Cardiology* 65(1990):1010.

deLateur, B. J., et al. "Footwear and Posture: Compensatory Strategies for Heel Height." *American Journal of Physical Medicine and Rehabilitation* 70(1991):246–54.

deLateur, B. J., and J. F. Lehmann. "Therapeutic Exercise to Develop Strength and Endurance." In *Krusen's Handbook of Physical Medicine and Rehabilitation.* 4th ed. Kotke and Lehman, Eds. Philadelphia: W. B. Saunders, 1990, pp. 480–95.

Delitto, R., and S. J. Rose. "An Electromyographic Analysis of Two Techniques for Squat Lifting and Lowering." *Physical Therapy* 72(June 1992):438–48.

DePiccoli, B., et al. "Anabolic Steroid Use in Body Builders: An Echocardiographic Study of Left Ventricle Morphology and Function." *International Journal of Sports Medicine* 4(1991):408–12.

Derosiers, "New Clues Found to How Some People Live with HIV." *Science* 270(1995):917.

DiClemente, R. J., et al. "Adolescents and AIDS: A Survey of Knowledge, Attitudes, and Beliefs about AIDS in San Francisco." *American Journal of Public Health* 76(1986):1443.

Dietary Guidelines and Your Diet. Hyattsville, MD: USDA, 1992, No. HG–232, 1–11.

DiPietro, L. "Physical Activity, Body Weight, and Adiposity: An Epidemiological Perspective." *Exercise and Sport Sciences Reviews* 23(1995):275.

Direct and Indirect Costs of Diabetes in the United States in 1987. Alexandria, VA: American Diabetes Association, 1988.

Direct Marketing Association. 6 East 43rd St., New York, N.Y. 10017.

Dishman, R. K., et al. "The Determinants of Physical Activity and Exercise." *Public Health Reports* 100(1985):158.

Dishman, R., et al. "Health Locus of Control Predicts Free-living, But Not Supervised, Physical Activity." *Research Quarterly for Exercise and Sport* 61(1990):383.

Dishman, R., and J. Sallis. "Determinants and Interventions for Physical Activity and Exercise." In C. Bouchard, et al., eds., *Physical Activity, Fitness, and Health.* Champaign, IL: Human Kinetics Publishers, 1994.

Dishman, R. K., ed. *Advances in Exercise Adherence.* Champaign, IL: Human Kinetics Publishers, 1994.

Dixon, A. E., et al. "Sudden Death in Sports Activities." *New England Journal of Medicine* 333(1995):1784.

Dondero, T. J., et al. "Monitoring the Levels and Trends of HIV Infection: The Public Health Service's HIV Surveillance Program." *Public Health Reports* 103(1988):213.

Dowdy, D. B., et al. "Effects of Aerobic Dance on Physical Work Capacity, Cardiovascular Fitness, and Body Composition of Middle-aged Women." *Research Quarterly* 56(1985):227.

"Drinking and Driving." *Alcohol Alert.* No. 31 PH362 January 1996. National Institute on Alcohol Abuse and Alcoholism.

"Drug Abuse and Pregnancy." *NIDA Capsules.* Washington, DC: National Institute on Drug Abuse; U.S. Department of Health and Human Services, Public Health Service; Alcohol, Drug Abuse and Mental Health Administration, June 1989.

"Drug Ecstasy Could Cause Brain Damage." *Orange County Register,* Sept. 15, 1995.

Duda, M. "Elite Lifters at Risk for Spondylolysis." *Physician and Sportsmedicine* 15(1987):57.

Duda, M. "The Medical Risks and Benefits of Sauna, Steam Bath and Whirlpool Use." *Physician and Sportsmedicine* 15(1987):170.

Duncan, P. W., et al. "Mode and Speed Specificity of Eccentric and Concentric Exercise Training." *Journal of Orthopaedic and Sports Physical Therapy* 11(1989):70–75.

Dunn, A., et al. "Exercise and the Neurobiology of Depression." *Exercise and Sport Sciences Reviews* 19(1991):41.

Durant, R. H., et al. "Use of Multiple Drugs Among Adolescents Who Use Anabolic Steroids." *New England Journal of Medicine* 328(1993):922.

Dye, C. *"Adam" & "Eve" & "Ecstasy":Facts about MDMA.* Tempe, AZ: D.I.N. Publications, 1988.

Dzewaltowski, D., et al. "Physical Activity Participation: Social Cognitive Theory Versus the Theories of Reasoned Action and Planned Behavior." *Journal of Sport and Exercise Psychology* 12(1990):388.

Early Signs of Addiction: Are the Illusions Taking Over? San Bruno, CA: Krames Communications, 1990.

"Ecstasy Causes Harm in Test Animals." *Orange County Register,* Aug. 15, 1995.

Eddy, D. M., et al. "The Value of Mammography Screening in Women under 50 Years." *Journal of the American Medical Association* 259(1988):187.

Eichner, E. R. "Does Running Cause Osteoarthritis?" *Physician and Sportsmedicine* 17(1989):147.

Eigen, L. D. "Alcohol Practices, Policies and Potentials of American Colleges and Universities: An OSAP White Paper." Washington, DC: Office for Substance Abuse and Prevention; Alcohol, Drug Abuse and Mental Health Administration; U.S. Department of Health and Human Services, 1991.

Ekoe, J. "Overview of Diabetes Mellitus and Exercise." *Medicine and Science in Sports and Exercise* 21(1989):353.

Elliot, D. L., et al. "Effect of Resistance Training on Excess Post-exercise Oxygen Consumption." *Journal of Applied Sport Science Research* 6(1992):77–81.

Elrick, H. "Exercise is Medicine." *The Physician and Sports Medicine* 24(1996):72.

Entyre, B. R., and L. D. Abraham. "Antagonist Muscle Activity during Stretching: A Paradox Reassessed." *Medicine and Science in Sports and Exercise* 20(1988):285–89.

Entyre, B. R., and E. J. Lee. "Comments on Proprioceptive Neuromuscular Facilitation Stretching Techniques." *Research Quarterly for Exercise and Sport* 58(1987):184–88.

Epidemiology of Inhalant Abuse: An Update. National Institute on Drug Abuse Research. Monograph Series no. 85, 1990.

Epstein, L., et al. "Ten-Year Follow-Up of Behavioral, Family-Based Treatment for Obese Children." *Journal of the American Medical Association* 264(1990):2519.

"Estimated U.S. Costs of Drug Abuse." Chapel Hill, NC: Research Triangle Institute, 1990.

Facts About Cigarette Smoking. New York: American Lung Association, n.d.

Facts About Nicotine Addiction and Cigarettes. New York: American Lung Association, 1990.

Facts About Secondhand Smoke. New York: American Lung Association, 1990.

Facts About the Nicotine Transdermal Patch. New York: American Lung Association, 1992.

Farley, D. "Making Sure Hype Doesn't Overwhelm Science." *FDA Consumer,* 56(1996):1.

"Fat Burning—Get the Facts," reported in *JOPERD* 66:8:12. Oct. '95.

"FDA Examines Danger of Patch Plus Cigarettes." Santa Ana, CA: *Orange County Register,* June 19, 1992.

Ferenchick, G. S., et al. "Steroids and Cardiomyopathy: How Strong a Connection?" *Physician and Sportsmedicine* 19(1991):107–10.

Fessel, W. J., et al. "Early Treatment of HIV Infections." *New England Journal of Medicine* 333(1995):1782.

Field, R. "How Humans Sit." *The American Way* (April 15, 1988):28–29.

Fields, R. *Drugs and Alcohol in Perspective.* Dubuque, IA: Brown & Benchmark Publishers, 1996.

Fisher, A. G. *Golf: Your Turn for Success.* Boston: Jones & Bartlett Publishers, 1992.

Fisher, H. R., et al. "Calculating Blood Alcohol Concentration (BAC) By Sex, Weight, Number of Drinks and Time." *Canadian Journal of Public Health* 78(5)(1987):300.

Fitness Canada. *Canada Fitness Survey—Highlights*. Ottawa, Ontario: Government of Canada, 1990.

Fitnessgram: Test Administration Manual. Dallas: Cooper Institute for Aerobics Research, 1992.

"Fitness Improves Driving," *Senior World of Orange Country* 17(Jan. 1991).

"Fitness: Working Out the Facts." *Consumer Reports Health Letter* 3(July 1991):49, 52.

Fleck, S. J. "Cardiovascular Adaptations to Resistance Training." *Medicine and Science in Sports and Exercise* 20(1988):Supplement, 146.

Fleck, S. J., and W. J. Kraemer. "Resistance Training: Basic Principles (Part 1 of 4)." *Physician and Sportsmedicine* 16(1988):160.

Fleck, S. J., and W. J. Kraemer. "Resistance Training: Physiological Responses and Adaptations (Part 2 of 4)." *The Physician and Sportsmedicine* 16(1988):108.

Fleck, S. J., and W. J. Kraemer. "Resistance Training: Physiological Responses (Part 3 of 4)." *The Physician and Sportsmedicine* 16(1988):63.

Fleck, S. J., and W. J. Kraemer. "Resistance Training: Exercise Prescription (Part 4 of 4)." *Physician and Sportsmedicine* 16(1988):68.

Flegal, K., et al. "The Influence of Smoking Cessation on the Prevalence of Overweight." *The New England Journal of Medicine* 333(1995):1166.

Fletcher, G. F., et al. "American Heart Association Medical/Scientific Statement on Exercise." *Circulation* 86(1992):340.

Flint, M., and J. Gudgell. "Electromyographic Study of Abdominal Muscular Activity during Exercise." *Research Quarterly* 36(1965):1.

Folkenberg, J. "Reporting Reactions to Additives." *FDA Consumer* 22(1988):16.

Food and Drug Administration. *Condoms and Sexually Transmitted Diseases*. Rockville, MD: U.S. Department of Health and Human Services, 1990.

"Foods, Drugs or Frauds?" *FDA Consumer*, May, 1985 (reprint).

Foreyt, J. "Factors Common to Successful Therapy for the Obese Patient." *Medicine and Science in Sports and Exercise* 23(1991):292.

Fox, K., et al. "The Physical Self-Perception Profile." *Journal of Sport and Exercise Psychology* 11(1989):408.

Fox, M., and D. Broide. *Molly Fox's Step On It*. New York: Avon Books, 1991.

Frankle, M., and D. Leffers. "Athletes on Anabolic-Androgenic Steroids: New Approach Diminishes Health Problems." *Physician and Sportsmedicine* 20(1992):75–87.

Franklin, B. "Exercise Training and Coronary Collateral Circulation." *Medicine and Science in Sport and Exercise* 23(1991):648.

Franklin, B., et al. "Exercise Testing Update." *Physician and Sportsmedicine* 19(1991):111.

Franks, B. D., et al. *Fitness Leader's Handbook*. Champaign, IL: Human Kinetics Publishers, 1989.

Freedman, A. M. "Philip Morris Draft Report May Help U.S. Case Against Tobacco." *Orange County Register*, Dec. 9, 1995.

Friden, J., and R. Lieber. "Structural and Mechanical Basis of Exercise Induced Muscle Injury." *Medicine and Science in Sports and Exercise* 5(1992):521.

Friedl, K., and R. J. Moore. "Steroid Replacers: Let the Athlete Beware." *National Strength and Conditioning Association Journal* 14(1992):14–19.

Friedman, J. M. W., et al. "Prevalence of Specific Suicidal Behaviors in a High School Sample." *American Journal of Psychiatry* 144(1987):1203.

Frisch, R. E. "Lower Prevalence of Breast Cancer and Cancers of the Reproductive System Among Former College Athletes Compared to Non-Athletes." *British Journal of Cancer* 52(1985):885.

Frisch, R. E., et al. "Lower Lifetime Occurrence of Breast Cancer and Cancers of the Reproductive System Among Former College Athletes." *American Journal of Clinical Nutrition* 45(1987):328.

Fuchs, C. S., et al. "Alcohol Consumption and Mortality Among Women." *New England Journal of Medicine* 332(1995):1245.

Gabel, S., et al. "Homovanillic Acid and Monoamine Oxidase in Sons of Substance Abusing Fathers: Relationship to Conduct Disorder." *Journals of Studies of Alcohol* 56(1995):135–39.

Gajdosik, R. L. "Effects of Static Stretching on the Maximal Length and Resistance to Passive Stretch of Short Hamstring Muscles." *Journal of Orthopaedic and Sports Physical Therapy* 14 (Dec. 1991):250–55.

Gallagher, W. "The Looming Menace of Designer Drugs." *Discover* (August 1986):24.

Gallup, G. "Importance of Social Values." *Gallup Report* (March 1989):282.

Gallup, G. "Leisure: Swimming, Fishing, Bicycling Are Top Sports Activities." *Gallup Report* 281(1989):28.

Gallup, G., and F. Newport. "Americans Have Love-Hate Relationship with Their TV Sets." *The Gallup Poll Monthly* 301(1990):2.

Gallup, G., and F. Newport. "Americans Now Drinking Less Alcohol." *Gallup Poll Monthly* (Dec. 1990):2–6.

Gallup, G., and F. Newport. "Despite Dissatisfaction with Way Things Are Going, Americans Remain Positive." *The Gallup Poll Monthly* 298(1990):10.

Gallup, G., and F. Newport. "Football Remains America's Number One Spectator Sport." *Gallup Poll Monthly* 325, 36(1992).

Gallup, G., and F. Newport. "Gallup Leisure Audit." *The Gallup Poll Monthly* 295(1990):27.

Gallup, G., and F. Newport. "Gallup Leisure Poll." *The Gallup Poll Monthly* 295(1990):27.

Gallup, G., and F. Newport. "Many Americans Favor Restrictions on Smoking in Public Places." *Gallup Poll Monthly* 301(1990):19.

Gammon, M. D., et al. "Abortion and the Risk of Breast Cancer: Is There a Believable Association?" *Journal of the American Medical Association* 275(1996):321.

Garbutt, G., et al. "Running Speed and Spinal Shrinkage in Runners With and Without Low Back Pain." *Medicine and Science in Sports and Exercise* 22(1990):769–72.

Garcia, A., et al. "Predicting Long-term Adherence to Aerobic Exercise: A Comparison of Two Models." *Journal of Sport and Exercise Psychology* 13(1991):394.

Garhammer, J. *Sports Illustrated Strength Training*. New York: Harper & Row, Publishers, 1986.

Garnica, R. A. "Muscular Power in Young Women After Slow and Fast Isokinetic Training." *Journal of Orthopaedic and Sports Physical Therapy* 8(1986):1.

Garrett, W. E. "Muscle Strain Injuries: Clinical and Basic Aspects." *Medicine and Science in Sports and Exercise* 22(1990):436–43.

Gauthier, M. M. "Can Exercise Reduce the Risk of Cancer?" *Physician and Sportsmedicine* 14(1986):171.

Gauthier, M. M. "Continuous Passive Motion: The No-Exercise Exercise." *Physician and Sportsmedicine* 15(1987):142.

Gauthier, M. M. "Soda Pop May Increase Fracture Risk." *Physician and Sportsmedicine* 17(1989):46.

Gerhardsson, M., et al. "Sedentary Jobs and Colon Cancer." *American Journal of Epidemiology* 123(1986):775.

Gillette, T. M., et al. "Relationship of Body Core Temperature and Warm-Up to Knee Range of Motion." *Journal of Orthopaedic and Sports Physical Therapy* 13(Mar. 1991):126–31.

Glantz, S. A., and W. W. Parmley. "Passive Smoking and Heart Disease: Mechanism and Risk." *Journal of the American Medical Association* 273(1995):1047.

Gleim, G. W., et al. "Influence of Flexibility on Economy of Walking and Jogging." *Journal of Orthopaedic Research* 8(1990):814–23.

Godges, J. J., et al. "The Effects of Two Stretching Procedures on Hip Range of Motion and Gait Economy." *Journal of Orthopaedic and Sports Physical Therapy* 11(1989):350–57.

Goldfine, H., et al. "Exercising to Health." *Physician and Sportsmedicine* 19(1991):81.

Goldstein, D. "Clinical Applications for Exercise." *Physician and Sportsmedicine* 17(1989):83.

Goode, E., ed. *Annual Editions: Drugs, Society and Behavior.* Guilford, CT: Dushkin Publishing Company, 1991.

Goodman, C. E. "Low Back Pain in the Cosmetic Athlete." *Physician and Sportsmedicine* 15(1987):97.

Gorman, C. "Invincible AIDS." *Time* 140(1992):30.

Gorman, D., and B. Brown. "Fitness and Aging: An Overview." *Journal of Physical Education, Recreation and Dance* 57(1986):50.

Gorman, M., et al. "Position of the American Dietetic Association: Health Implications of Dietary Fiber." *Journal of the American Dietetics Association* 88(1988):216.

Grabiner, M. D., and R. M. Enoka. "Changes in Movement Capabilities with Aging." *Exercise and Sport Sciences Review* 23(1995):65.

Grahame, R., and J. M. Jenkins. "Joint Hypermobility—Asset or Liability." *Annals of Rheumatic Disease* 31(1972):109.

Graves, J. E., et al. "Physiological Responses to Walking with Hand Weights, Wrist Weights and Ankle Weights." *Medicine and Science in Sports and Exercise* 20(1988):265.

Graves, J. E., et al. "The Effect of Hand-Held Weights on the Physiological Responses to Walking Exercise." *Medicine and Science in Sports and Exercise* 19(1987):260.

Greenberg, E. R., et al. "Mortality Associated with Low Plasma Concentration of Beta Carotine and the Effect of an Oral Supplementation." *Journal of the American Medical Association* 275(1996):699.

Greenberg, J. S. *Comprehensive Stress Management.* 5th ed. Dubuque, IA: Brown & Benchmark Publishers, 1996.

Greenberg, J. S. *Coping With Stress: A Practical Guide.* 3d ed. Dubuque, IA: Wm. C. Brown Publishers, 1990.

Greenberg, J. S. et al. "A Clinical Trial of Antioxidant Vitamins to Prevent Colorectal Adenoma." *The New England Journal of Medicine* 331(1994):141.

Griffith, D. "It's Not the Creep in a Trench Coat. . . ." *The Cutting Edge.* Riverside, CA: Teen Challenge 3(1992):1.

Grigg, W. "Quackery: It Costs More Than Money." *FDA Consumer* 22(1988):30.

Groves, D. "Is Childhood Obesity Related to TV Addiction?" *Physician and Sportsmedicine* 11(1988):117.

Guilland, J., et al. "Vitamin Status of Young Athletes Including the Effects of Supplementation." *Medicine and Science in Sports and Exercise* 21(1989):441.

Gulliver S., et al. "Interrelationship of Smoking and Alcohol Dependence, Use and Urges to Use." *Journals of Studies on Alcohol* 56(1995):202–6.

Gunderson, E., and R. Rahe, eds. *Life Stress and Illness.* Springfield, IL: Charles C Thomas, 1979.

Gunn, C. C. "Fibromyalgia—What Have We Created?" (Letter to the Editor) *Pain* 60 March 1995.

"Gymnastics Might Put a Nasty Twist on Back Problems." *Orange County Register,* Jan. 4, 1990.

Haennel, R., et al. "Effects of Hydraulic Circuit Training on Cardiovascular Function." *Medicine and Science in Sports and Exercise* 21(1989):605–11.

Hammond, K., et al. "Occupational Exposure to Environmental Tobacco Smoke." *Journal of the American Medical Association* 274(1995):956.

Hankinson, S. E. "All That Glitters is NOT Beta Carotine." *Journal of the American Medical Association* 272(1994):1455.

Hardy, L., and D. Jones. "Dynamic Flexibility and Proprioceptive Neuromuscular Facilitation." *Research Quarterly for Exercise and Sport* 57(1986):150.

Harman, E. A., et al. "Effects of a Belt on Intra-Abdominal Pressure during Weight Lifting." *Medicine and Science in Sports and Exercise* 21(1989):186.

Harmer, P. A. "The Effect of Pre-Performance Massage on Stride Frequency in Sprinters." *Athletic Training* 26(1991):55–59.

Harris, L. *Inside America.* New York: Vintage Books, 1987.

Harris, L. "Sports." *Harris Poll* (April 1989):1.

Hartz, A. J., et al. "The Association of Girth Measurements with Disease in 32,856 Women." *American Journal of Epidemiology* 119(1984):71.

Harvey, J., and S. Tanner. "Low Back Pain in Young Athletes: A Practical Approach." *Sports Medicine* 12(1991):394–406.

Haskell, W., et al. "Cardiovascular Benefits and Assessment of Physical Activity and Physical Fitness in Adults." *Medicine and Science in Sports and Exercise* 24(1992):S201 (Supplement).

Haskell, W. L. "Physical Activity in the Prevention and Management of Coronary Heart Disease." *Physical Activity and Fitness Research Digest* 2(1995):1.

Hauri, P., et al. "Slumber Strategies." *Health* 22(1990):57.

Haymes, E. M. "Nutritional Concerns: Need for Iron." *Medicine and Science in Sports and Exercise* 19(1987):Supplement, 197.

Haywood, K. *Lifespan Motor Development.* 2d ed. Champaign, IL: Human Kinetics Publishers, 1993.

"Health Behavior Modification—A Commitment to Change," reported in *JOPERD* p. 12 Oct. `95 Vol. 66 no. 8, from: Natl. Exercise For Life Institute, Excelsior, MN.

Health Hazards of Nitrite Inhalants. National Institute on Drug Abuse Research. Monograph Series no. 83, 1990.

Health Letters Associates. *Wellness Made Easy: 101 Tips for Better Health.* Berkeley: University of California, Berkeley, Wellness Letter, 1990.

"Health Spas, Exercise Clubs, etc." *Information For Prudent Consumers.* National Council Against Health Fraud. Loma Linda, CA 1994.

1995 Heart Facts Reference Sheet. Dallas: American Heart Association, 1995.

Heath, R. G. "Marijuana and the Brain." Reprint. Topsfield, MA: Committees of Correspondence, Inc., n.d.

Hebert, H. J. "Secondhand Smoke Hurts Children, EPA Says." Santa Ana, CA: *Orange County Register,* June 18, 1992.

Heino, J. G., et al. "Relationship Between Hip Extension Range of Motion and Postural Alignment." *Journal of Orthopaedic and Sports Physical Therapy* 12(1990):243–48.

Heinrich, C., et al. "Bone Mineral Content of Cyclically Menstruating Female Resistance and Endurance Trained Athletes." *Medicine and Science in Sports and Exercise* 22(1990):558.

Helmrich, S., et al. "Physical Activity and Reduced Occurrence of Non-Insulin-Dependent Diabetes Mellitus." *New England Journal of Medicine* 325(1991):147.

Hennekins, C. H. "Lack of Effect of Long-Term Supplementation with Beta Carotene on the Incidence of Malignant Neoplasms and Cardiovascular Disease." *The New England Journal of Medicine* 334(1996):1145.

"Herbal Roulette." *Consumers Report* 60(1995):689.

Hiatt, W., et al. "Benefits of Exercise Conditioning for Patients with Peripheral Arterial Disease." *Circulation* 81(1990):602.

Higgins, M., et al. "Rectus Femoris and Erector Spinae Activity During Simulated Knees-Bent and Knees-Straight Lifting." (Abstract of platform presentation at 1991 Section Meeting of APTA). *Journal of Orthopaedic and Sports Physical Therapy* 13(May 1991):257.

Hingson, R., et al. "Acquired Immunodeficiency Syndrome Transmission: Changes in Knowledge and Behaviors Among Teenagers." *Pediatrics* 85(1990):24.

Hoeger, W., and D. Hopkins. "Assessing Muscular Flexibility." *Fitness Management* 6(20):34–36, 42, 1990.

Hoeger, W. W. K., and D. R. Hopkins. "A Comparison of the Sit-and-Reach and the Modified Sit-and-Reach in the Measurement of Flexibility in Women." *Research Quarterly for Exercise and Sport* 31(June 1992):191–95.

Hoffman, J. "Growth Hormone." *National Strength and Conditioning Association Journal* 12(1990):78–81.

Holbrook, T., et al. "The Association of Lifetime Weight and Weight Control Patterns with Diabetes among Men and Women in an Adult Community." *International Journal of Obesity* 13(1989):723.

Holmstrom, E., et al. "Trunk Muscle Strength and Back Muscle Endurance in Construction Workers With and Without Low Back Disorders." *Scandinavian Journal of Rehabilitation Medicine* 24(1992):3–10.

"Hooked on Tobacco: The Teen Epidemic." *Consumer Reports.* 60:3(1995):142.

Hooper, P. L. "Aerobic Dance Program Improves Cardiovascular Fitness in Men." *Physician and Sportsmedicine* 12(1984):132.

Hopkins, D. R., and W. W. K. Hoeger. "A Comparison of the Sit-and-Reach Test and the Modified Sit-and-Reach Test in the Measurement of Flexibility for Males." *Journal of Applied Sport Science Research* 6(1992):7–10.

Hortobagyi, T., et al. "Effects of Simultaneous Training for Strength and Endurance on Upper and Lower Body Strength and Running Performance." *Journal of Sports Medicine and Physical Fitness* 31(1991):20–30.

Houmard, J. "The Effects of Warm-Up on Responses to Intense Exercise." *International Journal of Sports Medicine* 12(1991):480.

Hubbard, R. W., and L. E. Armstrong. "Hyperthermia: New Thoughts on an Old Problem." *Physician and Sportsmedicine* 17(1989):97.

Hueber, G. "Americans Report High Levels of Environmental Concern." *The Gallup Poll Monthly* 307(1991):6.

Hugick, L., et al. "The Perfect Meal: Something Old, Something New." *The Gallup Poll Monthly* 314(1991):35.

Hugick, L., and J. Leonard. "Job Dissatisfaction Grows; 'Moonlighting' on the Rise." *The Gallup Poll Monthly* 312(1991):2.

"Human Growth Hormone." *Sports Medicine Digest* 6(1984):13.

Ice: The Cold Hard Facts. Skill Builder. St. Rose, LA: SYNDISTAR INC., n.d.

Ike, R. W. "Arthritis and Aerobic Exercise: A Review." *Physician and Sportsmedicine* 17(1989):128.

Inhalant Abuse: A Volatile Research Agenda. National Institute on Drug Abuse Research. Monograph Series no. 129, 1992.

Inhofe, P. D., et al. "The Effects of Anabolic Steroid on Rat Tendon." *The American Journal of Sports Medicine* 23(1995):227.

International Federation of Sports Medicine. "Physical Exercise: An Important Factor for Health." *Physician and Sportsmedicine* 18(1990):155.

International Society of Sport Psychology. "Physical Activity and Psychological Benefits: Position Statement." 20(1992):179.

Is There a Safe Tobacco? Take a Look at the Facts. New York: American Lung Association, 1990.

Ivy, J. L., et al. "Muscle Glycogen Synthesis after Exercise: Effect of Time of Carbohydrate Ingestion." *Journal of Applied Physiology* 64(1988):1480.

Jackson, A. S., et al. "Generalized Equations for Predicting Body Density of Women." *Medicine and Science in Sports and Exercise* 12(1980):175.

Jacobson, B. "Effects of Amino Acids on Growth Hormone Release." *Physician and Sportsmedicine* 18(1990):63.

Jacobson, E. *You Must Relax.* New York: McGraw-Hill, 1978.

James, J. *Peyote and Mescaline: History and Use of the "Sacred Cactus."* Tempe, AZ: D.I.N. Publications, 1990.

James, J. "Smokeless Tobacco." *DATAFAX.* Tempe, AZ: Do It Now Foundation, 1990.

Janatuinen, E. K., et al. "A Comparison of Diets With and Without Oats." *New England Journal of Medicine* 333(1995):1033.

Jeffrey, R., et al. "Weight Cycling and Cardiovascular Risk Factors in Obese Men and Women." *American Journal of Clinical Nutrition* 55(1992):641.

Jenkins, W. L., et al. "Speed Specific Isokinetic Training." *Journal of Orthopaedic and Sports Physical Therapy* 6(1984):181–84.

Jinot, J., and S. Bayard. "Respiratory Health Effects of Passive Smoking: EPA's Weight of Evidence Analysis." *Journal of Clinical Epidemiology* 47(1994):339.

Johnson, E. (Magic). *What You Can Do To Avoid AIDS.* New York: Times Books, 1992.

Johnson, J. D., and P. Xanthos. *Tennis.* 6th ed. Dubuque, IA: Brown & Benchmark Publishers, 1993.

Jone, D. A., et al. "Physiological Changes in Skeletal Muscles as a Result of Strength Training." *Quarterly Journal of Experimental Physiology* 74(1989):233–56.

Jones, L. "The Pulling Movement." *National Strength and Conditioning Association Journal* 13(1991):14–17.

Jones, R., et al. "A Study of Worksite Health Promotion Programs and Absenteeism." *Journal of Occupational Medicine* 32(1990):95.

Kamwendo, K., et al. "Neck and Shoulder Disorders in Medical Secretaries. Part I: Pain Prevalence and Risk Factors." *Scandinavian Journal of Rehabilitation Medicine* 23(1991):127–33.

Kamwendo, K., et al. "Neck and Shoulder Disorders in Medical Secretaries: Part II. Ergonomical Work Environment and Symptom Profile." *Scandinavian Journal of Rehabilitation Medicine* 23(1991):135–42.

Kanders, B., et al. "Interaction of Calcium Nutrition and Physical Activity on Bone Mass in Young Women." *Journal of Bone Mineral Research* 3(1988):145.

Kanter, M. "Free Radicals and Exercise: Effects of Nutritional Antioxidant Supplementation." *Exercise and Sport Sciences Reviews* 23(1995):375.

Karkowsky, N. "Exercise with Care—Fitness Is Not Risk Free." *FDA Consumer* 23(1989):25.

Katch, F. I., and W. D. McArdle. *Nutrition, Weight Control, and Exercise.* Philadelphia: Lea & Febiger, 1988.

Kavanaugh, T. "Does Exercise Improve Coronary Collateralization? A New Look at an Old Belief." *Physician and Sportsmedicine* 17(1989):96.

Keefe, C. "Body Miracles Aren't Found All Bottled Up." *Orange County Register,* April 2, 1995.

Keeler, E., et al. "The External Costs of a Sedentary Life-Style." *American Journal of Public Health* 79(1989):975.

Kelleher, S. "R.S.I.: Treating Repetitive Motion Injuries is Fledgling Science." *Orange County Register,* March 1, 1995.

Kellie, S. E. "Tobacco Use: Women, Children and Minorities." In E. M. Blakeman, ed., *Final Report and Recommendations from the Health Community to the 101st Congress and the Bush Administration.* From the Tobacco Use in America Conference, Houston, Texas. Washington, DC: American Medical Association, 1989.

Kemnitz, J. W. "Body Weight Set Point Theory." *Contemporary Nutrition* 10(1985):2.

Kendall, F. P., and E. K. McCreary. *Muscles: Testing and Function.* 4th ed. Baltimore: Williams & Wilkins, 1993

Kennedy, J. F. "The Soft American." *Sports Illustrated* 13(1960):15.

Kenyon, G. S. "Six Scales for Assessing Attitudes Toward Physical Activity." *Research Quarterly* 39(1968):566.

Kibele, A. "Stress Factors in Leg Strength Training with Maximal Loads." *International Journal of Sports Medicine* 12(1991):93.

Kibler, W. "Musculoskeletal Adaptations and Injuries Due to Overtraining." *Exercise and Sport Sciences Reviews* 20(1992):99.

Kicman, A. T., et al. "Human Chorionic Gonadotrophin and Sport." *British Journal of Sports Medicine* 25(1991):73–78.

Kimiecik, J. "Predicting Vigorous Physical Activity of Corporate Employees." *Journal of Sport and Exercise Psychology* 14(1992):192.

King, A. C., et al. "Determinants of Physical Activity and Interventions in Adults." *Medicine and Science in Sports and Exercise* 24(1992):S221 (Supplement).

Kisner, C., and L. A. Colby. *Therapeutic Exercise: Foundations and Techniques.* 2d ed. Philadelphia: F. A. Davis, Company, 1990.

Klatz, R. M., et al. "Effects of Gravity Inversion on Hypertensive Subjects." *Physician and Sportsmedicine* 13(1985):85.

Klein, K. K. "The Deep Squat as Utilized in Weight Training for Athletics and Its Effect on the Ligaments of the Knee." *Journal of Physical and Mental Rehabilitation* 15(1961):10.

Kleiner, S. "Fiber Facts." *Physician and Sportsmedicine* 18(1990):19.

Kleiner, S. "Vegetarian Vitality." *Physician and Sportsmedicine* 20(1992):15.

Klerman, G. L. "Clinical Epidemiology of Suicide." *Journal of Clinical Psychiatry* 48(1987):33.

Klingshirn, L. A., et al. "Iron Status of Habitual Female Aerobic Dancers." *Medicine and Science in Sports and Exercise* 21(1989):Supplement, 78.

Kluka, D., and P. Dunn. *Volleyball.* 3d ed. Dubuque, IA: Brown & Benchmark Publishers, 1996.

Knox, R. A. "Smoke Gets in Your Eyes— Along with Cataracts." Santa Ana, CA: *Orange County Register,* August 26, 1992.

Kohrt, W., et al. "Body Composition of Healthy Sedentary and Trained, Young and Older Men and Women." *Medicine and Science in Sports and Exercise* 24(1992):832.

Koplan, J. P., et al. "The Risk of Exercise: A Public Health View of Injuries and Hazards." *Public Health Reports* 199(1985):189.

Koss, L. G. "The Papanicolaou Test for Cervical Cancer Detection: A Triumph and a Tragedy." *Journal of the American Medical Association* 261(1989):737.

Koszuta, L. E. "Low Impact Aerobics: Better Than Traditional Aerobic Dance?" *Physician and Sportsmedicine* 14(1986):156.

Kottke, F. J., et al. *Krusen's Handbook of Physical Medicine and Rehabilitation.* 4th ed. Philadelphia: W. B. Saunders Co., 1990.

Kraemer, W. J. "Endocrine Responses to Resistance Exercise." *Medicine and Science in Sports and Exercise* 20(1988):S152.

Kraus, H., and W. Raab. *Hypokinetic Disease.* Springfield, IL: Charles C. Thomas, 1961.

Krebs-Smith, S., et al. "U.S. Adults' Fruits and Vegetable Intakes, 1989 to 1991: A Revised Baseline for the Healthy People 2000 Objective." *American Journal of Public Health* 85(1995):1623.

Kreighbaum, E., and K. M. Barthels. *Biomechanics.* 3d ed. Minneapolis: Macmillan Publishing Co., 1990.

Krotkiewski, M. "Can Body Fat Patterning Be Changed." *Acta Medica Scandinavica* (Supplement) 723(1988):231.

Kuipers, H., et al. "Influence of Anabolic Steroids on Body Composition, Blood Pressure, Lipid Profile and Liver Functions in Body Builders." *International Journal of Sports Medicine* 12(1991):413–18.

Kushi, L. H., et al. "Dietary Antioxidant Vitamins and Death from Coronary Heart Disease in Postmenopausal Women." *The New England Journal of Medicine* 334(1996):1156.

Kusserow, R. P. "Do They Know What They Are Drinking?" *Youth and Alcohol: A National Survey.* Washington, DC: Office of Inspector General, Department of Health and Human Services, June 1991.

Kusserow, R. P. "Drinking Habits, Access, Attitudes and Knowledge." *Youth and Alcohol: A National Survey.* Washington, DC: Office of Inspector General, Department of Health and Human Services, June 1991.

LaBree, M. "A Review of Anabolic Steroids: Uses and Effects." *Journal of Sports Medicine and Physical Fitness* 32(1991):618–26.

LaChance, P. F., and T. Hortobagyi. "Influence of Cadence on Muscular Performance During Push-ups and Pull-up Exercise." *Journal of Strength and Conditioning Research* 8(1994):76–79.

Lagakos, S. W. "Comparison of Immediate with Deferred Zidovudine Therapy for Asymptomatic HIV-infected Adults with CD4 Counts of 500 or More per Cubic Millimeter." *New England Journal of Medicine* 333(1995):1782.

Laitner, B. "Doctors Criticize Tanning Salons." Santa Ana, CA: *Orange County Register* (Mar. 18 1991):E6.

Lake, D. A. "Neuromuscular Stimulation: An Overview and Its Implications in the Treatment of Sports Injuries." *Sports Medicine* 13(1992):320–36.

Lamanaca, J., and E. Haymes. "Effects of Dietary Iron Supplementation on Endurance." *Medicine and Science in Sports and Exercise* 21(1989):Supplement, 22.

Lampman, R., et al. "Effects of Exercise Training on Glucose Control, Lipid Metabolism, and Insulin Sensitivity in Hypertriglyceridemia and Non-Insulin Dependent Diabetes Mellitus." *Medicine and Science in Sport and Exercise* 23(1991):703.

Lander, J. E., et al. "The Effectiveness of Weight-Belts During the Squat Exercise." *Medicine and Science in Sports and Exercise* 22(1990):117–26.

Laseter, J. T., and J. A. Russell. "Anabolic Steroid-Induced Tendon Pathology: A Review of the Literature." *Medicine and Science in Sports and Exercise* 23(1991):1–3.

Lauderman, S. H., and D. Burns. "Quantifying HIV." *Journal of the American Medical Association* 275(1996):640.

Leach, R. "The Impingement Syndrome." In B. Zarins, et al., eds., *Injuries to the Throwing Arm.* Philadelphia: W. B. Saunders Co., 1985.

Leaf, D. A. "Omega-3 Fatty Acids and Coronary Artery Disease." *Postgraduate Medicine* 85(1989):237.

Leatt, P., et al. "Seven-year Follow-up of an Employee Fitness Program." *Canadian Journal of Public Health* 79(1988):20.

Leatz, C. A. *Unwinding.* Englewood Cliffs, NJ: Prentice-Hall, 1981.

Lee, I. "Exercise and Physical Health: Cancer and Immune Function." *Research Quarterly for Exercise and Sport* 66(1995):286.

Lee, I., et al. "Change in Body Weight and Longevity." *Journal of the American Medical Association* 268(1992):2045.

Lee, I., et al. "Physical Activity and Risk of Developing Colorectal Cancer Among College Alumni." *Journal of the National Cancer Institute* 83(1991):1324.

Lee, I., et al. "Time Trends in Physical Activity Among College Alumni 1962–1988." *American Journal of Epidemiology* 135(1992):915.

Lee, I., and R. S. Paffenbarger. "Do Physical Activity and Physical Fitness Avert Premature Mortality?" *Exercise and Sport Sciences Reviews* 24(1996):135.

Lemann, J. Jr. "Composition of the diet and calcium." *New England Journal of Medicine* 328(1993):880.

Lemonick, M. D. "Are We Ready for Fat Free Fat?" *Time* 4(Jan. 22, 1996), 40.

Lentell, G., et al. "The Use of Thermal Agents to Influence the Effectiveness of a Low Load Prolonged Stretch." (Platform presentation 1992 APTA Combined Sections Meeting, San Francisco.) Abstract. *Journal of Orthopaedic and Sports Physical Therapy* 15(Jan. 1992):48.

Leon, A., et al. "Leisure-time Physical Activity Levels and Risk of Coronary Health Disease and Death." *Journal of the American Medical Association* 258(1987):2388.

Lerman, C. "Reducing Avoidable Cancer through Prevention and Early Detection Regimens." *Cancer Research* 49(1989):4955.

Levy, M., et al. *Life and Health: Targeting Wellness.* New York: McGraw Hill, 1992.

Liehmohn, W. "Choosing the Safe Exercise." *Certified News* 2(1991):1.

Liemohn, W., et al. "Criterion Related Validity of the Sit and Reach Test." *Journal of Strength and Conditioning Research* 8(1994):91.

Liemohn, W. S., et al. "Unresolved Controversies in Back Management." *Journal of Orthopaedic and Sports Physical Therapy* 9(1988):239.

Lightsey, D. M. "Deceptive Tactics Used in Marketing Purported Ergogenic Aids." *National Strength and Conditioning Association Journal* 14:2(1992):26.

Lightsey, D., and J. Attaway. "Deceptive Tactics Used in Marketing Purported Ergogenic Aids." *National Strength and Conditioning Association Journal* 14(1992):26.

Lindeman, A. "Eating for Endurance or Ultraendurance." *Physician and Sportsmedicine* 20(1992):87.

Lindsey, R. "Figure Wrapping: Would You Believe It?" *Fitness For Living,* March/April 1972.

Lindsey, R., and C. Corbin. "Questionable Exercise—Some Alternatives." *Journal of Physical Education, Recreation and Dance* 60(1989):26.

Lindsey, R., and D. D. Gorrie. *Survival Kit for Those Who Sit.* Laguna Beach, CA: Publictec Editions, 1989.

Little, D. R. *Easy Stress-Reducing Strategies.* North Hollywood, CA: D. R. Little and Health Fair Expo, 1992.

Little, J. C. "The Athlete's Neurosis—A Deprivation Crisis." In M. H. Sacks, and M. L. Sachs, *Psychology of Running.* Champaign, IL: Human Kinetics Publishers, 1981.

Lohman, T. G., et al., eds. *Abridged Edition: Anthropometric Standardization Reference Manual.* Champaign, IL: Human Kinetics Publishers, 1991.

Long, B. C., and C. J. Haney. "Long-Term Follow-Up of Stressed Working Women: A Comparison of Aerobic Exercise and Progressive Relaxation." *Journal of Sport and Exercise Psychology* 10(1988):461.

Lord, J. P., et al. "Isometric and Isokinetic Measurement of Hamstring and Quadriceps Strength." *Archives of Physical Medicine and Rehabilitation* 73(1992):324–30.

Lubell, A. "Potentially Dangerous Exercises: Are They Harmful to All?" *Physician and Sportsmedicine* 17(1989):187.

Lucas, A. "Update and Review of Anorexia Nervosa." *Contemporary Nutrition* 14(1989):9.

Lucas, D. B. "Biomechanics of the Shoulder Joint." *Archives of Surgery* 107(1973):425.

Lundin, P., and W. Berg. "A Review of Plyometric Training." *National Strength and Conditioning Association Journal* 13(1991):22–30.

Macfarlane, P. "Out With the Sit-up, in With the Curl-up!" *Journal of Physical Education, Recreation and Dance* (August 1993):62.

Madding, S. W., et al. "Effect of Duration of Passive Stretch on Hip Abduction Range of Motion." *Journal of Orthopaedic and Sports Physical Therapy* 8(1987):409–16.

Magill, R. A. *Motor Learning: Concepts and Applications.* 4th ed. Dubuque, IA: Wm. C. Brown Publishers, 1993.

Malmivaara, A., et al. "The Treatment of Acute Low Back Pain—Bed Rest, Exercise or Ordinary Activity." *New England Journal of Medicine* 332(1995):351.

Manson, J. E. "Body Weight and Mortality Among Women." *New England Journal of Medicine* 333(1995):677.

Marcus, B. H. "Exercise Behavior and Strategies for Intervention." *Research Quarterly for Exercise and Sport* 66(1995):319.

Marcus, B., et al. "Motivational Readiness, Self-Efficacy and Decision-making for Exercise." *Journal of Applied Social Psychology* 22(1992):3.

Marcus, B., et al. "Self-Efficacy and the Stages of Exercise Behavior Change." *Research Quarterly for Exercise and Sport* 63(1992):60.

Marcus, B., et al. "Using the Stages of Change Model to Increase the Adoption of Physical Activity Among Community Participants." *American Journal of Health Promotion* 6(1992):424.

Marcus, R., et al. "Osteoporosis and Exercise in Women." *Medicine and Science in Sports and Exercise* 24(1992):S301 (Supplement).

Markowitz, M. "A Preliminary Study of Ritonavir, an Inhibitor of HIV-1 Protease, to Treat HIV." *New England Journal of Medicine* 333(1995):1534.

Martin, J. "Controlled Trial of Aerobic Exercise in Hypertension." *Circulation* 81(1990):1560.

Massara G., and F. Scoppa. "Proprioceptive Muscle Stretching." ICHPER. SD 31(Winter 1994–95):38.

McAtee, R. *Facilitated Stretching.* Champaign, IL: Human Kinetics Publishers, 1993.

McAuley, E., et al. "Self-Efficacy and Exercise Participation in Adult Females." *American Journal of Health Promotion* 5(1991):185.

McCarthy, P. "How Much Protein Do Athletes Really Need?" *Physician and Sportsmedicine* 17(1989):170.

McCunney, R. J. "Fitness, Heart Disease, and High-Density Lipoproteins: A Look at Relationships." *Physician and Sportsmedicine* 15(1987):67.

McDermott, R. J., and P. J. Marty. "Dipping and Chewing Behavior Among University Students: Prevalence and Patterns of Use." *Journal of School Health* 56:5(1986):175.

McGee, D., et al. "Leg and Hip Endurance Adaptations to Three Weight Training Programs." *Journal of Applied Sport Science Research* 6(1992):92–95.

McGinnis, J. M. "The Public Health Burden of a Sedentary Lifestyle." *Medicine and Science in Sports and Exercise* 24(1992):S196 (Supplement).

McGinnis, J. M., and P. R. Lee. "Healthy People 2000 at Mid Decade." *Journal of the American Medical Association* 273(1995):1123.

McGovern, P., et al. "Trends in Mortality, Morbidity and Risk Factor Levels for Stroke from 1960 to 1990." *Journal of the American Medical Association* 268(1992):753.

McIntosh, M. *Lifetime Aerobics.* Dubuque, IA: Wm. C. Brown Publishers, 1990.

McKenzie, R. *The Lumbar Spine: Mechanical Diagnosis and Therapy.* Upper Hutt, New Zealand: Spinal Publications, Ltd., 1981.

McKenzie, R. *Treat Your Own Back.* Waikanae, New Zealand: Spinal Publications, 1980.

McKenzie, R. *Treat Your Own Neck.* Waikanae, New Zealand: Spinal Publications, 1983.

Meacham, A. "Potent Pot Causes More Health Problems." *U.S. Journal of Drug and Alcohol Dependence* 14:1(1990):13.

"Media Action Alert. Issue: Industry Touts Alcohol as Heart Disease Cure-All." San Rafael, CA: The Marin Institute for the Prevention of Alcohol and Other Drug Problems, February 4, 1992.

"Medical Update: Kick Those Butts." *Golden Years* (Nov./Dec. 1991):34.

Melton, L., et al. "Epidemiology of Age-Related Fractures." In L. Avioli, ed., *The Osteoporetic Syndrome.* New York: Grune & Stratton, 1987.

Meredith, M. D. "Activity or Fitness: Is the Process or the Product More Important for Public Health?" *Quest* 40(1988):180.

Merten, T., and J. A. Potteiger. "Strength Training: Proper Techniques for the Big Three." *Athletic Training* 26(1991):295–309.

Mest, A., et al. "Long-term Morbidity and Mortality of Overweight Adolescents." *New England Journal of Medicine* 327(1992):1350.

"Methamphetamine Abuse on Rise." *Orange County Register,* Nov. 30, 1995.

Miko, C., et al., eds. *Opinions 90.* Detroit: Gale Research Inc., 1991.

Miller, R. W. "Critiquing Quack Ads." *FDA Consumer.* November 1982 (reprint).

Miller, W. "Introduction: Obesity, Diet Composition, Energy Expenditure, and Treatment of the Obese Patient." *Medicine and Science in Sports and Exercise* 23(1991):273.

"Miracle Cures and Other Frauds." *Johns Hopkins Medical Letter* 1(1990).

Misner, J. E., et al. "Sex Differences in Static Strength and Fatigability in Three Different Muscle Groups." *Research Quarterly for Exercise and Sport* 61(1990):238–42.

Mitchell, J. "Bulimia Nervosa." *Contemporary Nutrition* 14(1989):10.

Mitchell, J. B., et al. "Effects of Carbohydrate Ingestion on Gastric Emptying and Exercise Performance." *Medicine and Science in Sports and Exercise* 20(1988):110.

Mochizuki, R. M., and K. J. Richter. "Cardiomyopathy and Cerebrovascular Accident Associated with Anabolic-Androgenic Steroid Use." *Physician and Sportsmedicine* 16(1988):109.

Moffatt, R. J., et al. "Effects of Anabolic Steroids on Lipoprotein Profiles of Female Weight Lifters." *Physician and Sportsmedicine* 18(1990):106–15.

Moffet, B. "Smoking: Implications for Lipids." San Francisco, CA: NASPE Session, AAHPERD National Convention, 1991.

Moffroid, M. T., and J. E. Kusial. "The Power Struggle—Definition and Evaluation of Power and Muscular Performance." *Physical Therapy* 55(1975):1098.

Moffroid, M. T., and R. H. Whipple. "Specificity of Speed of Exercise." *Journal of Orthopaedic and Sports Physical Therapy* 12(1990):72–78.

Mole, P. A., et al. "Exercise Reverses Depressed Metabolic Rate Produced by Severe Caloric Restriction." *Medicine and Science in Sports and Exercise* 21(1989):29.

Monahan, T. "Exercise and Depression: Swapping Sweat for Serenity." *Physician and Sportsmedicine* 14(1986):192.

Monahan, T. "Perceived Exertion: An Old Exercise Tool Finds New Applications." *Physician and Sportsmedicine* 16(1988):174.

Morgan, W. P. "Affective Beneficence of Vigorous Physical Activity." *Medicine and Science in Sports and Exercise* 17(1985):94.

Morgan, W. P., and S. E. Goldston, eds. *Exercise and Mental Health.* New York: Hemisphere, 1987.

Morgan, W. P., and P. J. O'Connor. "Exercise and Mental Health." In R. K. Dishman, *Exercise Adherence.* Champaign, IL: Human Kinetics Publishers, 1988.

Morris, D. L. "Serum Cartinoids and CHD." *Journal of the American Medical Association* 272(1994):1439.

Morris, J., et al. "Exercise in Leisure Time: Coronary Attack and Death Rates." *British Heart Journal* 63(1990):325.

Morton, M. B. *Growing Up Drug Free: Teachers' Manual and Resource Book.* Glenview, IL: Scott, Foresman and Company, 1991.

Mosher, P., et. al, "Effects of 12 Weeks of Aerobic Circuit Training on Aerobic Capacity, Muscular Strength and Body Composition in College-Age Women." *Journal of Strength and Conditioning Research* 8(3):144–48.

Munnings, F. "Exercise and Estrogen in Women's Health: Getting a Clearer Picture." *Physician and Sportsmedicine* 16(1988):152.

Munson, W. W., and F. E. Pettigrew. "Cooperative Strength Training." *Journal of Physical Education, Recreation and Dance* 59(1988):61.

Murphy, E., and R. Schwarzkoph. "Effects of Standard Set and Circuit Weight Training on Excess Post-exercise Oxygen Consumption." *Journal of Applied Sport Science Research* 6(1992):88–91.

Murphy, P. "Office Stress: Is a Solution Shaping Up?" *Physician and Sportsmedicine* 12(1984):114.

Mutoh, Y., et al. "Aerobic Dance Injuries among Instructors and Students." *Physician and Sportsmedicine* 16(1988):81.

Myburgh, K. H., et al. "Factors Associated with Shin Soreness in Athletes." *Physician and Sportsmedicine* 16(1988):129.

Myers, J. L., and J. L. Knight. "General and Specific Habituation to Electrical Muscle Stimulation during Three Weeks of Training." (Abstracts) *Athletic Training* 24(1989):115.

Nafziger, N. A., et al. "Passive Exercise System: Effect on Muscle Activity, Strength, and Lean Body Mass." *Archives of Physical Medicine and Rehabilitation* 73(1992):184–89.

National Goals for Education. Washington, DC: U.S. Department of Education, 1990.

"National High School Senior Survey: Trends in Drug Use by High School Seniors." Washington, DC: National Institute on Drug Abuse; U.S. Department of Health and Human Services; Public Health Service; Alcohol, Drug Abuse and Mental Health Administration, Spring 1991.

National Institute of Health. "Consensus Statement: Preventing the Kidney Disease of Diabetes Mellitus." *American Journal of Kidney Disease* 13(1989):2.

National Institute of Health. "Optimal Calcium Intake." *Consensus Development Conference Statement, June 1994.* Available from NIH Office of Medical Applications Research.

National Institute of Occupational Safety and Health. *National Strategies for the Ten Leading Work-Related Diseases and Injuries.* Washington, DC: Department of Health and Human Services, 1989.

National Institute on Alcohol Abuse and Alcoholism. *Seventh Special Report to the U.S. Congress on Alcohol and Health.* Washington, DC: U.S. Department of Health and Human Services, 1990.

National Research Council. *Diet and Health: Implications for Reducing Chronic Disease Risk.* Washington, DC: National Academy of Sciences, 1989.

National Strength Coaches Association. "The Squat Exercise in Athletic Conditioning: A Position Statement." *National Strength and Conditioning Association Journal* 13(1991):51.

"Natural Products for Athletic Performance." *Annals of Pharmacotherapy* 27(1993):607.

NCAF Newsletter The New Dietary Supplement Laws. *NCAF Newsletter* 17(1994):1.

NCAHF Asks FTC to Stop Antioxidant Supplement Advertising." *National Council Against Health Fraud Newsletter* 17(July–August 1994):1.

Neck Exercises for a Healthy Neck. Daly City, CA: Krames Communications, 1990.

Nelson, A. G., et al. "Consequences of Combining Strength and Endurance Training Regimens." *Physical Therapy* 70(1990):287–94.

Nelson, K. C., and W. L. Cornelius. "The Relationship Between Isometric Contraction Durations and Improvement in Shoulder Joint Range of Motion." *Journal of Sports Medicine and* Physical Fitness 63(Sept. 1991):385–88.

Newport, F., and L. DeStefano. "Football Top Sport Among Fans; Basketball Gains Support." *The Gallup Poll Monthly* 295(1990):17.

Nigg, B., et al. "Biomechanical and Orthopedic Concepts in Sport Shoe Construction." *Medicine and Science in Sports and Exercise* 24(1992):595.

Nirschl, R. P. "Health Clubs Are a Great Source of Business for Orthopedists." *Physician and Sportsmedicine* 14(1986):54.

Noble, E. P. "What the Doctor Orders." San Rafael, CA: The Marin Institute for the Prevention of Alcohol and Other Drug Problems (Summer 1991):7.

Norkin, C., and P. Levangie. *Joint Structure and Function: A Comprehensive Analysis.* Philadelphia: F. A. Davis, Co., 1983.

North, T., et al. "Effect of Exercise on Depression." *Exercise and Sport Sciences Reviews* 18(1990):379.

Novello, A. "Another Disease of Women: AIDS." *Arizona Republic,* July 22, 1992:A9.

"O^2 Max or Percent Body Fat." *Medicine and Science in Sports and Exercise* 20(1988):150.

O'Connor, P. J., and S. D. Youngstedt. "Influence of Exercise on Human Sleep." *Exercise and Sport Sciences Reviews* 23(1995):105.

O'Keefe, J. H. "Dietary Prevention of Coronary Artery Disease." *Postgraduate Medicine* 85(1989):243.

Oakley, G. P., and J. D. Erickson. "Vitamin A and Birth Defects: Continuing Caution is Needed." *New England Journal of Medicine* 333(1995):1414.

Oja, P. "Descriptive Epidemiology of Health-Related Physical Activity and Fitness." *Research Quarterly for Exercise and Sport* 66(1995):303.

Oldridge, N., et al. "The Health Belief Model: Predicting Compliance and Dropout in Cardiac Rehabilitation." *Medicine and Science in Sports and Exercise* 22(1990):678.

Omenn, G. S., et al. "Effects of Combination of Beta Carotine and Vitamin A on Lung Cancer and Cardiovascular Disease." *The New England Journal of Medicine* 334(1996):1150.

"One in Nine American Women Will. . . ." *The University of California at Berkeley Wellness Letter.* Fernandina Beach, FL: Health Letter Associates, 8(1992):1.

Oscai, L. B. "Exercise or Food Restriction: Effect of Adipose Cellularity." *American Journal of Physiology* 27(1974):902.

Osternig, L. R., et al. "Differential Responses to Proprioceptive Neuromuscular Facilitation (PNF) Stretch Techniques." *Medicine and Science in Sports and Exercise* 22(1990):106–11.

Otten, A. "Women's Growing Role in the Workforce." *Wall Street Journal* 7(1989):B1.

"Our Vitamin Prescription: The Big Four." *University of California at Berkeley Wellness Letter* 10 (July 1994):1.

Owen, M. D., et al. "Effects of Ingesting Carbohydrate Beverages during Exercise in the Heat." *Medicine and Science in Sports and Exercise* 18(1986):568.

Pacelli, L. C. "To Fortify Bones, Use Calcium and Exercise." *Physician and Sportsmedicine* 17(1989):27.

Pacelli, L. S. "Straight Talk on Posture." *Physician and Sportsmedicine* 19(Feb. 1991):124–27.

Paffenbarger, R., et al. "Changes in Physical Activity and Other Lifeway Patterns Influencing Longevity." *Medicine and Science in Sports and Exercise* 26(1994):857.

Paffenbarger, R., et al. "Physical Activity and Physical Fitness as Determinants of Health and Longevity." In C. Bouchard, et al., *Exercise, Fitness and Health.* Champaign, IL: Human Kinetics Publishers, 1990.

Paffenbarger, R. S. "Contributions of Epidemiology to Exercise Science and Cardiovascular Health." *Medicine and Science in Sports and Exercise* 20(1988):426.

Paffenbarger, R. S., and R. T. Hyde. "Exercise Adherence, Coronary Heart Disease, and Longevity." In R. K. Dishman, *Exercise Adherence.* Champaign, IL: Human Kinetics Publishers, 1988.

Paffenbarger, R. S., et al. "The Association of Changes in Physical-Activity Level and Other Lifestyle Characteristics with Mortality Among Men." *The New England Journal of Medicine* 328(1993):538.

Paffenbarger, R. S., et al. "Physical Activity, All-Cause Mortality, and Longevity of College Alumni." *New England Journal of Medicine* 314(1986):605.

Paffenbarger, R. S., et al. "Physical Activity and Incidence of Cancer in Diverse Populations: A Preliminary Report." *American Journal of Clinical Nutrition* 45(1987):312.

Paliwal, Y., et al. "Stress and Cardiovascular Disease." *Hospital Medicine* n.d., 12, 16.

Parish, S., et al. "Cigarette Smoking, Tar Yield and Non-Fatal Myocardial Infarction." *British Medical Journal* 333(1995):471.

Parker, D., et al. "Juvenile Obesity." *Physician and Sportsmedicine* 19(1991):113.

Parrott, A. C., et al. "Anabolic Steroid Use by Amateur Athletes: Effects upon Psychological Mood States." *Journal of Sports Medicine and Physical Fitness* (1994):292.

Pate, R., et al. "Physical Activity and Associated Behaviors in American Adolescents." *Medicine and Science in Sports and Exercise* 24(1992):Supplement, 124.

Pate, R., et al. "Physical Activity and Public Health." *Journal of the American Medical Association* 273(1995):402.

Pate, R. R. "The Evolving Definition of Physical Fitness." *Quest* 40(1988):174.

Pate, R. R. "Physical Activity and Health: Dose-Response Issues." *Research Quarterly for Exercise and Sport* 66(1995):313.

Pedersen, T. R. "Lowering Cholesterol with Drugs and Diet." *New England Journal of Medicine* 333(1995):1350.

People Magazine, "Impossible Mission." 45(June 3, 1996):65.

Peota, C. "Studies Counter Myths about Iron in Athletes." *Physician and Sportsmedicine* 17(1989):26.

Perrine, J. J., and R. V. Edgerton. "Muscle Force-Velocity and Power Velocity Relationships under Isokinetic Loading." *Medicine and Science in Sports and Exercise* 10(1978):159.

Perry, P. J. "Illicit Anabolic Steroid Use in Athletes: A Case Series Analysis." *American Journal of Sports Medicine* 18(1990):422–28.

Petersen, S. R., et al. "The Effects of Concentric Resistance Training on Eccentric Peak Torque and Muscle Cross-Sectional Area." *Journal of Orthopaedic and Sports Physical Therapy* 13(1991):132–33.

Petersen, S. R., et al. "The Influence of Velocity-Specific Resistance Training on the In Vivo Torque-Velocity Relationship and the Cross Sectional Area of the Quadriceps Femoris." *Journal of Orthopaedic and Sports Physical Therapy* 10(1989):456.

Peterson, J. A., et al. *Strength Training for Women.* Champaign, IL: Human Kinetics Publishers, 1995.

Peterson, P. *Drug Facts.* Santa Cruz, CA: ETR Associates, n.d.

Peterson, P. G. *About Steroids.* Santa Cruz, CA: ETR Associates, Network Publications, 1990.

Peterson, S. "Cal-Ban 3000 Diet Aid Labeled a Health Risk." *Orange County Register,* July 27, 1992.

Peterson, S., et al. "Influence of Concentric Resistance Training on Concentric and Eccentric Strength." *Archives of Physical Medicine and Rehabilitation* 71(1990):101–5.

Petruzzello, S. J., et al. "A Meta-Analysis on the Anxiety-Reducing Effects of Acute and Chronic Exercise: Outcomes and Mechanisms." *Sports Medicine* 11(1991):143–82.

Philen, R., et al. "Survey of Advertising for Nutritional Supplements in Health and Body Building Magazines." *Journal of the American Medical Association* 268(1992):1008.

Physical Activity and Cardiovascular Health: NIH Consensus, *Online,* 1995 December 18–20; 13(3):1–13.

Physical Medicine Research Foundation. "Seventh International Symposium on Repetitive Strain Injuries, Fibromyalgia and Chronic Fatigue Syndrome." Vancouver, B.C. Canada. June 10–12, 1994.

Pickett, B., et al. "Bench Aerobics." *Strategies* 4(1990):28.

Pinner, R. W., et al. "Trends in Infectious Diseases Mortality in the U.S." *Journal of the American Medical Association* 275(1996):189.

Plowman, S. "Physical Activity, Physical Fitness, and Low Back Pain." *Exercise and Sport Sciences Reviews* 20(1992):221.

Plowman, S. A. "Physical Fitness and Healthy Low Back Function." *Physical Activity and Fitness Research Digest* 1(1993):1.

Pollock, C. "Breaking the Risk of Falls: An Exercise Benefit for Older People." *Physician and Sportsmedicine* 20(1992):146.

Pollock, M. L., et al. "Measurement of Cardiorespiratory Fitness and Body Composition in the Clinical Setting." *Comprehensive Therapy* 6(1980):12.

Ponte, D. J., et al. "A Preliminary Report on the Use of the McKenzie Protocol versus Williams Protocol in the Treatment of Low Back Pain." *Journal of Orthopaedic and Sports Physical Therapy* 6(1984):130.

Powell, K. E. "Habitual Exercise and Public Health: An Epidemiological View." In R. K. Dishman, *Exercise Adherence.* Champaign, IL: Human Kinetics Publishers, 1988.

Powell, K. E., et al. "An Epidemiological Perspective on the Cause of Running Injuries." *Physician and Sportsmedicine* 14(1986):100.

Powell, K. E., et al. "Physical Activity and Chronic Diseases." *American Journal of Clinical Nutrition* 49(1989):999.

Powell, K. E., et al. "Physical Activity and the Incidence of Coronary Heart Disease." *Annual Review of Public Health* 8(1987):253.

Powell, K. E., et al. "The Status of the 1990 Objectives for Physical Fitness and Exercise." *Public Health Reports* 101(1986):15.

Powers, S. K., and E. T. Howley. *Exercise Physiology.* 2d ed. Dubuque, IA: Brown & Benchmark Publishers, 1994.

Prapavessis, H., and A. V. Carron. "Learned Helplessness in Sport." *The Sport Psychologist* 2(1988):189.

Prendergast, M. L. "Substance Abuse Among College Students: A Review of Recent Literature." *Journal of College Health* 43(1994):99.

Prevention Resource Guide: College Youth Put on the Brakes. Rockville, MD: National Clearinghouse for Alcohol and Drug Information, 1991. Produced for the Office for Substance Abuse Prevention; U.S. Department of Health and Human Services; Public Health Service; Alcohol, Drug Abuse and Mental Health Administration.

Public Health Service. *Healthy People 2000: National Health Promotion and Disease Prevention Objectives.* Washington, DC: U.S. Government Printing Office, 1991. (DHHS Pub. No. PHS 91-50212.)

Public Health Service. *The Surgeon General's Report on Nutrition and Health.* Washington, DC: Department of Health and Human Services, 1988, Pub. No. 88-50210.

Public Health Service. *Surgeon General's Report on Physical Activity and Health.* Washington, DC: U.S. Government Printing Office, 1996.

Pugliese, M. T., et al. "Fear of Obesity: A Cause of Short Stature and Delayed Puberty." *New England Journal of Medicine* 309(1983):513.

"Pyramid Scheme Foiled." *Nutrition Action Health Letter* 19(1992):3.

Raithel, K. S. "Chronic Pain and Exercise Therapy." *Physician and Sportsmedicine* 17(1989):203.

Ramsey, M. L. "Pseudomonas Folliculitis Associated with Use of Hot Tubs and Spas." *Physician and Sportsmedicine* 17(1989):150.

Ransdell, L. B., et al. "Syndrome X: A Postmenopausal Woman's Hidden Nemesis." *Journal of Women and Aging,* in press.

Rapola, J. M., et al. "Effects of Vitamin E and Beta Carotine on the Incidence of Angina Pectoris: A Randomized Double Blind Controlled Trial." *Journal of the American Medical Association* 275(1996):693.

Rasch, P. J. *Weight Training.* 5th ed. Dubuque, IA: Wm. C. Brown Publishers, 1990.

Recker, R., et al. "Bone Gain in Young Adult Women." *Journal of the American Medical Association* 268(1992):2403.

"Red Wine No 'Magic Bullet' for Heart Disease." *Health Digest* (July/August 1992):9.

Reid, I. R., et al. "Effects of Calcium Supplementation of Bone Loss in Post Menopausal Women." *New England Journal of Medicine* 328(1993):460.

Reiger, D. A., et al. "One-Month Prevalence of Mental Disorders in the United States." *Archives of General Psychiatry* 45(1988):977.

Reiken, G. B. "Negative Effects of Alcohol on Physical Fitness and Athletic Performance." *Journal of Physical Education, Recreation and Dance* 62(October 1991):64.

Rejeski, W. J., and E. A. Kenney *Fitness Motivation: Preventing Participant Dropout.* Champaign, IL: Human Kinetics Publishers, 1988.

Rejeski, W. J., et al. "Physical Activity and Health-Related Quality of Life." *Exercise and Sport Sciences Reviews* 24(1996):71.

Richie, D. H. "Aerobic Dance Injuries: A Retrospective Study of Instructors and Participants." *Physician and Sportsmedicine* 13(1985):130.

Rider, R. A., and J. Daly. "Effects of Flexibility Training on Enhancing Spinal Mobility in Older Women." *Journal of Sports Medicine and Physical Fitness* 31(1991):213–17.

Riebe, D., et al. "The Blood Pressure Response to Exercise in Anabolic Steroid Users." *Medicine and Science in Sports and Exercise* 24(1992):633–37.

Rimer, B., et al. "Why Women Resist Screening Mammography." *Radiology* 172(1989):243.

Rimm, E. B. et al. "Vegetable, Fruit, and General Fiber Intake and Risk of CHD Among Men." *Journal of the American Medical Association* 275(1996):447.

Rippe, J., et al. "Walking for Health and Fitness." *Journal of the American Medical Association* 259(1988):2720.

Rizzo, T. H. "Join the Office Ergonomic Revolution." *Idea Today* (Mar. 1992):42.

Roach, K., et al. "The Use of Patient Symptoms to Screen for Serious Back Problems." *Journal of Sports Physical Therapy* 21(1995):1.

Robbins, S., et al. "Athletic Footwear: Unsafe Due to Perceptual Illusions." *Medicine and Science in Sports and Exercise* 23(1991):217.

Roberts, M. "The Well Done Stretch." *U.S. News and World Report* (Mar. 5, 1990):65–67.

Roberts, R., et al. "Effects of Warm-Up on Muscle Glycogenesis During Intense Exercise." *Medicine and Science in Sports and Exercise* 23(1991):37.

Roberts, W. "Managing Heatstroke." *Physician and Sportsmedicine* 20(1992):17.

Robertson, J. "Preventing Heat Injury in Sports." *Physician and Sportsmedicine* 19(1991):31.

Robertson, L., et al. "Influence of Job and Personal Risk Factors on Safety Limits for Kinesiotherapists Performing a Stressful Clinical Lifting Task." *Clinical Kinesiology* (Spring. 1993):7.

Robinson, W., et al. "Competing With the Cold." *Physician and Sportsmedicine* 20(1992):61.

Roper, W. L. "Current Approaches to Prevention of HIV Infections." *Public Health Reports* 106(1991):111.

Rosenberg, P. S. "Scope of the AIDS Epidemic in the U.S." *Science* 270(1995):1372.

Rossi, F., and S. Dragoni. "Lumbar Spondylolysis Occurrence in Competitive Athletes." *Journal of Sports Medicine and Physical Fitness* 30(Dec. 1990):450–52.

Rousseau, P. "Exercise in the Elderly." *Postgraduate Medicine* 85(1989):113.

Rovere, G. D. "Low Back Pain among Athletes." *Physician and Sportsmedicine* 15(1987):105.

Roy, S. H., et al. "Fatigue, Recovery, and Low Back Pain in Varsity Rowers." *Medicine and Science in Sports and Exercise* 22(1990):463–69.

Royal Canadian Air Force. *Exercise Plans for Physical Fitness.* Ottawa, Ontario, Canada: Queen's Printer. Rev. U.S. ed. published by Simon and Schuster, Inc., by special arrangement with *This Week Magazine.* Copies available from *This Week Magazine,* P.O. Box 77-E, Mt. Vernon, NY.

Rozenek, R., et al. "Physiological Responses to Resistance-Exercise in Athletes Self-Administering Anabolic Steroids." *Journal of Sports Medicine and Physical Fitness* 30(1990):354–60.

"Running Shoes: The Sneaker Grows Up." *Consumer Reports* 57(1992):308.

Runyan, C., et al. "Epidemiology and Prevention of Adolescent Injury." *Journal of the American Medical Association* 262(1989):2273.

Ryan, B. E., and J. F. Mosher. "Media Action Alert. Issue: Study Finds Reduced Alcohol Industry Presence on College Campuses: Some Promotions Persist." *Progress Report: Alcohol Promotion on Campus.* San Rafael, CA: The Marin Institute for the Prevention of Alcohol and Other Drug Problems, December 16, 1991.

Ryan, L. M., et al. "Velocity Specific and Mode Specific Effects of Eccentric Isokinetic Training of the Hamstrings." *Journal of Orthopaedic and Sports Physical Therapy* 13(1991):33–39.

Ryan, M. E., et al. "A Research-Based HIV/AIDS Education Program via the University Computer System: Bridge to Prevention." *Health Education* 23(1992):198.

Saad, L. "Children, Hard Work Taking Their Toll on Baby Boomers." *The Gallup Poll Monthly* 355, 21, 1995.

Saal, J. A. "Rehabilitation of Football Players with Lumbar Injuries." *Physician and Sports Medicine* 16:9, 10 Sept., Oct. (1988).

Saavedra, T. "Would-Be Quitters Learn That Patch Is No 'Magic Bullet' For Smoking." Santa Ana, CA: *Orange County Register,* Aug. 23, 1992.

Sady, S. P., et al. "Flexibility Training: Ballistic, Static or Proprioceptive Neuromuscular Facilitation." *Archives of Physical Medicine and Rehabilitation* 63(1982):261.

Safran, M., et al. "Warm-Up and Muscle Injury Prevention." *Sports Medicine* 8(1989):239.

Safran, M. R., et al. "The Role of Warm-up in Muscular Injury Prevention." *American Journal of Sports Medicine* 16(1988):123.

Safrit, M., et al. "The Difficulty of Sit-up Tests: An Empirical Investigation." *Research Quarterly for Exercise and Sport* 63(1992):277.

Sallis, J. "Influences on Physical Activity of Children, Adolescents, and Adults or Determinants of Active Living." *Physical Activity and Research Digest* 1(1994):1.

Sallis, J., et al. "Determinants of Exercise Behavior." *Exercise and Sport Sciences Reviews* 18(1990):307.

Sallis, J., et al. "Determinants of Physical Activity and Interventions in Youth." *Medicine and Science in Sports and Exercise* 24(1992):S248 Supplement.

Sallis, J. F., and K. Patrick. "Physical Activity Guidelines for Adolescents: Consensus Statement." *Pediatric Exercise Science* 53(1994):302.

Sambrook, P. N. "Treatment of Post Menopausal Osteoporosis." *New England Journal of Medicine* 333(1995):1495.

Samford, B. "Creeping Obesity." *Physician and Sportsmedicine* 16(1988):143.

Sandvik, L., et al. "Physical Fitness as a Predictor of Mortality Among Healthy, Middle Aged Norwegian Men." *New England Journal of Medicine* 328(1993):533.

Saudek, C. E., and K. A. Palmer. "Back Pain Revisited." *Journal of Orthopaedic and Sports Physical Therapy* 8(1987):556.

Sawka, M. "Current Concepts Concerning Thirst, Dehydration, and Fluid Replacement: An Overview." *Medicine and Science in Sports and Exercise* 24(1992):643.

Schatz, M. P. "Exercises You Can Take to Work." *Physician and Sportsmedicine* 20(Jan. 1992):165–66.

Schenkman, M., and V. R. DeCartaya. "Kinesiology of the Shoulder Complex." *Journal of Orthopaedic and Sports Physical Therapy* 8(1987):438.

Schettler, J. *HIV: Get the Answers.* Santa Cruz, CA: ETR Associates, 1992.

Schipplein, O. D., et al. "Relationship Between Moments at the L5/S1 Level, Hip and Knee Joints When Lifting." *Journal of Biomechanics* 23(1990):907–12.

Schmidt, G., et al. "Sport Commitment: A Model Integrating Enjoyment, Dropout, and Burnout." *Journal of Sport and Exercise Psychology* 13(1991):254.

Schneider, D., et al. "Choice of Exercise: A Predictor of Behavioral Risks." *Research Quarterly for Exercise and Sport* 63(1992):231.

Schon, L., et al. "Chronic Exercise-Induced Leg Pain in Active People." *Physician and Sportsmedicine* 20(1992):100.

Seaborg, E., and E. Dudley. *Hiking and Backpacking.* Champaign, IL: Human Kinetics Publishers, 1994.

"Secondhand Smoke: Is it a Hazard?" *Consumer Reports* 60:1(1995):142.

Sedlock, D. A., et al. "Accuracy of Subject-Palpated Carotid Pulse after Exercise." *Physician and Sportsmedicine* 11(1983):106.

Seiger, L. H., and J. Hesson. *Walking for Fitness.* 2d ed. Dubuque, IA: Wm. C. Brown Publishers, 1994.

Sekiya, C. *Help Your Child Succeed.* Los Angeles: Asian American Drug Abuse Program, 1991.

Selby, G. "When Does an Athlete Need Iron?" *Physician and Sportsmedicine* 19(1991):96.

Selby, G. B., and E. R. Eichner. "Age-Related Increases of Iron Stores in Athletes." *Medicine and Science in Sports and Exercise* 21(1989): Supplement, 78.

Sellers, J. S. *Steroids in Athletes.* Phoenix, AZ: Center for Sports Medicine and Orthopedics, 1992.

Sellers, T., et al. "Effect of Family History, Body-Fat Distribution, and Reproductive Factors in the Risk of Postmenopausal Breast Cancer." *New England Journal of Medicine* 326(1992):1323.

Selye, H. "Secret of Coping with Stress." *U.S. News and World Report,* March 21, 1977, p. 51.

Selye, H. *The Stress of Life.* 2d ed. New York: McGraw-Hill, 1978.

Seward, B. L. *Managing Stress.* Boston: Jones & Bartlett Publishers, 1994.

Shaffers, D., et al. *Prevention in Child and Adolescent Psychiatry: The Reduction of Risk of Mental Disorders.* Washington, DC: American Academy of Child and Adolescent Psychiatry, 1990.

Sharpe, G. L., et al. "Exercise Prescription and the Low Back." *Journal of Physical Education, Recreation and Dance* 59(1988):74.

Shaw, J. M., and C. Snow-Harter. "Osteoporosis and Physical Activity." *Physical Activity and Fitness Research Digest*. Washington, DC: President's Council on Physical Fitness and Sports, 1995.

"Shearing the Suckers." *Consumer Reports* (February 1986):87.

Sheehan, G. "Running Away from Smoking." *Physician and Sportsmedicine* 19(1991):55.

Shephard, R. "Par-Q, Canadian Home Fitness Test and Exercise Screening Alternatives." *Sports Medicine* 5(1988):185.

Shephard, R. "Physical Activity, Health and Well-Being at Different Life Stages." *Research Quarterly for Exercise and Sport* 66(1995):298.

Shephard, R., et al. "The Canadian Home Fitness Test." *Sports Medicine* 11(1991):358.

Shephard, R. J. *Physical Activity and Health-Related Fitness*. Champaign, IL: Human Kinetics Publishers, 1993.

Shephard, R. J. "Readiness for Physical Activity." *Physical Activity and Fitness Research Digest* 1(1994):1.

Sheridan, M. J. "A Psychometric Assessment of Children of Alcoholics Screening Test (CAST)," *Journal of Studies on Alcohol* 56(1995):156.

Shockey, G. L. "Hydration and Health: Meeting the Athletes' Fluid Needs." *Sportcare and Fitness* 3(1988):43.

Shore, S. "Coors Product Zima Under Fire. . . . *Orange County Register*, Feb. 9, 1995.

Siegel, B. S. *Love, Medicine, and Miracles*. New York: Harper and Row, 1986.

Siff, M. C. "Modified PNF as a System of Physical Conditioning." *National Strength and Conditioning Association Journal* 13(1991):73–77.

Signorile, J., et al. "An Electromyographical Comparison of the Squat and Knee Extension Exercises." *Journal of Strength and Conditioning Research* 8(1994):178.

Sihvonen, T., et al. "Electric Behavior of Low Back Muscles During Lumbar Pelvic Rhythm in Low Back Pain Patients and Healthy Controls." *Archives of Physical Medicine and Rehabilitation* 72(Dec. 1991):1080–84.

Silverman, J. L., et al. "Quantitative Cervical Flexor Strength in Healthy Subjects and in Subjects with Mechanical Neck Pain." *Archives of Physical Medicine and Rehabilitation* 72(Aug. 1991):679–81.

Silvester, L. J. *Weight Training for Strength and Fitness*. Boston: Jones & Bartlett Publishers, 1992.

Simon, H. B. "Exercise and Infection." *Physician and Sportsmedicine* 15(1987):135.

Simons-Morton, D. G., et al. "Health-Related Physical Fitness in Childhood: Status and Recommendations." *Annual Review of Public Health* 9(1988):403.

Simons-Morton, D. G., et al. *Promoting Physical Activity among Adults*. Atlanta, GA: Centers for Disease Control, 1988.

Singh, A., et al. "Chronic Multivitamin-Mineral Supplementation Does Not Enhance Physical Performance." *Medicine and Science in Sports and Exercise* 24(1992):726.

Slava, S., et al. "The Long-Term Effects of a Conceptual Physical Education Program." *Research Quarterly for Exercise and Sports* 55(1984):161.

Slavin, J. L., et al. "Amino Acid Supplements: Beneficial or Risky?" *Physician and Sportsmedicine* 16(1988):221.

Smith, E. L., and S. L. Zook. "The Aging Process: Benefits of Regular Physical Activity." *Journal of Physical Education, Recreation and Dance* 57(1986):32.

Smith, L. "Acute Inflammation: The Underlying Mechanism in Delayed Onset Muscle Soreness." *Medicine and Science in Sports and Exercise* 23(1991):542.

Smith, L. L., et al. "The Effects of Static and Ballistic Stretching on Delayed Onset Muscle Soreness and Creatine Kinase." *Research Quarterly for Exercise and Sport* 64(1993):103.

"Smoking Deaths Likely to Triple in 25 Years." *Orange County Register*, Dec. 9, 1995.

Snow-Harter, C., et al. "Exercise, Bone Mineral, and Osteoporosis." *Exercise and Sport Sciences Reviews* 19(1991):351.

Snyder, A. C., et al. "Influence of Dietary Iron Sources on Measures of Iron Status among Female Runners." *Medicine and Science in Sports and Exercise* 21(1989):7.

Solomon, M. Z., and W. DeJong. "Preventing AIDS and Other STDs Through Condom Promotion: A Patient Education Intervention." *American Journal of Public Health* 79(1989):453.

Spence, W. R. *Drugs and You: A Guide for Teenagers*. Waco, TX: Health EDCO, 1991.

Spence, W. R. *Hallucinogens: Trip or Trap?* Waco, TX: Health EDCO, 1991.

Spence, W. R. *Heroin: Highway to Oblivion*. Waco, TX: Health EDCO, n.d.

Spence, W. R. *Smokeless Tobacco: A Chemical Time Bomb*. Waco, TX: Health EDCO, n.d.

Spence, W. R. *Substance Abuse in the Workplace: Strung Out on the Job*. Waco, TX: Health EDCO, n.d.

Stamford, B. "Caffeine and Athletes." *Physician and Sportsmedicine* 17(1989):193.

Stamford, B. "The Differences between Strength and Power." *Physician and Sportsmedicine* 13(1985):155.

Stamford, B. "Exercise and Air Pollution." *Physician and Sportsmedicine* 18(1990):153.

Stamford, B. "Saunas, Steam Rooms and Hot Tubs." *Physician and Sportsmedicine* 17(1989):188.

Stanton, P., and C. Purdam. "Hamstring Injuries in Sprinting—The Role of Eccentric Exercise." *Journal of Orthopaedic and Sports Physical Therapy* 10(1989):343–49.

Steiner, M. E. "Hypermobility and Knee Injuries." *Physician and Sportsmedicine* 15(1987):159–68.

Stephens, T. "Exercise and Mental Health in the United States and Canada: Evidence from Four Population Surveys." *Preventive Medicine* 17(1988):195.

Stephens, T., et al. "A Descriptive Epidemiology of Leisure-Time Physical Activity." *Public Health Reports* 100(1985):147.

Sternfeld, B. "Cancer and the Protective Effect of Physical Activity." *Medicine and Science in Sports and Exercise* 24(1992):1195.

Stone, M. H., et al. "Health and Performance-Related Potential of Resistance Training." *Sports Medicine* 11(1991):210–31.

Stone, M. H., et al. "Muscle Conditioning and Muscle Injuries." *Medicine and Science in Sports and Exercise* 22(1990):457–61.

Stratton, J., et al. "Effects of Physical Conditioning of Fibrinolytic Variables and Fibrinogen in Young and Old Healthy Subjects." *Circulation* 83(1991):1692.

Straus, R. H. "Spittin' Image: Breaking the Sports-Tobacco Connection." *Physician and Sportsmedicine* 19(1991):46.

"Stress on Job Affects Health." *Orange County Register*, Jan. 1, 1990.

Strickler, T., et al. "Effects of Passive Warming on Muscle Injury." *American Journal of Sports Medicine* 18(1990):141.

Stunkard, A., and R. Berkowitz. "Treatment of Obesity in Children." *Journal of the American Medical Association* 264(1990):2550.

"Substance Abuse Quiz." Downey, CA: Department of Health Services, Rancho Los Amigos Medical Center, n.d.

Substance Abuse Report. Washington, DC: National Institutes on Drug Abuse; U.S. Department of Health and Human Services; Public Health Service; Alcohol, Drug Abuse and Mental Health Administration, January 1, 1992:4.

Summerfield, L. M. "Adolescents and AIDS." *ERIC Digest.* Washington, DC: ERIC Clearinghouse on Teacher Education, 1992. EDO-SP:8–89.

Summerfield, L. M. "Drug and Alcohol Prevention Education." *ERIC Digest.* Washington, DC: ERIC Clearinghouse on Teacher Education, 1991.

Superko, H. R. "Exercise Training, Serum Lipids, and Lipoprotein Particles: Is There a Change Threshold?" *Medicine and Science in Sport and Exercise* 23(1991):677.

Superko, H. R. "The Role of Diet, Exercise, and Medication in Blood Lipid Management of Cardiac Patients." *Physician and Sportsmedicine* 16(1988):65.

Surgeon General's Office. *Surgeon General's Report on Physical Activity and Health.* Washington, DC: U.S. Government Printing Office, (1996).

Tanji, J. "Hypertension: How Exercise Helps." *Physician and Sportsmedicine* 18(1990):77.

Taylor, D. C., et al. "Viscoelastic Properties of Muscle-Tendon Units: The Biomechanical Effects of Stretching." *American Journal of Sports Medicine* 18(1990):300–309.

Taylor, W. N. *Hormonal Manipulation: A New Era of Monstrous Athletes.* Jefferson, NC: McFarland and Co., Inc., Publishers, 1985.

"Teenagers and AIDS." *Newsweek* (August 3, 1992):44.

Teitz, C. C., and D. M. Cook. "Rehabilitation of Neck and Low Back Injuries." *Clinics in Sports Medicine: Rehabilitation of Injured Athletes* 4(1985):456.

Thanepohn, S. G. "How to Kick the Butts." *U.S. Journal of Drug and Alcohol Dependence* 14:1(1990):1.

The Alcoholism Report. Newsletter for Professionals in the Fields of Alcoholism and Drug Dependence. Washington, DC: N.p., Vol. 9, No. 8. (March 1991).

"The Antioxidant Scare." *National Council Against Health Fraud Newsletter* 17(May–June 1994):1.

The Rockport Company. *The Rockport Guide to Fitness Walking.* Marlboro, MA: The Rockport Company, 1990.

"The Squat Exercise in Athletic Conditioning: A Position Statement and Review of the Literature." *National Strength and Conditioning Association Journal* 13(1991):51.

"The Supplement Story: Can Vitamins Help?" *Consumer Reports* 57(1992):12.

The Wellness Way: Managing Stress. Daly City, CA: Krames Communications n.d.

The World of Rope Jumping. Rothstein, M. Video Series. 1–800–368–JUMP.

Thein, L. A. "Impingement Syndrome and Its Conservative Management." *Journal of Orthopaedic and Sports Physical Therapy* 11(Nov. 1989):183–90.

"Thigh Cream Fails Test." *National Council Against Health Fraud Newsletter* 18(1995).

Thompson, M. L. *Growing Up Drug Free.* Glenview, IL: Scott, Foresman & Co., 1991.

Thompson, P. D., et al. "Incidence of Death during Jogging in Rhode Island from 1975 through 1980." *Journal of the American Medical Association* 247(1982):2535.

Tichauer, E. R. *Biomechanical Basis of Ergonomics.* New York: John Wiley & Sons, 1978.

Tipton, C. "Exercise, Training, and Hypertension: An Update." *Exercise and Sport Sciences Reviews* 19(1991):447.

Tittel, K. "The Loadability and Relievability of the Lumbo-sacral Transition in Sports." *Journal of Sports Medicine and Physical Fitness* 30(June 1990):113–21.

"Tobacco Use Among Youth." *Tobacco Free America.* Washington, DC: Legislative Clearinghouse, August 1989.

"Toning Tables Fail Test." *NCAF Newsletter* 13(Nov./Dec. 1990).

Travell, J., and D. G. Simons. *Myofascial Pain and Dysfunction: The Trigger Point Manual.* Baltimore: Williams & Wilkins, vol. 1, 1983; vol. 2, 1992.

Trzaskoma, Z., et al. "Investigation of an Experimental Weight-Training Program." *Journal of Sports Sciences* 10(1992):109–17.

Tucker, L. A., and G. M. Friedman. "Television Viewing and Obesity in Adult Males." *American Journal of Public Health* 79(1989):516.

Understanding Anabolic Steroids: For Parents, Teachers and Coaches. San Diego, CA: San Diego County Office of Education, n.d.

University of California at Berkeley Wellness Letter, "The Breathtaking Promises of Melatonin." *University of California at Berkeley Wellness Letter* 12(1996):1.

University of California at Berkeley Wellness Letter, "Strength in One Third the Time." *University of California at Berkeley Wellness Letter* 12(1996):3.

University of California at Berkeley Wellness Letter, "Thin Thighs in a Bottle." *University of California at Berkeley Wellness Letter* 10(1994):1.

University of California at Berkeley Wellness Letter, "Weight, Fate, Set Point and Counterpoint." *University of California at Berkeley Wellness Letter* 11(1995):1.

U.S. Department of Agriculture and U.S. Department of Health and Human Services. *Nutrition and Your Health: Dietary Guidelines for Americans* (4th ed.). Washington, DC: U.S. Department of Agriculture and U.S. Department of Health and Human Services, 1995.

U.S. Department of Health and Human Services. *Alcohol and Health.* Seventh Special Report to the U.S. Congress from the Secretary of Health and Human Services. NIAAA, Rockville, MD: 1990.

"USDA Adopts New Pyramid Graphic for Nutrition Guide." *Food Production Management* 115(1992):8.

Vakos, J., et al. "EMG Activity of Selected Trunk and Hip Muscles During a Squat Lift: Effect of Varying the Lumbar Posture." (Abstract of platform presentation at the 1991 Section Meeting of APTA.) *Journal of Orthopaedic and Sports Physical Therapy* 13(May 1991):257.

Van De Graaff, K. M., and S. I. Fox. *Concepts of Human Anatomy and Physiology.* 3d ed. Dubuque, IA: Wm. C. Brown Publishers, 1992.

Van Duser, B. L., and P. B. Raven. "The Effects of Oral Smokeless Tobacco on the Cardiorespiratory Response to Exercise." *Medicine and Science in Sports and Exercise* 24(1992):389.

Van Itallie, T. B. "Topography of Body Fat: Relationship to Risk of Cardiovascular and Other Diseases." In T. G. Lohman, et al., eds., *Anthropometric Standardization Reference Manual.* Champaign, IL: Human Kinetics Publishers, 1988.

Vena, J. E., et al. "Occupational Exercise and Risk of Cancer." *American Journal of Clinical Nutrition* 45(1987):318.

Vickers, B., and W. Vincent. *Swimming.* 6th ed. Dubuque, IA: Brown & Benchmark Publishers, 1994.

"Vitamins: New RDAs." *Newsweek* (November 6, 1989):84.

Volski, R. V., et al. "Lower Spine Screening in the Shooting Sports." *Physician and Sportsmedicine* 14(1986):101.

Voy, R. O. "Water-Soluble Vitamins Not Safe in Megadoses." *Physician and Sportsmedicine* 14(1986):52.

Vuori, I. "Exercise and Physical Health: Musculoskeletal Health and Functional Capacities." *Research Quarterly for Exercise and Sport* 66(1995):276.

Wallberg-Henriksson, H. "Exercise and Diabetes Mellitus." *Exercise and Sport Sciences Reviews* 20(1992):339.

Weinhouse, S., et al. "American Cancer Society Guidelines on Diet, Nutrition and Cancer." *CA-A Cancer Journal for Clinicians* 41(1991): 334.

Weinstock, C. P. "The Grazing of America: A Guide to Healthy Snacking." *FDA Consumer* 23(1989):8.

Weitman, A., and B. Stamford. "Is Excessive Sweating Healthy?" *Physician and Sportsmedicine* 11(1983):195.

Wells, K. B., et al. "The Functioning and Well-Being of Depressed Patients." *Journal of the American Medical Association* 262(1989):914.

"We're Sticking by Our Beta-Carotene." *University of California at Berkeley Wellness Letter* 10(July 1994):1.

Wescott, W. L. *Strength Fitness: Physiological Principles and Training Techniques.* 4th ed. Dubuque, IA. Brown & Benchmark, 1995.

Wessel, H. *Basketball: Steps to Success.* Champaign, IL: Human Kinetics Publishers, 1994.

What Is Your Alcohol I.Q.? Skill Builder. St. Rose, LA: SYNDISTAR, INC., 1991.

What You Should Know About Smoking and Cancer. New York: American Lung Association, n.d.

White, G. W., et al. "Preventing Steroid Abuse in Youth: The Health Educator's Role." *Health Education* 18:4(1987):32.

White, M. *Water Exercise.* Champaign, IL: Human Kinetics Publishers, 1995.

Wichmann, S. "Exercise Excess: Treating Patients Addicted to Fitness." *Physician and Sportsmedicine* 20(1992):193.

Wichmann, S., and D. Martin. "Athletic Shoes: Finding the Right Fit." *Physician and Sportsmedicine* 21(1993):204.

Wichmann, S. A., and D. R. Martin. "Sports and Tobacco: The Smoke Has Yet to Clear." *Physician and Sportsmedicine* 19(1991):125–31.

Wilks, B. "Stress Management for Athletes." *Sports Medicine* 11(1991):289–99.

Willett, W. C. "Weight, Weight Change and CHD." *Journal of the American Medical Association* 273(1995):461.

Willet, W. C., et al. "Coffee Consumption and CHD in Women." *Journal of the American Medical Association* 275(1996):458.

Willett, W., et al. "Dietary Fat and Fiber in Relation to Risk of Breast Cancer." *Journal of the American Medical Association* 268(1992):2037.

Williams, M. H. *Nutrition for Fitness and Sport.* 4th ed. Dubuque, IA: Wm. C. Brown Publishers, 1995.

Williams, P. C. *Low Back and Neck Pain: Causes and Conservative Treatment.* Springfield, IL: Charles C. Thomas, 1974.

Williford, H. N., et al. "Is Low-Impact Aerobic Dance an Effective Cardiovascular Workout?" *Physician and Sportsmedicine* 17(1989):95.

Willis, J. "About Body Wraps, Pills and Other Magic Wands for Losing Weight." *FDA Consumer,* November 1982 (reprint).

Willis, J. "Diet Books Sell Well But. . . ." *FDA Consumer,* March 1985 (reprint).

Wilmore, J. "Exercise, Obesity, and Weight Control." *Physical Activity and Fitness Research Digest* 1(1994):1.

Wilmore, J., and D. Costill. *Physiology of Sport and Exercise.* Champaign, IL: Human Kinetics Publishers, 1994.

Wilmore, J. H., and D. L. Costill. *Training for Sport and Activity: The Physiological Basis of the Conditioning Process.* 3d ed. Dubuque, IA: Wm. C. Brown Publishers, 1988.

Wilmore, J. H., et al. "Body Breadth Equipment and Measurement Techniques." In T. G. Lohman, et al., eds. *Anthropometric Standardization Reference Manual.* Champaign, IL: Human Kinetics Publishers, 1988.

Wilmore, J. H., et al. "Body Composition: A Round Table." *Physician and Sportsmedicine* 14(1986):144.

Wilson, G. J., et al. "Stretch Shorten Cycle Performance Enhancement Through Flexibility Training." *Medicine and Science in Sports and Exercise* 24(1992):116–23.

Wilson, G. J., et al. "The Relationship Between Stiffness of the Musculature and Static Flexibility: An Alternative Explanation for the Occurrence of Muscular Injury." *International Journal of Sports Medicine* 12(1991):403–7.

Wilterdink, E. "Amount of Exercise Per Day and Weeks of Training: Effects on Body Weight and Daily Energy Expenditure." *Medicine and Science in Sports and Exercise* 24(1992):396.

Winningham, M.L., and M. G. MacVicar. "Response of Cancer Patients on Chemotherapy to a Supervised Exercise Program." (abs.) *Medicine and Science in Sports and Exercise* 17(1985):292.

Winningham, M. L., et al. "Exercise for Cancer Patients: Guidelines and Precautions." *Physician and Sportsmedicine* 14(1986):125.

Wooden, M. J., et al. "Effects of Strength on Throwing Velocity and Shoulder Muscle Performance in Teenage Baseball Players." *Journal of Orthopaedic and Sports Physical Therapy* 15(1992):223–27.

Woodhouse, M. L. "Isokinetic Trunk Rotation Parameters of Athletes Utilizing Lumbar/Sacral Supports." *Athletic Training* 25(1990):240–43.

Woodhouse, M. L., et al. "Selected Isokinetic Lifting Parameters of Adult Male Athletes Utilizing Lumbar/Sacral Supports." *Journal of Orthopaedic and Sports Physical Therapy* 11(1990):467–72.

Work, J. "Exercise for the Overweight Patient." *Physician and Sportsmedicine* 18(1990):113.

Work, J. A. "How Healthy Are Corporate Fitness Programs?" *Physician and Sportsmedicine* 17(1989):226.

Work, J. A. "Is Weight Training Safe During Pregnancy?" *Physician and Sports Medicine* 17(1989):257.

Wright, J. E., and V. S. Cowart. *Anabolic Steroids.* Carmel, IN: Benchmark Press, 1990.

Wynder, E. L., et al. "High Fiber Intake: Indicators of a Healthy Lifestyle." *Journal of the American Medical Association* 275(1996):486.

Yarber, W. L. *AIDS: What Young Adults Should Know. Instructor's Guide.* 2d ed. Reston, VA: AAHPERD, 1989.

Yesalis, C. *Anabolic Steroids in Sport and Exercise.* Champaign, IL: Human Kinetics Publishers, 1993.

Yesalis, C. E. "Winning and Performance-Enhancing Drugs: Our Dual Addiction." *Physician and Sportsmedicine* 18(1990):161–67.

Yessis, M. "Latest Strength Techniques You Can Offer Your Clients." *Fitness Management* 5(1989):36.

Yessis, M. "Speaking of Strength." *Fitness Management* (1989):36.

Zamula, E. "Back Talk: Advice for Suffering Spines." *FDA Consumer* 23(1989):28.

Zelasko, C. J. "Exercise for Weight Loss: What Are the Facts?" *Journal of American Dietetics Association* 95(1995):1414.

Zeni, A. I., et al. "Energy Expenditure With Indoor Machines." *Journal of the American Medical Association* 275(1996):1424.

CREDITS

Illustrations

Anatomy Chart, page 49, From Kent M. Van De Graaff, *Human Anatomy,* 3rd edition. Copyright © 1992 Times Mirror Higher Education Group, Inc., Dubuque, Iowa. All Rights Reserved. Reprinted by permission. **Anatomy Chart, page 50,** From Kent M. Van De Graaff and Stuart Ira Fox, *Concepts of Human Anatomy and Physiology,* 4th edition. Copyright © 1995 Times Mirror Higher Education Group, Inc., Dubuque, Iowa. All Rights Reserved. Reprinted by permission. **Anatomy Chart, page 51,** From John W. Hole, Jr., *Human Anatomy and Physiology,* 6th edition. Copyright © 1993 Times Mirror Higher Education Group, Inc., Dubuque, Iowa. All Rights Reserved. Reprinted by permission.

Concept 2
Figure 2.4 From Kent M. Van De Graaff and Stuart Ira Fox, *Concepts of Human Anatomy and Physiology,* 4th edition. Copyright © 1995 Times Mirror Higher Education Group, Inc., Dubuque, Iowa. All Rights Reserved. Reprinted by permission.

Concept 3
Figure 3.1 From David Shier, *Hole's Human Anatomy and Physiology,* 7th edition. Copyright © 1996 Times Mirror Higher Education Group, Inc., Dubuque, Iowa. All Rights Reserved. Reprinted by permission.

Concept 4
Figure 4.2 From *Fitness for Life,* 4th edition, by Charles B. Corbin and Ruth Lindsey. Copyright © 1997 by Scott Foresman and Company, a division of Addison-Wesley Educational Publishers, Inc. Reprinted by permission.

Concept 5
Figure 5.1 From David Shier, *Hole's Human Anatomy and Physiology,* 7th edition. Copyright © 1996 Times Mirror Higher Education Group, Inc., Dubuque, Iowa. All Rights Reserved. Reprinted by permission. **Figure 5.5** From *Fitness for Life,* 4th edition, by Charles B. Corbin and Ruth Lindsey. Copyright © 1997 by Scott Foresman and Company, a division of Addison-Wesley Educational Publishers, Inc. Reprinted by permission.

Concept 6
Figure 6.1 From *Fitness for Life,* 4th edition, by Charles B. Corbin and Ruth Lindsey. Copyright © 1997 by Scott Foresman and Company, a division of Addison-Wesley Educational Publishers, Inc. Reprinted by permission.

Concept 9
Figure 9.2 From *Fitness for Life,* 4th edition, by Charles B. Corbin and Ruth Lindsey. Copyright © 1997 by Scott Foresman and Company, a division of Addison-Wesley Educational Publishers, Inc. Reprinted by permission.

Concept 15
Figure 15.1 From *Fitness for Life,* 4th edition, by Charles B. Corbin and Ruth Lindsey. Copyright © 1997 by Scott Foresman and Company, a division of Addison-Wesley Educational Publishers, Inc. Reprinted by permission.

Photographs

Section Openers
SO 1: © David Stoecklein/Adstock; **SO 2:** © Rick Rusing/Leo de Wys, Inc.; **SO 3:** © Tim Davis/Photo Researchers; **SO 4:** © Bill Bachmann/Adstock; **SO 5:** © Randy Taylor/Leo de Wys, Inc.

Concept 1
Concept 1 Opener: David Frazier Photolibrary; **p. 5T:** © David R. Laurie; **p. 5B:** © Vic Bider/PhotoEdit; **p. 6TL:** David Frazier Photolibrary; **p. 6BL:** David Frazier Photolibrary; **p. 6TR:** Digital Stock; **p. 6BR:** David Frazier Photolibrary; **p. 7TL:** David Frazier Photolibrary; **p. 7BL:** Digital Stock; **p. 7TR:** © D. McDonald/Unicorn Stock Photos; **p. 7BR:** © Scott Stallard/The Image Bank-Chicago; **p. 8L:** David Frazier Photolibrary; **p. 12:** David Frazier Photolibrary; **p. 13:** © David Young-Wolff/PhotoEdit.

Concept 2
Concept 2 Opener: © Kari Weatherly/Corbis; **p. 27:** David Frazier Photolibrary.

Concept 3
Concept 3 Opener: PhotoDisc; **p. 39:** Photo Disc.

Concept 4
Concept 4 Opener: © David Young-Wolff/PhotoEdit; **p. 45:** PhotoDisc; **p. 48:** © David Madison.

Concept 5
Concept 5 Opener: David Frazier PhotoLibrary; **Figures 5.7A and 5.7B:** © David R. Laurie; **p. 66:** © David R. Laurie.

Concept 6
Concept 6 Opener: Charles Corbin; **p. 70:** © Ken Akers/First Image West; **p. 73:** © Karl Weatherly/Corbis.

Concept 7
Concept 7 Opener: © Vic Bider/PhotoEdit; **p. 80:** Charles B. Corbin.

Concept 8
Concept 8 Opener: © Bob Krist/Leo DeWys.

Concept 9
Concept 9 Opener: © Sue Bennett/Adstock; **p. 105:** © David R. Laurie; **p. 109:** David Frazier Photolibrary.

Concept 10
Concept 10 Opener: © David Stoecklein/Adstock; **p. 122:** © David R. Laurie.

Concept 11
Concept 11 Opener: © David R. Frazier Photolibrary.

Concept 12
Concept 12 Opener: © David R. Laurie.

Concept 13
Concept 13 Opener: © David R. Laurie; **Figure 13.1:** © David R. Laurie.

Concept 14
Concept 14 Opener: Digital Stock Professional; **p. 178:** Charles Corbin.

Concept 15
Concept 15 Opener: PhotoDisc; **p. 187:** © James Marshall/First Image West; **p. 192:** David Frazier Photolibrary.

Concept 16
Concept 16 Opener: © James W. Kay/Adstock.

Concept 17
Concept 17 Opener: © Tony Freeman/PhotoEdit; **p. 217:** David Frazier Photolibrary.

Concept 18
Concept 18 Opener: PhotoDisc; **p. 225:** © James L. Shaffer.

Concept 19
Concept 19 Opener: David Frazier Photolibrary; **p. 241:** David Frazier Photolibrary.

Concept 20
Concept 20 Opener: David Frazier Photolibrary; **p. 250:** PhotoDisc.

Concept 21
Concept 21 Opener: © Tony Freeman/PhotoEdit; **p. 259:** © Kevin Syms/David Frazier Photolibrary; **p. 261:** © David R. Laurie; **p. 262:** Charles Corbin.

Concept 22
Concept 22 Opener: Charles Corbin; **p. 268:** Charles Corbin; **p. 269:** © D. Bunde/Unicorn Stock Photos; **p. 270:** © M. McBride/Unicorn Stock Photos.

Concept 23
Concept 23 Opener: © Myrleen Ferguson/PhotoEdit; **p. 276:** David Frazier Photolibrary.

·INDEX·